CHILDREN
with VISUAL
IMPAIRMENTS

A Parents' Guide

Edited by M. Cay Holbrook, Ph.D.

Woodbine House ▪▪ 2006

© 2006 Woodbine House
Second edition

All rights reserved under International and Pan American copyright laws. Published in
the United States of America by Woodbine House, Inc., 6510 Bells Mills Road, Bethesda,
MD 20817. 800-843-7323.
www.woodbinehouse.com

Cover art by Nancy Bea Miller (www.nancybeamiller.com)

Library of Congress Cataloging-in-Publication Data

Children with visual impairments : a parents' guide / edited by M. Cay Holbrook.
— 2nd ed.
   p. cm.
 Includes bibliographical references and index.
 ISBN-13: 978-1-890627-40-9
 ISBN-10: 1-890627-40-2
 1. Children with visual disabilities. 2. Children, Blind. 3. Parents of children with
disabilities. I. Holbrook, M. Cay, 1955-
 HV1596.2.C55 2006
 649'.1511—dc22   2006019585

Published in the United States of America

10   9   8   7   6   5   4   3   2   1

Dedicated to the memory of

Carl Holbrook

and

Alan Koenig

TABLE

OF

CONTENTS

Acknowledgements

During the past several years I have been thinking a great deal about the concepts of "family" and "home." It is easy to long for a traditionally defined family (like the families represented on television shows such as *Father Knows Best* or *Happy Days*) and "home" (with the white picket fence). But these pictures of family and home are almost never reality for us. Many of us live in tightly packed urban areas, in high rises or condos, and if we do have a picket fence, we realize that we have to paint it! And the concept of family is just as complex! But what I believe now is that opening up my definition of home and family actually enriches my life in ways that give me strength and support.

I am deeply grateful for people who have given me a sanctuary (home) and who have supported and loved me (family). My mother continues to be an important source of support for me, as do my brother and sister and their families. I appreciate the way that their ongoing love has had an impact on how I understand the love of parents for their children. I hope that this understanding is reflected in the chapters of this book because there can be no more important relationship for young children.

The authors who contributed chapters to this book have tried their best to provide compassionate and meaningful information that will allow parents to learn from those who have walked this path before while respecting their own instincts. I am grateful that these parents, teachers, doctors, and other professionals agreed to contribute their thoughts and expertise to help new parents as they grow in understanding and love for their child who is blind or visually impaired.

INTRODUCTION

All parents learn about parenting one day at a time. Some of their days are filled with joy and warm feelings as they learn how to encourage their child's innate talents and enjoy watching their son or daughter learn and grow. Others are filled with questions and challenges as parents learn how to balance support and discipline and how to care for their children through childhood illnesses, routine cuts and scrapes, and temper tantrums. As the parent of a child with a visual impairment, your experiences will be more like than unlike every other parent's experiences. As for most parents, most of the time, your instincts will take over and you will do what is right for your child in the context of the complex needs of your family. Other times, you will turn to trusted family and friends for advice. Still other times, you will want to gather information from other sources like the Internet and books like this one.

Of course, no one resource can provide all the information you need, and you are the best judge of what is right for you and your child. In this second edition of *Children with Visual Impairments,* however, we have tried to pull together information that might help you on your journey to parent a child who is visually impaired. This book has been written by people with a variety of perspectives about visual impairments, including parents, teachers, doctors, and other professionals who have a deep, personal or professional understanding of children with visual impairments and their families. These authors rely on their own experiences and their connection with many other people to bring a range of ideas and opinions into each chapter. This second edition incorporates much of the new knowledge that has become available in the past ten years. Important information about new legal regulations related to educational services for children with disabilities is included. In addition, this edition provides parents with up-to-date information about the best practices in advocacy and educational service for young children with visual impairments.

The focus of this book is on the needs of very young children (birth to age five), but a great deal of information will also be helpful to parents of older children. We have included information that we hope will be helpful to parents of children with a wide range of visual impairments—from children with "low vision" (those who have a level of vision but who are not able to see as clearly as a child with typical vision) to children who are totally blind. We also address the concerns of parents whose child has one or more other disabilities in addition to a visual impairment. The second edition of *Children with Visual Impairments* will also be helpful to extended family members, teachers of students with visual impairments, preschool teachers, medical professionals and therapists, and others who work directly and indirectly with young children with visual impairments and their families.

It is our hope that parents will benefit from the information in this book and that it might be a starting point for gathering information and becoming informed advocates. Not everything included in this book will apply to all children; likewise not all available information is included within these pages. *Children with Visual Impairments* is intended to serve as a beginning. You may be reading this book before reading anything else, or you may already have a wealth of knowledge and information before reading it. In any case, the information contained in these pages will be most helpful if you trust yourself and your knowledge of your child to find the relevant and helpful parts. The following chapters in the book will help point you in the right direction:

- Chapter 1 addresses very basic information about the nature of visual impairments, how the degree of visual impairment is assessed, and the impact of visual impairment on the life of a child and a family.
- Chapter 2 focuses on medical aspects, including the most common causes of visual impairment and how they are treated. This chapter was co-written by an ophthalmologist and optometrist, combining the best of information from both professionals.

- Chapter 3 addresses the experiences that families have as they begin to understand and come to terms with a child's visual impairment and possible additional disabilities. It is written by a teacher of students with visual impairments, and incorporates the personal stories of several families.
- Chapter 4 provides information about child development and how a visual impairment may have an impact on development.
- Chapter 5 is written by an author who is both a teacher and a parent of a young man who is visually impaired with additional disabilities and covers issues related to helping your child learn self-help and other skills needed in daily life.
- Chapter 6 focuses on family life and how having a child who is visually impaired may enrich and challenge family activities and dynamics, while Chapter 7 is devoted to encouraging positive self-esteem for your child throughout his life.
- Chapter 8 contains an overview of special education issues, including what you can expect in early intervention and school-age programs. This chapter outlines and explains the expanded core curriculum for students with visual impairments; that is, the skills students with visual impairment need in addition to the core curriculum.
- Chapter 9 gives a brief overview of legal issues related to education, discrimination, accessibility, and other areas.
- Chapter 10 offers information about reading and writing and will give you some help in supporting your child as he develops literacy skills.
- Chapter 11 discusses orientation and mobility skills—the skills that enable a child with a visual impairment to know where he is in the environment and travel independently from one place to another.
- Chapter 12 provides information relevant to parents of children who have disabilities in addition to a visual impairment, focusing on differences in development and how developmental problems can be minimized.
- Chapter 13 looks to the future and provides some insight into what educational, social, travel, self-help, and other issues your child might face in the years to come.

At the end of the book are additional resources (lists of organizations, schools, helpful publications, and a glossary). We hope that these resources will help you get started in gathering information and support.

Throughout this book we have alternated the use of the personal pronouns "he" and "she" to simplify the awkwardness of "he/she" and "his/her" wording. We have also chosen to use the term "visual impairment" rather than such variations as "visual disabilities" or "visual handicaps." The term visual impairment is widely used and accepted to refer to all levels of vision loss. Please note, however, that the word "blind" is perfectly acceptable and should be freely and comfortably used.

Gathering information that will help you and your child is an ongoing process. You are beginning a journey that will take you through a lifetime of successes and failures. The more prepared you are and the more prepared your child is, the more successful you will be. Most of the time you won't need a book to guide you through the process of parenting or to help you solidify what your family means to each other. However, sometimes it helps to gather information and learn from other people's experiences. This book is for those sometimes.

1

WHAT IS
VISUAL
IMPAIRMENT?

M. Cay Holbrook, Ph.D.

Most people believe that they know the answer to the question "What is visual impairment?" Maybe this is because blindness is one of the few disabilities that we believe that we can simulate. From the time we are children, we play games that involve wearing a blindfold. We close our eyes and believe that this is "what it is like" to be blind. In reality, however, visual impairments are seldom like this. Most children and adults who are considered visually impaired have some vision that is useful to them. In fact, even children who are considered blind often have some visual perception of light and dark that will assist them as they learn about their world.

This chapter will give you a basic understanding of the great variability in visual impairments. It introduces and explains some of the terminology used to describe different types and degrees of visual impairment. It also explains how a visual impairment is diagnosed and provides an idea of what the future may hold for your child.

Throughout this chapter and this book you will find general information about children who have visual impairments. Some of this information and some of the suggestions may be useful to you right

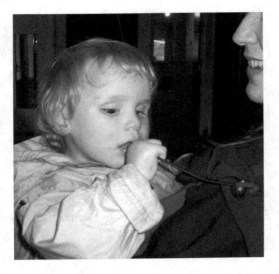

now. Other information may not be useful to you now, but may help you in the future. Still other information may seem as if it is just not applicable to your child. This is to be expected. Children with visual impairments, like all children, are individuals, first and foremost. There is no one accurate picture of what "the child with a visual impairment" is like. Remember that you are now and will always be the best judge of your child's needs, abilities, and challenges. This book can give you a general idea of what to expect for your child, but only your child can show you his true capabilities.

:: What Is Visual Impairment?

The term *visual impairment* can refer to any condition in which eyesight cannot be corrected to what is considered "normal." In this book, the term is used to refer to a loss of vision that makes it difficult or impossible to complete daily tasks without specialized adaptations. This visual impairment is often due to a loss of *visual acuity.* That is, the eye is not able to see objects as clearly—to make out as much detail—as usual. Visual impairments may also be due to a loss of *visual field*—the total area that can be seen without moving the eyes or head. A child with a visual field loss may or may not be able to see objects clearly within his smaller field of vision.

There are three underlying reasons for impairment of vision. First, there may be damage to one or more parts of the eye essential to vision. This damage may interfere with the way the eye receives or processes visual information. Second, the eyeball may be proportioned incorrectly (have different dimensions than usual), making it harder to focus on objects. And third, the part of the brain that processes visual information may not work properly. The eye itself may work well, but the brain is not able to analyze and interpret visual information so that the child can see. Chapter 2 discusses the most common conditions that cause these problems with the eye or the brain.

A visual impairment may be present at birth, or it may develop during infancy or childhood. Some visual impairments get worse over time, some stay about the same, and a few may even get better. Some children have "fluctuating vision"—or visual functioning that is different at different times of the day. (See below.)

The same eye condition can sometimes affect two children's vision very differently. One may have a slight vision loss, while the other may have a more significant loss. Chapter 2 will give you some specific information about various eye conditions and typical effects of the conditions. You must remember, however, that every child is unique. Your child's vision may be quite different from that of another child with the same condition. Your ophthalmologist or optometrist will be the best source of information about the nature and extent of your child's visual impairment.

∷ The Diagnosis of a Visual Impairment

Sometimes visual impairments are detected at birth, before the baby leaves the hospital. Other times, parents may be the first to notice that something is different about their child's eyes. They may notice that their baby doesn't watch them as they walk across the room. Maybe his eyes are crossed or he seems startled when someone picks him up without talking to him first. No matter how strong a parent's suspicions are, however, the diagnosis of a visual impairment is not "official" until an eye care professional confirms that there is a significant loss of visual acuity or field. This section introduces the professionals who may evaluate your child's sight and explains how they determine whether your child has a significant loss of vision.

Professionals Qualified to Make a Diagnosis

Two different professionals are qualified to measure your child's vision and determine whether he has a visual impairment. The first is an *ophthalmologist,* a medical doctor who has specialized training in diagnosing and treating diseases and conditions of the eye. When an ophthalmologist's name is written, the letters M.D. follow it, because he or she is a medical doctor who has completed basic medical training and specialization in the study and treatment of disorders of the eye. This doctor is qualified to prescribe medications, perform surgery on the eye, and address medical problems relating to the eyes. He or she can also measure visual acuity and visual fields and prescribe eye glasses.

The other professional who can evaluate vision is an *optometrist*. The optometrist is a "doctor of optometry" (O.D.), who has completed four years of study at an accredited optometry school but is not a medical doctor. This eye care professional is qualified to examine eye health, measure visual acuity and visual fields, test depth and color perception, and to prescribe eye glasses.

Either an ophthalmologist or optometrist can make the initial determination of whether your child has a visual impairment. Both are qualified to prescribe corrective lenses and should be able to discuss your child's visual impairment with you. If, however, your child needs medical attention because of his eye condition, it is advisable for him to be under the care of an ophthalmologist. Chapter 2 discusses some additional considerations to keep in mind when choosing an eye care professional for long-term care of your child's visual impairment.

Sometimes eye doctors use abbreviations to describe a child's visual impairment. Listed in the Glossary are the most common abbreviations that are used in eye

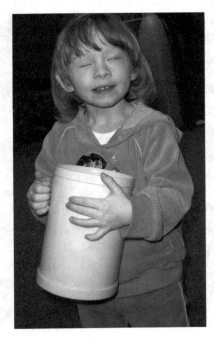

reviations that are used in eye reports from ophthalmologists and optometrists. You should not hesitate to ask questions if your child's eye doctor uses terminology you do not understand. The professionals working with you should be willing to explain anything that you do not understand. In the same vein, let professionals know that you *do* understand what they are trying to explain and that they can give you more complicated information. You will have to set the tone for your interactions with professionals. See Chapter 2 for more information on dealing with eye care professionals.

How Vision Is Measured

To understand how visual impairments are diagnosed, you need to understand how vision is measured. Most of us have had our vision checked at one time or another, but what does it really mean if we are told that we do or do not have 20/20 vision?

Measuring Acuity

The phrase "20/20 vision" is a measurement of how well someone is able to read a chart that contains letters and/or numbers of different sizes. The most common chart used by eye care professionals has a large E at the top and is sometimes called the "E Chart," but its official name is the "Snellen Chart." Visual acuity (how clearly you see) is determined by the size of letters that you can read and the distance at which you can read them. The typical testing distance is 20 feet from the chart, because at 20 feet your eye is relaxed; the lens of your eye is in its natural position instead of trying to focus (or *accommodate*).

People with normal visual acuity can clearly read 3/8 inch letters or numbers at a distance of 20 feet. They are said to have 20/20 vision because at 20 feet from the chart they see what a normally sighted person sees at 20 feet. When someone's visual acuity is not as clear as normal, the second number will be larger than 20. Someone with 20/80 vision, for example, sees at 20 feet what a normally sighted person sees at 80 feet. Someone with 20/400 vision sees at 20 feet what a normally sighted person sees at 400 feet. When someone's acuity is better than normal, the second number will be smaller than 20. For instance, someone with 20/15 vision sees at 20 feet what a normally sighted person sees at 15 feet. (Note: to convert the Snellen Notation used in the United States to Metric Notation, divide both the top and the bottom numbers by 3.25—for example, 20/200 equals 6/60 in Metric Notation.)

You should note the use of the phrase *normally sighted*. There is no such thing as "perfect" sight. A visual acuity of 20/20 only indicates that the person, while sitting in the eye doctor's office, was able to read certain letters on a chart. This acuity measurement does not carry with it a judgment of how someone uses the information that his eyes are gathering.

Naturally, the Snellen Chart is only used to measure visual acuity in those who are able to read letters and numbers. For young children and nonreaders, there are other ways that visual acuity can be measured. One of the most common is through a test known as the *Lighthouse Flash Card Test for Children*. This test works the same way as the Snellen Chart except that there are bold line drawings of a circle, an apple, a house, and a square instead of letters and numbers. Even very young preschoolers can identify these shapes (especially after a little practice), so acuity can be measured at a very young age. Approximate visual acuities can also be obtained by using toys and household objects of various sizes and determining the child's ability to see the objects at various distances. If the child wears glasses, acuity is measured both with and without glasses.

It is very difficult or impossible to determine an accurate acuity for infants or for children with communication difficulties. One way to attempt to determine approximate visual acuities is through *preferential looking*. A doctor using this technique shows two cards to the child at the same time. One card has black and white stripes, and the other has a large gray area. The doctor watches the child to determine whether he fixates (focuses) on the striped card, which is presumed to be more interesting for him to look at. The doctor continues to present cards with stripes that are smaller and closer together until the child no longer focuses on them. This gives a general idea of visual acuity until a more accurate measurement can be made.

Typically, your child's eye doctor will measure acuity in each eye and in both eyes working together. It is possible to have a visual acuity of 20/20 in one eye, and 20/40 in the other eye, and still see with an acuity of 20/20 with both eyes together. As the doctor measures your child's visual acuity, he or she will give you information on the visual acuity of each eye and also a visual acuity of both eyes working together.

Measuring Visual Field

The eye doctor may also conduct an assessment of your child's visual field. This assessment will help your doctor determine how much of the space around him your child can see without moving his eyes or head. Visual field is expressed in degrees. "Normal" visual fields are obstructed by facial features such as the nose and eyebrows, but are approximately 160 to 170 degrees horizontally.

Testing your child's visual field may be difficult because in order to get accurate results, your child must keep his head straight and still and focus his eyes for an extended period of time on a spot directly in front of him. As you might guess, small children are rarely able to do this! Instead, your doctor may ask you or someone else to help do a less precise but more dependable assessment. You will sit on a chair or on the floor with your child in your lap and the doctor sitting right in front of you. Usually, the doctor holds an interesting toy or object and draws your child's attention to him while you slowly bring a toy, bright object, or penlight from in back of your child to in front of him. By watching your child's eyes, the doctor will be able to see when your child's gaze shifts to something new coming into his visual field. You will repeat this procedure several times, bringing the toy into your child's visual field at different locations—sometimes from above, sometimes from the sides, sometimes from below.

If you participate in the assessment process, you may find that you become more aware of shifts in your child's gaze as he uses his peripheral vision throughout the day. For example, as your child is sitting at the kitchen table eating lunch, his gaze may shift as the family cat walks by. He is demonstrating an awareness of movement outside his central vision.

When your child gets older and is able to sit still for longer periods of time, your doctor will probably want to conduct a more sophisticated assessment of your child's visual field. This test will be able to provide more complete information including, in some situations, information on the existence and location of scotomas (partial loss of vision or "blind-spots" within a person's visual field). Until then, informal assessments provide very useful information.

Degrees of Vision Loss

After your child's visual acuity and visual field have been measured, the ophthalmologist or optometrist will be able to tell you:

1. whether your child has a visual impairment, and, if so,
2. how significant it is.

If your child has a visual impairment, you may find that additional labels are used to describe the amount of vision he has. In fact, there have been many debates over labels and terminology to be used when referring to individuals with impaired vision. In part, this debate continues because of a need or desire to use terminology which accurately reflects the person's visual ability, but also because of an unfortunate sensitivity over the use of the words "blind" and "blindness." Historically, the word "blind" has not been used positively in our society. No one sitting at the ballpark would mistake the angry cry, "What? Are you blind, ump?"

with a compliment of the umpire's officiating skills. Likewise, someone who is said to "blindly follow his peers" is pegged as a person with little independence and poor judgment. But truly, the word "blind" is accurate when describing significant loss of vision and does not carry with it a judgment of a person's worth or his ability. We must be diligent in our insistence that there is no shame attached to the word "blind."

Still, in order to accurately describe individuals with different degrees of vision loss, additional terms may be used. For instance, individuals who have vision that can be used to read print (either regular print, enlarged print, or magnified print) may be referred to as being *"partially sighted"* or having *"low vision."* You will probably also hear the term *legal blindness.* When this term is used, it does not necessarily mean that the person is totally blind. This term has a specific definition. It is: "a visual acuity of 20/200 or less in the better eye after correction and/or a visual field of no greater than 20 degrees." In other words, even with glasses or contact lenses on, this person would see at 20 feet what a normally sighted person sees at 200 feet, and/or would have a visual field of no greater than 20 degrees.

There are children whose vision is so limited that it cannot be expressed in 20/XX terms. These children are not able to see any of the letters on the eye chart as they sit or stand 20 feet away. The first thing an eye doctor will probably do is to try to test the child closer than 20 feet away from the chart. If this is the case, the top number of the acuity measurement will indicate the distance at which the testing is done. The bottom number still indicates what the child is able to see at that distance. You may see an acuity like 10/200 or 5/200. Theoretically, these acuity measurements can be mathematically converted into more standard acuities (for example, 10/200 can be converted to 20/400; 5/200 to 20/800). As mentioned below, however, these numbers often don't tell us much about how a child uses his vision and so are not as valuable as an examination of his functional vision. (See the section on Functional Vision below.)

Some children's acuity cannot be measured using the eye chart at all. In these cases, the eye doctor may try alternative methods for testing vision. Here are some terms that might be used:

> ***Counts Fingers (or CF) at _____ feet (or inches)***
> This simply means that the doctor holds up his fingers and asks the child to count them (or for very young chil-

dren, to point at them or touch them) and takes note of the distance at which the child is able to do this.

Hand Movement (or HM) at _____ *feet (or inches)*
This measurement indicates the distance at which the child can recognize the movement of a hand in front of his eyes.

Light Projection
This term refers to the ability to tell where light is coming from and can be tested by asking the child to point to the light coming from the window or an open door.

Light Perception
This term refers to the ability to tell the presence or absence of light (whether the light is on or off) without being able to tell where the light is coming from.

As you can see, there are many terms to describe different visual abilities. Rarely do we assume that a child has absolutely no vision, unless his eyes have been *enucleated* (removed) for some reason. If the child has some level of visual ability, it may be used for important tasks such as orientation and mobility and daily living skills.

It is sometimes difficult for people who are sighted to understand what is referred to as *"total blindness."* This term refers to a total lack of visual information. Children who are totally blind have no light perception and gather information about their world completely through other senses. The reason it is so difficult for people who are sighted to understand this term is that sight is such a pervasive sense. The first thing we do when we get up in the morning is to open our eyes. It is easier to understand conditions that result in decreased visual functioning than total blindness because we have all had experiences in which our vision has been decreased (for example looking at a foggy mirror or out our car window before the defroster starts to work). As you learn more about how your child experiences the world, you will probably find yourself more aware of information available through hearing, touch, smell, or taste.

Some services or benefits are only available to individuals with a measured acuity of a certain level or less. Often this level is 20/200, after the best possible correction. For this reason, you may hear about legal blindness a lot. Maybe you will hear it because a camp offers summer scholarships for children with a visual acuity of no greater than 20/200. Or maybe you might need your eye doctor to sign a form certifying that your child's visual acuity is no greater than 20/200 so that you can get books on cassette tape or in braille from the Library of Congress/Library for the Blind and Physically Handicapped.

Some school districts have a visual acuity level which must be documented prior to a child being admitted into a special education program. More commonly, though, school districts consider each child individually to determine eligibility for special education services. A child would be eligible if it is determined that his visual impairment has had or will have an impact on his learning.

Although it is important to know what your child's visual acuity or visual field is, you must remember that 20/200 (or any measurement) is not a magic number. What is much more important is *how* your child uses the vision he has to accomplish daily tasks at home and in his community. Your child has his own unique abilities and needs, strengths and weaknesses. Learning about the general characteristics of children with visual impairments, as well as your child's particular eye condition, can be useful and helpful. It is most important, however, that your child be allowed to develop in his own way without preconceived expectations based on what is considered "typical."

❚❚ Your Child's Functional Vision

Sometimes two children who have the same visual acuity have different abilities to use their vision to accomplish everyday activities. One six-year-old with 20/400 vision may be able to walk independently to the corner bus stop using his vision to help him, while another child with the same visual acuity may not. One twelve-year-old with 20/600 vision might effectively use his vision to examine maps in his social studies book, while another student with the same visual acuity might struggle with the same task. To help you and the adults who interact with your child know how well your child uses his vision to function in his world, he should be given a functional vision assessment. A professional who has special training in the area of visual impairments should conduct this assessment.

There are many different types of functional vision assessments. In general, however, information about how your child uses his vision will be gathered by observing him in a variety of settings. The person conducting the assessment should observe your child during inside and outside activities, during structured activities (such as calendar time at preschool) and unstructured activities (such as play time when your child is deciding what activities to do and how to accomplish tasks). The functional vision assessment should yield such information as:

- How well does your child use his eyes to scan across the environment to locate something or someone?
- What lighting is best for your child? Does he easily move from a light room into a dark room (or from dark to light) without visual difficulties? Although it is a common belief that children with decreased vision require more or brighter lights, this is not always true. Children with albinism, for example, are often bothered by bright lights.
- What size objects is your child able to identify at what distance?
- Does your child get tired easily when trying to accomplish visual tasks such as reading, writing, coloring, and looking at pictures?
- What natural compensations does your child use when he is having difficulty accomplishing a task? Does he squint, place the object closer to him, tilt his head?
- What postures and positions are best for your child? Does he need to have toys, food, etc. presented to him on the right? On the left?
- What does your child enjoy looking at? Bright lights? Colorful toys? Objects with black and white patterns?
- How does your child use his vision to move around? Can he avoid large objects by using sight alone, or does he need to touch them?

By gathering this type of information, a teacher of students with visual impairments can help you create a safe environment for your child that is stimulating and visually interesting for him. Regardless of the level of visual impairment, a child can be taught to move safely and efficiently throughout his world.

Some states and provinces require that every child with a visual impairment have a functional vision assessment to be eligible for special education. Some states do not require this. Even if your state does not require that your child be given a functional vision assessment, however, your child's teacher of students with visual impairments should do one to learn how best to arrange his environment. By examining how well your child uses his vision, his teachers will be able to begin teaching him strategies to use it more efficiently. The goal of this instruction is not to improve visual acuity, but to encourage your child to maximize the use of his vision.

Even before your child has a functional vision assessment, you may be able to recognize situations in which he can use vision to gather information, and situations in which he will find his other senses more

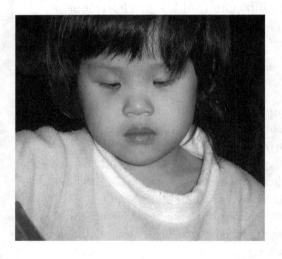

useful. It is important that you begin to communicate how your child functions visually with people who work with him. For example, let the Sunday School teacher know that your child will enjoy looking at the brightly colored illustrations in the Sunday School book, but will not be able to color in the faint lines of the workbook. Or, tell the babysitter that he needs to say something when he enters or leaves a room so that your child will know where he is. The more time you spend caring for, playing with, and observing your child, the more you will understand how he is able to use his vision for daily activities.

■■ Fluctuating Vision

Not all children who have a visual impairment have fluctuating vision, but it is important to recognize if your child does. Fluctuating vision may be due to factors such as changes in lighting, familiarity and complexity of the task, fatigue, and/or characteristics of some medical conditions. If your child's vision is fluctuating, you may notice that he is able to accomplish a visual task more easily at some times than others. You may see him get frustrated or angry, or he may rub his eyes or complain of headaches. By watching your child carefully, you will begin to notice which factors affect his ability to use his vision. You will also be better able to help control these factors wherever your child is—at home, at school, at a friend's house, or at other places in the community.

A rheostat control on lights in your house can allow you to alter the illumination to meet your child's needs, even if those needs change throughout the day. Encouraging your child to close his eyes and rest for a few minutes between activities may help alleviate fatigue. Likewise, helping your child learn to wait patiently when he moves from sunlight into a darker inside room (or from an inside room into the sun) while his eyes adjust to the change may be useful. Your child may or may not independently learn how to compensate for these changes in visual functioning. By teaching him some of these "tricks," you help him to be safer and more efficient. Just as importantly, you also show him that making these kinds of adaptations is a normal part of his life and completely accepted, even though they may take a little more time.

▪▪ Is My Child the Only One?

It is likely that before the diagnosis of your child's visual impairment you had little or no experience with vision loss. You may have known *adults* with a visual impairment, as blindness is most common in those over 65 years old. You probably didn't know parents of a *child* with visual impairments, however. Even now you may not yet have met other families with children with visual impairments. It may feel as if your child is the only child who has a visual impairment, and that your family is the only one with questions and concerns about visual impairments.

Although your child is *not* the only one with a visual impairment, there are legitimate reasons for you to feel somewhat isolated. Blindness or visual impairment is considered a "low incidence disability" among children. This means that compared to other disabilities, visual impairments occur in fewer numbers among children. Approximately one-tenth of a percent of the children in the United States are visually impaired. In other words, 1 in 1000 children have a severe visual impairment. Of these children, approximately 80 to 85 percent have some useable vision. Although estimates about the number of children with visual impairments may vary according to definitions used, it is clear that the number is relatively small.

To help you cope with feelings you may have of being alone, here are some initial suggestions.

- *Realize that being a good parent of a child with a visual impairment is very similar to being a good parent of a child without disabilities.* Your child needs your love, your support, and your consistency: the same things that any child needs.

- *Trust yourself.* There will be times when you would love to call a neighbor, friend, or relative and ask, "What did *you* do when your child. . . ." Feel comfortable asking those questions, even when the issues revolve around vision loss. But don't think that you must wait for solutions from others. Trust yourself, your instincts, and your own solutions.

- *Look for support.* There are a number of resources you can use for support. Family and friends can provide a special kind of help; let them know when you need them.

- *Find ways to connect with helpful blind adults and parents of other children with visual impairments.* Building a strong community of knowledgeable supporters will help throughout your child's life. There are many groups of parents of children with visual impairments (at the local, state, and national levels). It is even easier these days to access these groups, thanks to the Internet. Some of these groups are listed in the Resource Guide at the back of this book. Medical and educational professionals in the area of visual impairment can also provide support, including helping you find resources to answer your specific questions. More specific information about the need for and availability of support can be found in Chapter 3 and throughout this book.

- *Look for your child's unique talents, and try to understand that visual impairment is only one of your child's characteristics.* Perhaps your child is very affectionate or has a great sense of humor. Maybe he is mischievous or adventurous or creative. By focusing on all of your child's characteristics, you will begin to realize that in many ways your parenting challenges parallel those faced by all parents.

■■ When a Visual Impairment Is Not the Only Disability

It is estimated that up to 50 to 60 percent of children with visual impairments also have other disabilities. They may, for example, also have a hearing impairment, developmental delay, or cerebral palsy.

One reason that visual impairments so often go hand in hand with other disabilities is that more and more premature babies are surviving, due to improved medical technology. As Chapter 2 explains, prematurity can lead to problems such as bleeding in the brain or loss of oxygen to the brain. These complications can not only damage the visual system, but also parts of the brain that govern movement, hearing, or thinking. Other causes of visual impairment, such as viruses or maternal infections like rubella, can also damage more than one part of the brain, leading to multiple disabilities.

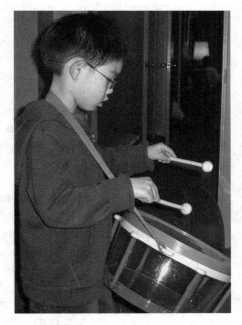

If your child has two or more disabilities, there is a good chance he will be considered "multiply disabled." Schools often label children multiply disabled if they have two or more disabilities which each make it more difficult for them to learn in a regular classroom setting.

If your child has multiple disabilities, it will be especially important to pay close attention to his individual strengths, weaknesses, needs, and abilities. The combination of your child's disabilities will be unique to your child. You will need to gather information from a wide variety of sources and learn to apply the information to your unique situation. Many professionals will be able to help you, but you will become the first and most important expert on your child. See Chapter 12 for information on some of the most important issues associated with children with visual impairments and other disabilities.

▪▪ What about Future Children?

The decision to have children is highly personal for all parents. Parents must take many factors into account, including financial, home, and lifestyle considerations. Parents may also weigh the impact that a new baby will have on other children in the family. Parents of children with disabilities have a couple of special considerations on top of these typical concerns. When trying to decide whether to have additional children, these parents need to think about the energy, time, and money they have available, since children with disabilities often take more of all three.

Perhaps the biggest concern for many parents of children with any disability is that future children may also have a disability. Many eye conditions that result in visual impairments are genetic, meaning that they are passed on by one or both parents. Chapter 2 contains information about specific eye conditions and whether or not they are considered genetic.

There is a great deal that we do not understand about genes and how traits are passed on from generation to generation, but there is also a great deal that we do understand. Parents who want to know their chances of having another child with the same visual impairment can consult a geneticist or genetic counselor. These professionals usually cannot tell you with any certainty whether your next child will have a visual impairment. Instead, the probability will be expressed in terms like "you have a 1 in 4 chance that your next child will have a similar visual impairment," or "you have a 50–50 chance that future children will have this same condition."

Parents in the process of making this decision may receive unasked-for advice from family members, friends, and total strangers. Consider the example of a young mother who was grocery shopping with her son Tony, who was blind. The cashier, noticing that the mother was pregnant, pointed to Tony and asked, "Aren't you afraid that your baby will be like him?" The mother replied, "I'd have a dozen if I knew they would all have Tony's sense of humor and easy-going personality!"

In another example, a thoughtful father expressed well his family's decision *not* to have additional children: "We've decided to keep our family small so that we will have the time and energy to do all of those special family activities we have been looking forward to."

Remember that this decision is an important one, but only you can know what is best for your family. By gathering all the information possible, including genetic information, you will be able to make a more knowledgeable decision.

∷ Your Child's Future

As a parent, you are naturally concerned about your child's future. You are also naturally worried about the effect that your child's visual impairment will have on his future. At this point, it is impossible for anyone to predict exactly how your child's visual impairment will affect his life. But it may reassure you to know that with each passing year the quality of life is generally improving for *all* people with disabilities.

We have come a long way from the days when people who were blind were placed in institutions or hidden from sight. Your child will have opportunities that were only dreamed about even a generation ago. For example, the printed word has become increasingly accessible to blind children since the invention of braille in the nineteenth century. There are computers with speech output that can "read" printed matter aloud, as well as braille printers that can be attached to word processors to allow almost instant translation of print to braille and braille to print.

There are new devices as well as tried-and-true techniques for orientation and mobility that can enable your child to move about independently in his environment. And in 1990, an important law—the Americans with Disabilities Act—was passed in the United States to prohibit discrimination against people with disabilities in a number of areas. As a result, your child will be able to become more a part of his community than ever before. He will grow up knowing that employers cannot discriminate against him simply because he has a visual impairment, and that public buildings have braille labels on their elevators and restaurants have braille menus.

The challenge for you as parents is to make sure that your child receives the training and services he needs to become an independent, productive, and happy individual. The following chapters of this book should help to point you in the right direction.

∷ Conclusion

If you have just learned that your child has a visual impairment, your questions and concerns may be overwhelming. Bear in mind, however, that you don't have to learn everything about your child's condition at once. Over time, you will meet others—parents, teachers, doctors—who can help answer your questions, offer advice about caring for your child, and refer you to helpful resources. Gradually, as your child grows, you will realize that some information is relevant to your child, and some is not, and you will get better at separating the important information from the unimportant. Like other parents, you will learn the best ways to take care of your child's needs, play with him, and enjoy his company. More importantly, you will learn that despite your child's visual impairment, he is really much more like other children than different.

With time, your early focus on your child's visual impairment will shift so that it is no longer your overriding concern. As difficult as it may be to believe today, there *will* come a day when your family's situation will seem manageable again and you and your child will be able to get on with your lives.

:: Parent Statements

I am so glad to live in these days when it is easier to get information about blindness. I've talked to parents of older children who have told me about how difficult it used to be to find out basic information. Now, it is just a click of the mouse and I can get answers to my questions.

❧

Sometimes I just sit and close my eyes to try to understand what it is like not to be able to see.

❧

The best thing to happen to us was linking up with a blind adult almost from the very beginning. She has helped all of us so much. We have a sense of what Sarah's life will be like in the future.

❧

As soon as I found out my son had a visual impairment, I got on the phone. I called everyone I could. I would ask people to send me information and sometimes it would take weeks to get it. After a few calls I realized that I was the only one in a hurry.

❧

I'm a little surprised that we have so much energy for this. My entire family has embraced the challenges and the joys of watching Jennifer grow into a funny, sweet, happy little girl.

❦

Before Kevin was born, I had never met anyone who was blind.

❦

We have to keep this all in perspective. Michael is healthy and happy. His visual impairment will have an impact on his life, but it won't ruin it.

❦

I never really noticed before how much I use my vision during the course of the day. Now I think about it all the time.

❦

I've spent so much time just trying to find out very basic things. I've been to the library, I've spent hours on the phone, I've even gone to a conference. Every time I get more information I feel better and more powerful.

❦

The other day I saw a character who was blind on a television show. I realized that I was watching everything about that character and laughed when I thought about it being "just a fictional character." But later I was talking with my wife and we discussed how good it was that the character was strong and complete. I don't think the media always shows realistic portrayals of people with disabilities.

❦

I called the school for the blind and they were able to help me immediately even though my child was only a few months old.

❦

I have always been a "self-help junkie." Any time I have a problem or question I look everywhere for information about it. When Samantha was diagnosed with Leber's Congenital Amaurosis I tried to find out everything I could about it. I looked in the library and spent hours looking things up on the Internet.

MEDICAL ISSUES, TREATMENTS, AND PROFESSIONALS

Steven Stiles, O.D., & Robert Knox, M.D.*

Most children with visual impairments are just as healthy as other children. They are no more likely to catch routine childhood illnesses, develop allergies, or need to visit the pediatrician than any other child. They do, however, need specialized medical care to diagnose and treat their eye condition. Consequently, you may find yourself spending more time in doctors' offices than you would otherwise. You will also need to spend more time learning about selected medical issues in order to understand your child's condition and feel comfortable talking to doctors about it.

This chapter provides the basic information you need to get started talking with your ophthalmologist or optometrist. It explains how the eye ordinarily works, as well as the most common eye conditions that can cause visual impairments in children. It also covers important considerations in choosing and working with eye care professionals and gives you an idea of what to expect during a complete eye examination. Over the months and years, it will, of course, be important for you to focus more on the issues directly related to your child. But at

---

* *Editor's note: Special thanks to Darick Wright, Perkins School for the Blind, for assistance with the revision of this chapter.*

least in the beginning, a basic knowledge of general ophthalmology and medical terms will help boost your confidence in dealing with eye care professionals.

▪▪ Basic Anatomy of the Eye

When you talk with your child's eye care specialist, you may hear references to different parts of the eye as they relate to your child's visual impairment. Nobody expects you to have a complete medical knowledge of the eye. However, a general understanding of the parts of the eye and how they work is essential to understanding your child's visual impairment.

The eye is small, but complex. It contains many of the tiniest parts of the body, and the way it works is still not completely understood. Knowledge about the parts of the eye and their function, however, has greatly increased during the past century. The parts of the eye have been assigned to three different groups, based on the role they play in vision. These groups are known as:

1. the optical system,
2. the nervous system, and
3. the eye movement system.

This section explains how these three systems work together to enable us to see. You may want to refer to the drawing of the eye on the next page as the different parts of the eye are described.

The Eye's Optical System

Sometimes the eye is referred to as a light receptor organ. This means that the eye receives light rays, which are then interpreted by the brain. The optical system is the part of the eye that receives the light rays and focuses them before they are relayed to the brain. The optical system consists of the following parts of the eye:

The **cornea** is the clear dome on the front of the eye. To function properly, the cornea needs to be smooth, evenly curved, and clear so that light can pass through it. The cornea is the only part of the eye that can currently be transplanted.

The **anterior chamber** is the space between the cornea and the iris. It is filled with fluid called **aqueous.**

The **iris** is the colored part of the eye. The amount of pigment in the iris may vary from minimal in the light blue eye to densely pigmented in

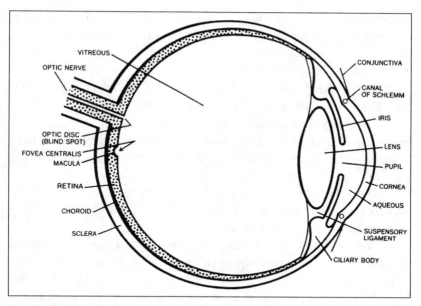

Reprinted with permission by Prevent Blindness America. © 1995

the dark brown eye. The function of the iris is to regulate the amount of light that enters the eye. A healthy or normal iris is circular and controls the size of the pupil, which looks like a black dot in the center of the eye, but is really a hole, created by the doughnut-like shape of the iris. The iris allows the **pupil** to contract or expand (get smaller or larger) and thus let the correct amount of light into the eye.

Behind the iris is the **lens** of the eye, sometimes called the crystalline lens. The lens must be clear so that light will pass through it. The lens changes shape, getting fatter or thinner in order to help focus the light on the back of the eye. This focusing ability of the eye is called *accommodation*. Children have the maximum ability to accommodate for near reading or activities at a close distance. This is why some children can hold reading materials very close to their eyes without fatigue. The ability to accommodate diminishes with age.

The back of the eye consists of three main layers. The outer layer (covering the outside of the eye) is called the **sclera.** It is the white part of the eye, and extends from the back of the eye to the cornea. It helps the eye maintain its shape. The second layer is called the **choroid.** It is rich in blood vessels, which carry nourishment to the eye. The final, inner layer is known as the retina. The **retina** consists of millions of specialized cells that serve as light receptors. The signal initiated in these light receptors is then transported to the brain via the optic nerve.

The Eye's Nerve System

As explained above, the retina consists of millions of light receptors. There are two types of light receptors: cones and rods.

The cones are located in the center of the retina, in an area on the retina called the **macula.** Thus, the cones are sometimes referred to as central or macular receptors. The cones enable us to see detail and color. They are what enable us to see details for reading.

The rods are primarily responsible for peripheral, or "side," vision, and are therefore sometimes referred to as peripheral receptors. They also enable us to see movement and to see in dimmer light.

The nature and severity of many visual impairments is determined by which of the two types of retinal receptors is affected and to what extent (damaged or non-functional). It is not currently possible to repair retinal receptors or optic nerve fibers once they have been damaged or failed to function.

The **optic nerve,** which consists of millions of nerve fibers, carries the message from the light receptors to the area of the brain associated with vision.

The Eye's Movement System

Each eye's movement system consists of six muscles connected to the outside of the eye. These muscles, called the *extraocular* muscles, allow the eyes to aim, search, follow, converge (come together), diverge, and fixate. When these muscles align properly, the eyes can then fuse their separate images into one single three-dimensional image. This is what allows *depth perception* (binocular vision).

◫ How We See

The process of seeing begins when the movement system directs the eyes to aim at and fixate on something in the environment. The optical system then focuses the image in much the same way that a camera focuses an image on film. First, light rays reflected from an object enter the eye through the smooth, clear, curved cornea. The cornea begins the process of bending the light rays so that they will focus correctly on the back of the retina. The light rays then pass through the pupil to the lens. The muscles in the iris surrounding the pupil expand and contract so that the correct amount of light is available. The lens then focuses the light rays so that they form clear images on the retina. Light rays striking the receptors (rods and cones) of the retina are converted into nerve impulses by photochemical reaction. The nerve impulses are next carried to the brain via the optic nerve. Finally, the brain "develops" and interprets the image that was projected on the retina. When we perceive this interpreted image, we are doing what is commonly known as "seeing."

▪▪ Causes of Visual Impairment

Because so many parts of the eye and brain must work closely together in order for us to see well, there are many ways that vision can be impaired.

In children, there are a variety of reasons that one or more parts of the visual system may be damaged or may malfunction. In general, however, visual impairments are due to one of three broad causes:

1. structural impairments, or damage to one or more parts of the eye;
2. refractive errors, or an inability of the eye to sharply focus images on the back of the retina; or
3. cortical visual impairments, which are due to damage to the part of the brain that interprets visual information.

The section below describes the most common types of eye conditions that result from these broad causes. The descriptions are fairly basic; so, for additional information about your child's particular visual impairment, contact your family doctor or refer to one of the references listed in the Reading List at the back of this book.

Structural Impairments

When a child has a structural impairment, one or more parts of the eye's optical, movement, or nerve system is poorly developed, damaged, or does not function properly. Structural impairments may occur before birth or after birth. When they occur before birth, it may be because the baby has inherited a condition that causes structural impairments, or because something happened to disrupt the normal development of the visual system. After birth, structural damage may be caused by injury to the eye, disease, inherited conditions, or a variety of other causes. Regardless of when the damage occurred, the key is to identify the vision problem as soon as possible and promptly take steps to minimize its impact on your child's growth and learning. Listed below are explanations of some common structural impairments.

Cataracts

A cataract is a cloudiness of the crystalline lens of the eye. Since light cannot pass normally through the cataract, it obscures vision. The effect on vision may vary from no detectable visual impairment to a severe loss of vision. In severe cases, the child may only be able to detect light from dark. Some types of cataracts progressively worsen, while others remain unchanged throughout life. Cataracts may be found in only one eye (unilateral) or in both eyes (bilateral). Cataracts may be present at birth.

Cataracts vary in size and severity. Since the early months and years in childhood are critical in learning, prompt assessment and diagnosis are very important.

There are many causes of cataracts in children. They may be inherited, or they may result from an infection to the mother during pregnancy. They may also occur as part of a disease or syndrome that affects many parts of a child's body. Marfan syndrome, Turner syndrome, Cri du chat syndrome, Crouzon syndrome, Apert syndrome, Lowe syndrome, Down syndrome, osteogenesis imperfecta, and juvenile rheumatoid arthritis are examples of conditions associated with cataracts.

The definitive treatment involves surgically removing cataracts from the eyes. Cataracts that are sufficiently cloudy to obscure vision require prompt attention. Often surgery is needed within the first three months of life so that vision can develop properly. Cataract surgery in children is performed under general anesthesia, either on an outpatient or inpatient basis, depending on the child's overall health and age. Young infants are often kept in the hospital for an overnight stay; rarely is a more prolonged stay necessary. The operation is not usually painful.

Surgically removing the crystalline lens results in what doctors refer to as *aphakia* (an eye with no lens). Without a lens, the eye can no longer focus on its own. Consequently, your child will need either contact lenses or glasses to provide a clear image to the retina. Cataract surgery is usually very successful for all ages. If your child's eye is otherwise healthy, she could possibly develop normal vision after the operation.

Usually children become quite farsighted immediately after the operation and need strong corrective lenses. The farsightedness is corrected with one contact lens if only one eye underwent cataract surgery and with two contact lenses or eyeglasses if both eyes had surgery. The amount of farsightedness frequently decreases over several years as the child's eye grows, reaching normal adult size near puberty. As your child's eye grows, she will require frequent changes in her prescription for corrective lenses. Once her eyes have stopped growing, she may be able to have artificial lenses (intraocular lenses) permanently implanted. Your doctor might even suggest implanting lenses earlier.

Sometimes children who have had cataracts have trouble learning to use vision in one eye or both eyes. If so, your doctor may prescribe the use of an eye patch, as described in the section on Amblyopia, below. The road to maximal visual development following cataract removal requires long-term follow-up and much dedication. Be sure to follow your doctor's advice and schedule routine visits to make sure your child's visual development continues to progress.

Glaucoma

Glaucoma is a condition in which the pressure from fluid inside the anterior chamber of the eye is too high. If the condition is not promptly detected and treated, the excessive pressure can irreversibly damage the optic nerve. This nerve damage results in loss of peripheral (side) vision initially, and central vision if the damage continues.

If glaucoma is treated before severe nerve damage results, there can still be lasting visual impairments. Since the outer wall of an infant's eye is very elastic, continued high pressures cause the wall to stretch and the eye to enlarge. (Only in infancy does the eye actually enlarge due to glaucoma; once enlarged, the eye usually remains large even after surgery.) The effects of glaucoma result in high degrees of nearsightedness and astigmatism. (See "Refractive Errors," below.) As the eye enlarges, the cornea may also become stretched, which can lead to clouding and scarring of the cornea. Glaucoma in infants is usually not painful.

To prevent or minimize damage to the eye and the optic nerve, your child's doctor will try to decrease the pressure inside the eye. Sometimes prescription eye drops or oral medications may decrease the pressure. Usually, however, surgery is necessary. The surgery opens the "drainage channels" in the front chamber of the eye, allowing the fluid to drain out more readily. This operation is usually very successful in decreasing the pressure. As in cataract surgery, the glaucoma surgery is performed under general anesthesia on an outpatient or inpatient basis. When glaucoma occurs in infancy, surgery alone may control the pressure for life. Continued follow-up and monitoring of the intraocular pressure, however, is very important.

The degree of visual impairment resulting from glaucoma varies from no visual impairment to complete blindness. The amount of impairment depends on the age at onset of glaucoma, how soon the condition is diagnosed and treated, how well the condition responds to the treatment, and how severely the pressure is increased. Once the pressure is controlled, glaucoma usually does not cause further damage. Often, children need glasses to improve visual acuity that has been impaired by enlargement of the eyes. Many children also require patching treatment for amblyopia, as described below.

In approximately 1 out of 10,000 children born, glaucoma occurs in infancy and early childhood as an isolated inherited disorder. Glaucoma may also be associated with other conditions that affect the eyes or other parts of the body. These conditions include Sturge-Weber syndrome, aniridia, Lowe syndrome, neurofibromatosis, Marfan syndrome, Stickler syndrome, Rubinstein-Taybi syndrome, Trisomy 13, mucopolysaccharidosis, and retinopathy of prematurity.

Amblyopia

Amblyopia is a term derived from the Greek work for "dullness of vision." Colloquially, you may hear it called "lazy eye." Amlyopia refers to the visual impairment that results when a child's brain suppresses the image from one eye. It is important to note that amblyopia is *not* a turning or wandering eye, but may result *from* an eye that turns or wanders.

Ordinarily, the visual system continues to develop until a child is about nine years old. Sometimes, however, something interferes with normal visual development in one or both eyes. This most often happens:

1. when one eye has better acuity than the other (due to a refractive error, cataracts, corneal scarring, droopy eyelid, or tumor);
2. when one eye is crossed or turned due to strabismus (see "Strabismus," below).

To prevent blurred or double vision using both eyes, the child's brain may selectively ignore (suppress) vision in one eye. Over a period of time, this can result in a permanent visual loss in the unused eye. Vision loss may range from mild to severe, but not total blindness.

If amblyopia is detected and treated before the visual system has reached maturity (approximately age nine), the visual loss may be reversible. Just as the eye can become "lazy" with suppression or with a poorly focused image, so too can it regain vision with proper treatment.

The first step in treating amblyopia is generally to determine why the child isn't using one eye and to treat any underlying vision problem in that eye. For example, if one eye has a droopy eyelid, cataracts, or a large refractive error, these conditions would be treated first. Treatment for amblyopia itself consists of forcing your child to use the "lazy" eye. This is commonly done by covering the stronger eye with a patch. This patch may need to be worn for anywhere from a few months to over a year. Glasses are often also necessary to provide the eyes with a well-focused image. Early detection and treatment are essential, as the younger the child, the more rapidly her eyes respond to treatment.

Patching an eye is sometimes uncomfortable for children. It feels very different to see with only the "lazy" eye, and some children may protest. It is very important that you realize that the number one factor in the success of eye patching is to keep the patch on the eye as prescribed by the doctor. You will need to be diligent in your efforts to help your child keep the patch on. Think of ways to reinforce or reward her for keeping the patch on. These rewards should have nothing to do with the patch. In other words, allowing her to take the patch off for a reward is not a good idea. Instead, you might suggest a trip to the library for story hour or a visit to a favorite aunt. Remember, the best time for this treatment is early in your child's life. Damage to the eye caused by failure to wear the patch will likely be permanent.

If a child cannot tolerate patching, it is possible to use a special eye drop that blurs the vision in the better eye. This forces the child to use the "lazy" eye. These drops are seen as a last resort because they cannot be as easily controlled as a patch. Once the drops are administered, the vision will be blurred for several hours, which may not be as effective as being able to control the suppression of vision by taking a patch on and off.

Strabismus

Strabismus is a general term for misaligned ("crossed") eyes. One or both eyes may turn inward (*esotropia*) or turn outward (*exotropia*), or the gaze of one eye may be higher than the other (*hypertropia*).

Strabismus may become apparent within a child's first year of life, or may suddenly appear several years later. Strabismus is one of the most common eye conditions among children.

Treatment for strabismus depends on its cause. Sometimes children who are farsighted cross their eyes as they focus to see more clearly. Glasses that correct the farsightedness often also treat the strabismus. Other times strabismus results from paralysis of the extraocular muscles of the movement system, which creates an imbalance in the muscles' strength. Sometimes children are born with esotropia (congenital esotropia). In these instances, the cause of strabismus is not known. In congenital esotropia, surgery is necessary to correct the misalignment. The operation is performed under general anesthesia on an outpatient basis. About 70 percent of the time, one surgical procedure is enough to "fix" the misalignment. Additional surgery can be performed months or years later if further straightening is needed to improve binocular vision or the appearance of the eyes.

If strabismus is not promptly treated, your child may ignore or suppress the vision in one eye. As discussed above, this can prevent the suppressed eye from developing normal vision (amblyopia). Your child will also have reduced binocular ("3–D") vision if her eyes are not properly aligned. (Children with congenital esotropia may still have reduced binocular vision even with surgery.) Because the crucial period for the development of the visual system is approximately in the first ten years of life, strabismus should be treated as early as possible. This can maximize your child's development of binocular vision and minimize the risk of amblyopia.

Retinopathy of Prematurity

Retinopathy of prematurity (ROP) is a condition that can cause vision loss or blindness in infants born prematurely. As the name implies, it is caused by damage to the retina.

Ordinarily, the blood vessels of the retina complete their growth at the baby's approximate due date (9 months gestation). Premature infants are thus born before the retinal blood vessels have completed their growth. As the vessels continue to grow after a premature baby's birth, abnormal vessels, as well as scar tissue, can form inside the eye. In extreme cases, the retina may become scarred, distorted, or detached (separated from the back of the eye). This causes visual impairment ranging from a mild decrease in acuity to total loss of vision.

The more premature an infant is and the less she weighs at birth, the greater the risk of developing ROP. Infants who weigh at least 2500 grams (5 pounds, 8 ounces) are usually not at risk. Infants born at 28 weeks of gestation or earlier or with a birth weight of 1250–1500 grams or less (approximately 2 pounds, 12 ounces to 3 pounds, 5 ounces) have the greatest risk of developing ROP. One study found that 66 percent of infants who weighed 1250 grams or less at birth and 82 percent of infants who weighed 1000 grams or less (approximately 2 pounds, 3 ounces) developed some degree of ROP. Premature infants who are given oxygen treatment for respiratory problems are thought to be at increased risk for ROP.

Several types of treatment can often prevent ROP from reaching its most severe stages. Cryotherapy (freezing therapy) and laser therapy can be used to decrease the abnormal growth of blood vessels. The point at which either of these treatments is recommended is termed *threshold disease*. If a child's retinas have already become detached, complicated surgical procedures are necessary to try to reattach the retinas. If the retina is totally detached, surgery is much less likely to be successful and a significant visual impairment is more likely.

Children with ROP usually require long-term eye care. Some children have normal visual acuity, but amblyopia and significant refractive errors, including nearsightedness, farsightedness, and astigmatism, are common. Total blindness with no light perception may also occur. Strabismus and glaucoma may also develop and require additional treatment or surgery.

Nystagmus

Nystagmus is a rhythmic oscillation or "jiggling" of the eyes that cannot be controlled by the child. Most often, the eyes move back and forth, but they may also move up and down, in a rotary or bobbing fashion, or in a combination of these movements. Nystagmus is usually present in both eyes, but can also occur in one eye. Nystagmus may occur alone, or it may accompany another vision problem such as congenital cataracts, albinism, a neurological condition, or an abnormality of the cornea.

Although congenital nystagmus generally does not appear to make objects move, visual acuity is reduced. In children with congenital nystagmus, distance vision may be limited to 20/40 to 20/400. Often, however, children with nystagmus find a head position or eye position which diminishes the intensity of the nystagmus. This head position, called the *"null point,"* is strongly preferred by the child, as it gives her the best possible visual acuity. Sometimes this position or posture is so extreme that surgery to alter the alignment of the eyes and thus move the null point over may be beneficial. This type of operation usually succeeds in moving the null point, but does not eliminate the nystagmus. Frequently, nystagmus is dampened when a child focuses on a near object. Therefore, your child's vision when reading may be much better than her vision for distant objects. Some parents report that their child's nystagmus gets worse when her eyes are tired.

There is no single accepted treatment for nystagmus. The doctor should determine whether your child has nearsightedness, farsightedness, or astigmatism that could be improved with glasses. Attempts to decrease the intensity of the nystagmus through eye muscle surgery or by injecting botulinum toxins (poisons) around the eyes have been investigated with varying levels of success. These treatments are generally considered to be of questionable benefit. Your child's ophthalmologist can give you more information about the possible risks and benefits of these controversial treatments.

Albinism

Albinism is an inherited condition that causes decreased pigment either in the skin, hair, and eyes, or in the eyes alone. The lack of pigment in the front of the eye (iris) is most noticeable and leads to a very light blue color of iris. When a light is directed into the eye, the lack of pigment allows the red reflex to shine through the iris tissue as well as the pupil, giving the iris a "pink" appearance. Albinism is present at birth and does not become worse over time. Approximately 1 in 20,000 children is born with the condition.

Children with albinism have incompletely formed (hypoplastic) maculas—the central portion of the retina which provides the sharpest vision. They also have nystagmus and often have refractive errors (see below). As a result, they have reduced visual acuity. With corrective lenses, visual acuity usually measures around 20/100 to 20/200, although it may be as good as 20/40.

Because their eyes lack pigment to block or absorb light, children with albinism may be very sensitive to the light (*photophobic*). Tinted glasses or contact lenses can relieve sensitivity to light, and proper prescription lenses or low vision aids can help maximize vision.

Optic Nerve Atrophy

The optic nerve consists of approximately one million fibers that transmit signals from the retina to the brain. If fibers are damaged, they may die and atrophy (waste away). When fibers atrophy, transmission of information from the eye to the brain is impaired. The resulting visual impairment can range from minimal loss of acuity or visual field to total blindness.

Optic atrophy can result from a variety of disorders, including hydrocephalus, glaucoma, retinitis pigmentosa, or from trauma. How significantly vision is affected will depend on the severity of the damage. Depending on the cause of the atrophy, your child's vision may or may not continue to worsen. If possible, treatment is directed at the specific cause in an attempt to prevent further damage to the nerve. For example, if the damage is due to hydrocephalus, treatment involves treating the pressure around the brain; if the damage is due to glaucoma, treatment involves reducing the pressure in the eyes.

Refractive Errors

Refraction refers to the process by which the cornea and lens of the eye bend light rays so they are focused on the retina. For the light rays to be sharply focused, the eyeball must be the right length, the lens must have appropriate power, and the cornea must have the right shape. If any of these parts of the eye is *not* properly proportioned, then visual acuity is reduced. This type of visual impairment is known as a refractive error. Common varieties of refractive errors include nearsightedness, farsightedness, and astigmatism.

Refractive errors, especially nearsightedness, continue to change (usually for the worse) as a child grows. Usually, however, they do not change as much after the teenage years or early adulthood. Some refractive errors are inherited, or passed down from parent to child. There are also some specific eye conditions that may result in extreme refractive errors. These conditions include retinopathy of prematurity, aphakia, glaucoma, and microphthalmia.

Glasses can often compensate for refractive errors, improving vision at least to some degree when they are worn. Contact lenses may also be an option when your child is mature enough to handle the responsibility, or if she has had a lens removed during cataract surgery. See the discussion on "Corrective Lenses and Their Limitations" below for more information.

Myopia (Nearsightedness)

In myopia (nearsightedness), the cornea is excessively curved, the lens is too strong, or the eye is elongated. As a result, images of distant objects are not focused precisely *on* the retina, but in front of it. This makes them appear blurry. Usually, children with myopia can see nearer objects more clearly.

Myopia is quite common. It affects about 2 percent of children by age 6 and 10 percent by age 10. By age 20, approximately 20 percent of young adults have myopia.

The degree of myopia is measured with a unit called the *diopter,* which corresponds with the 20/XX formula explained in Chapter 1. The higher the bottom number in the fraction, the greater a child's myopia. A child with 20/100 vision, for example, can identify an object 20 feet away as well as someone with normal vision would identify it from a distance of 100 feet. A child with 20/600 vision sees at 20 feet as well as someone with normal vision sees at 600 feet. If your child is unable to identify the largest test symbol (which could be a letter, number, picture, or shape) on the regular chart at twenty feet, the examiner will test at a closer distance and note the distance at which your child is able to identify it. For instance, 6/400 would indicate that your child could identify a 20/400 size symbol at six feet. Similarly, 2/400 would mean that your child needed the 20/400 symbol to be placed at two feet before she could identify it.

Myopia may appear alone, or in combination with other eye conditions. Premature infants with retinopathy of prematurity, for instance, are more likely to have high (significant) refractive errors, including high myopia and/or high anisometropia (see below).

Hyperopia (Farsightedness)

Hyperopia (farsightedness) occurs when the cornea is relatively flat, the eye is not as long as normal, or the focusing power of the eye is too weak. Consequently, objects are focused at a point behind the eye's retina. As a result, the child must strain excessively to focus, especially on nearby objects. Children with relatively mild hyperopia, however, often can see both distant and near objects clearly. This is because children have a tremendous ability to increase the focusing power of their eyes and thereby "focus" objects on the retina. Children with a high degree of hyperopia generally cannot do this, though, and need glasses to see a clear, single image. Glasses are also needed if a child crosses her eyes when attempting to focus to keep them aligned.

The strength of correction for hyperopia is expressed in diopters, as with myopia. The greater the number of diopters in the prescription for corrective lenses, the more farsighted a child is.

Anisometropia

Usually a child's two eyes are very close in refractive power. Occasionally, however, there is a significant difference between the refractive power of each eye. For example, one eye may be nearsighted, while the other is farsighted. This disparity in refractive power is known as anisometropia.

Because the eyes may appear normal and straight when a child has anisometropia, the condition may go undetected. This can result in amblyopia and below normal "3–D vision" (*stereoacuity*) if the brain selectively ignores the image from one eye. Providing glasses to correct any significant difference between the eyes and treating the amblyopia as soon as possible can maximize a child's potential for clear, 3–D vision.

Astigmatism

In astigmatism, the shape of the cornea is not quite right, so light rays passing through it are not properly focused. Most often, the cornea is steeper (more curved) in one meridian (that is, vertically) than it is in the horizontal meridian. Consequently, each meridian has a different focusing power. Both near and far objects may appear blurry to a child with astigmatism, depending on the severity of the astigmatism. Astigmatism often appears in combination with nearsightedness or farsightedness.

Cortical Visual Impairment

In contrast to a structural impairment or refractive error, a cortical visual impairment ("cortical blindness") is not caused by any abnormality of the eyes. Instead, it results from damage within the brain, often within the visual cortex of the brain. (Hence the term "cortical.") This damage prevents the child from adequately receiving or interpreting messages from the eyes, even though the eyes may be quite capable of gathering visual information. This damage may result in a decrease in visual acuity or possibly total blindness. Causes of cortical visual impairment range from insufficient oxygen to the brain at birth or during heart surgery, to hydrocephalus, stroke, or trauma.

Children with cortical visual impairment often have other disabilities such as cerebral palsy, seizure disorders, developmental disabilities, or hydrocephalus. This is because the same injury that damages the brain's visual center can also cause damage that results in cognitive, motor, or other impairments. When cortical visual impairment occurs alone, it is often as the result of *anoxia* (no oxygen) or *hypoxia* (insufficient oxygen) during the birth process.

There is no medical treatment for cortical visual impairment. It is important, however, to rule out any ocular abnormality, such as cataracts or retinal or optic nerve abnormalities, which may contribute to the vision loss. Glasses should also be prescribed if your child has a significant refractive error in addition to cortical visual impairment. Cortical visual impairments do not usually worsen over the years. Occasionally, vision improves spontaneously over a period of months or years. In these instances, however, vision usually remains impaired to some degree.

☷ Searching for the Cause of Your Child's Impairment

Knowing the cause of your child's visual impairment is clearly very important in knowing how to treat it. Obviously, the treatments for structural problems such as glaucoma and cataracts are very different from treatments for refractive errors. And diagnosing and treating problems as early as possible is often vital to preventing further visual impairment or total blindness.

In this day and age, it is unusual that the cause for a child's visual impairment cannot be determined. Usually some explanation can be given as to the most likely cause for a visual loss. Although it is beyond the scope of this book to cover every possible cause of visual impairments, rest assured that eye care professionals are trained to recognize and diagnose many more conditions than are described here. If, for some reason, you have been told that the cause of your child's visual impairment is not known, it may be helpful to seek a second opinion.

☷ Choosing an Eye Care Professional

Chapter 1 introduced the ophthalmologist and the optometrist—the eye care professionals most often involved in diagnosing and treating visual impairments. As you may remember, the areas of expertise of these professionals overlap somewhat. But they also have special and unique areas of expertise. For this reason, many parents find that the most effective and beneficial approach to vision care is a team approach, using the services of both ophthalmology and optometry.

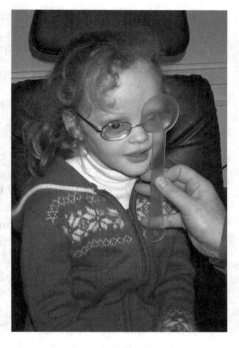

Using the team approach, your child would see an ophthalmologist for diagnosis and treatment of a visual loss with an underlying medical problem. For example, your child would need to see an ophthalmologist for surgical treatment of glaucoma or cataracts, and for medical follow-up of these conditions. Depending on the laws in your state, your child may also need to see the ophthalmologist for prescriptions she needs related to her visual impairment.

Using the team approach, your child would see an optometrist for treatment of refractive errors (or she could see the ophthalmologist). She would also see the optometrist for special treatment if she has "low vision." Many optometrists specialize in evaluating and treating children with low vision, prescribing specific low vision devices which may help the child live and perform up to her potential. These optometrists are often called low vision specialists or low vision consultants. Low vision specialists may be in practice by themselves, or may be associated with a larger clinic, low vision center, teaching institution, or child development center.

Low vision specialists prescribe, fit, adjust, and train patients to use low vision optical devices such as special magnifying glasses, special glasses for reading or distance vision, permanent or temporary "prism" lenses, or telescopic devices which are used to spot things at a distance (for example, a telescopic device your child could use to find a street sign or a house number). In addition, many new, high-tech devices are now available for use with computers in reading or even spotting objects at a distance. New technology is continually being developed.

If you are not sure whether your child should see an ophthalmologist or an optometrist, you may wish to ask whether the ophthalmologist or optometrist you are considering works with the other as a team.

Here are some suggestions to help you choose among the eye care professionals in your community:

- *Check the qualifications of the doctor.* Has he or she had special training in working with very young children? (Pediatric ophthalmologists are specially trained to work with young children and are interested in their unique conditions.) Has he had experience working with children who are visually impaired? Does he have a particular specialty, such as diseases of the retina? If your child has other disabilities, has he worked with other children with multiple disabilities? Is he involved in professional activities such as attending special conferences related to visual impairments? Has he published papers that you could read? If you think your child might benefit from low vision devices, does he have experience and a special interest in working with patients with low vision?

- *Consider carefully the geographic location of your doctor's office.* The location of your primary eye care professional will be important, especially if your child has an eye condition that should be closely monitored. While you may consult closely with eye care professionals at a distance, it is a good idea to have someone locally available to call in case of an emergency. Long trips to the doctor can also be burdensome, especially if your child's condition could be followed just as well by a local professional.

- *Talk with the doctor.* Tell him or her your concerns and questions about your child's eye condition. Note how he responds to you. Does he speak in medical jargon, or is he willing to explain things in language you can understand? Is he patronizing, or does he treat you like a respected member of your child's health care team? Make sure that you are comfortable with your interactions. There may be times when you and your doctor must discuss difficult issues and make difficult decisions about your child's care. It is very important to trust your doctor and be able to talk to him about the most sensitive issues.

- *Consider how your child responds to the doctor.* You will want to make sure that your child is comfortable with the doctor. You must also realize, however, that a visit to the eye doctor may not always be pleasant for your child, so she may sometimes react negatively. An understanding eye doctor will try to alleviate this difficulty as much as possible.

In searching for an eye care specialist, it is a good idea to ask friends, family members, your pediatrician, or others in your community for recommendations. Especially good sources of recommendations are local groups for parents of children with visual impairments. If you have difficulty locating an appropriate ophthalmologist, optometrist, or low vision specialist, you may contact The American Optometric Association (website: www.aoa.org; phone: 800-365-2219) or The American Academy of Ophthalmology (website: www.aao.org; phone: 415-447-0223).

⣿ What to Expect at an Eye Examination

Over the years, your child will have eye examinations for many different reasons: to monitor eye health, measure refractive errors, and, if she has a progressive disease, to monitor vision. In addition, low vision devices may need to be changed or prescribed to meet the changing needs of a growing child. It is beyond the scope of this chapter to describe every possible test and procedure that might be done on your child. Instead, this section explains in a general way what often happens at a complete eye examination. Your child may have some of these procedures done at some visits, but not others; she may or may not ever have them all performed on the same visit. Knowing how and why particular procedures are done, however, may help you and your child be more knowledgeable participants in the examination.

A complete eye examination is done by either an ophthalmologist or optometrist. Sometimes it is difficult to examine the eyes of infants and small children, as they cannot respond the way that adults can respond. A patient doctor will spend time with your child, trying to obtain the best information possible. Rarely, it may be necessary to medicate your child to sedate her or even to give a general anesthesia in order to fully evaluate her eyes.

Especially during early exams, the doctor will begin by getting a complete history from you. He will want to know about other family members with similar eye disorders. Since the growth of the eye begins very early in fetal development, the doctor will probably ask questions about events during pregnancy. For instance, he may ask which medications the mother took or whether she had any infections. The more specifically you can answer the doctor's questions, the more quickly an accurate diagnosis and plan for treatment can be made.

After discussing your child's and family's history, the doctor will measure distance and near visual acuities. As discussed in Chapter 1, the method he uses will depend on your child's age and her ability and willingness to respond. Testing of pupils, external facial appearance, motility/muscle balance, visual fields, and color perception is then performed. The doctor will dilate (widen) your child's pupils with eye drops in order to examine the inner structures of the eyes (lens, retina, optic nerve) and to make it easier to measure refraction. These eyedrops may be uncomfortable for your child, but the discomfort is very brief. You may be able to comfort or distract your child with a hug or a joke or by playing with a favorite toy. Your child's refractive error can be measured precisely by holding different lenses in front of her eye and measuring the eye's reflex with a special hand-held instrument. No input is required from the child; therefore, even a very young infant could be assessed for the need for glasses! The retina and optic nerve are examined with hand-held and head-mounted lights, as well as with special hand-held lenses.

A visit to the ophthalmologist or optometrist can give you valuable information. Listed below are some of the results you might expect from the doctor's exam:

1. Practical information concerning the size of materials your child is able to identify. This will help you choose appropriate toys and books. It may also help you know how best to modify your child's preschool classroom or your own home.

2. The best type of lighting for your child, especially if her eye condition is associated with difficulty in seeing in either dim or bright lighting.

3. A prescription for the best corrective lenses for your child. The doctor will also prescribe medication, if necessary.

4. A complete understanding of your child's visual condition, visual history, and prognosis, in both technical and

layman's terms. Having this is important not only for your knowledge of your child's impairment, but also in case you change doctors and another eye care professional becomes involved. Understanding all this information will also be helpful for sharing information with other professionals, especially school professionals and vision specialists.

5. Information about any secondary eye conditions your child has. Some eye conditions such as retinopathy of prematurity carry with them the likelihood that some other optical difficulty will develop as a result of the first or primary eye condition. Sometimes your doctor will let you know that your child should be followed closely and that warning signs should be carefully monitored. Sometimes your doctor might indicate that your child's physical activity should be limited. A thorough knowledge of your doctor's recommendations will be essential to help you monitor your child's visual difficulties.

Something you should *not* expect from your doctor is education or rehabilitation goals or recommendations regarding the frequency of specialized services. Eye care professionals are rarely qualified to make these recommendations. Decisions to teach braille, for example, should *not* be made by the ophthalmologist or optometrist based on what is found during the eye exam. These types of recommendations are best made by a teacher of students with visual impairments, O&M instructors, and rehabilitation teachers. See Chapter 8 for an overview of these special education issues.

Preparing for an Eye Exam

Unfortunately, a trip to the eye doctor may not always be pleasant for your child. As positive and encouraging as your eye care professional may be, your child will be asked to perform tasks during the exam that may be difficult for her. She will be required to respond, not just once but many times, to questions about what she can see. She may not understand what the "correct" response is and may become frustrated because she is not able to do as she is asked. In addition, an eye exam is time-consuming, and your child may become bored. Listed below are some suggestions that may help make visits to the eye doctor a little more pleasant:

- *Contact the doctor's office before your visit to find out if there are forms to complete or specific questions that the doctor may want to ask you.* By completing forms in advance and being prepared for your doctor's questions, you can limit the time your child must be at the doctor's office

- *Be careful not to communicate any negative emotions you may feel about the examination to your child.* Pay attention to the way that you talk about the eye doctor's office. Your child will reflect your attitude. Even if you think that your child is not paying attention to conversations between you and your spouse, you may find that she acts more on your attitudes than you expect. It is important, then, to talk positively, in a matter-of-fact manner about trips to the eye doctor.

- *As your child becomes older, discuss the procedures at the eye doctor's office in more detail.* When she is curious about her eye condition or about any part of the examination, be sure to answer her questions as completely as possible and encourage her to ask more questions when she is ready.

- *Bring some of your child's favorite toys, books, or tapes with you to the examination.* Even though the eye doctor

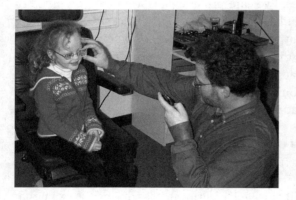

may have toys in the waiting room, familiar playthings may make your child feel more comfortable and help to pass the time. They will also give the doctor an idea of the type of toys and the size of objects your child likes to look at.

- *Help to make a trip to the eye doctor something to look forward to by planning a treat after the appointment.* This does not need to be an elaborate special event. A walk around the park or a visit to the ice cream parlor would be a pleasant reward for the work that your child has done at the doctor's office. It is a good idea to have several treats in mind and let your child select the one she would like. Your child does not have the choice of going to the eye doctor or not. By giving her a choice of what to do after her visit to the doctor, you allow her to have some control of the situation.

Besides preparing your child for a visit to the eye doctor, you may also want to prepare yourself so that you can help the doctor, yourself, and your child get the maximum benefit from an exam. Following are some suggestions to help you become a more effective participant:

- *Be observant.* Watch your child's behavior. For example, how does she handle toys? What kinds of head positions does she use when looking at objects? You may be the best "examiner," and your observations will be important. This is especially true during a functional vision assessment, as discussed in Chapter 1. It will also be helpful information, however, during a clinical examination (during testing performed by the doctor). Be sure to communicate your observations to your child's doctor.
- *Ask questions.* It is your right to have your questions answered in a clear, understanding, nonjudgmental way. However, some parents find it difficult to know the questions to ask. It may be helpful to make a list of questions before you go to the doctor. The more prepared you are, the more likely it is that your doctor will be able to give you the information you want and need. If you think of questions after you leave the doctor's office, do not hesitate to write or call your doctor for additional information. A caring doctor will be sympathetic to your needs and will welcome an open discussion.
- *Provide stimulation to your child.* Some people believe that children who are visually impaired do not need visually interesting environments. Nothing could be further from the truth. Most children with visual impairments do have some vision that they can use. Maybe they see light and shadows, or maybe they see colors. Regardless, it is important to provide your child with toys and room decorations that are visually motivating. If your child is used to examining things visually as well as tactually, she will be more prepared to respond to questions from her eye doctor.

- *Be positive.* Encourage your child to explore her world. Re-inforce her exploration through vision, touch, and hearing.
- *Put things in perspective.* Remember that 20/40, 20/200, or any visual acuity is not a magic number. Base your expectations on your child's abilities, not clinical numbers. Make sure that the doctor does the same—that he actually looks at what your child can do, without making assumptions that she's in every respects like a "typical" kid with 20/200 vision. Not all children adapt to visual impairment the same way, although most adapt very well.
- *Keep good records of your child's eye exams or know the names of doctors who have seen your child so you can readily obtain records.* Keep copies of reports, records of medications taken, and information about your child's operations so that you can readily answer doctors' questions. This is especially important if your child sees many different doctors.
- *Help your doctor.* Most doctors would welcome your help if your child is having trouble with the eye examination. You will know how to help your child in ways that the doctor may not know. Especially if your child is misbehaving or struggling or seems upset by the process, feel free to offer your help.

■■ Corrective Lenses and Their Limitations

Eyeglasses and contact lenses do not "cure" farsightedness, near-sightedness, or astigmatism. Instead, they actually compensate for these refractive errors by allowing a clear optical image to be focused on the retina. When the glasses or contacts are removed, the child is still farsighted, nearsighted, or astigmatic. The glasses or contacts do not permanently "fix" the refractive error. Normally, eyeglasses or contacts can only compensate for refractive errors. They cannot compensate for physical damage to the eye due to other causes, such as optic atrophy, glaucoma, or corneal scars.

Corrective lenses work by refocusing images so that they fall *on* the retina, rather than in front of, or behind it. They are ground to very precise curves based on the degree and type of refractive error your child has. The lens's total power is made up of a combination of the powers of the curves on the front and back surfaces of the lenses, and on the lens's thickness. A lens that compensates for nearsightedness is thinner in the center and thicker at the edges (concave). A lens that compensates for farsightedness is thicker in the center and thinner at the edges (convex). Generally, the higher the prescription, the thicker the lenses.

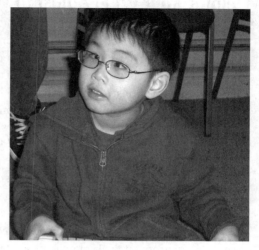

Parents frequently wonder why lenses can't be made stronger and stronger so that every child can have better vision or 20/20 vision. The purpose of prescription lenses is to compensate for the child's refractive error only and thus focus incoming images on the retina. There may be other factors limiting vision—such as glaucoma, optic atrophy, or amblyopia—that cannot be corrected simply with glasses or contact lenses. Any additional lens power would only over-compensate for the exact refractive error. It would not help visual acuity, because it would cause the image not to be focused on the retina.

Reading glasses for children with low vision are one exception to the rule that extra strong lenses are generally not helpful. Special higher-powered low vision reading glasses may be prescribed specifically to allow a child to read at a closer distance. These types of glasses magnify, rather than correct for refractive error.

Many parents wonder where they should go to have their child's glasses made. There are several different options, including the "one-hour" optical centers available in many communities. Although these may be fine for some prescriptions, other prescriptions are more complicated and require more extensive work. You should check with the ophthalmologist or optometrist who prescribed the glasses to find out the best place to get your child's glasses. Often your eye doctor can recommend a specific *optician,* the technician who grinds lenses to make glasses. An optician is not qualified to prescribe glasses, but once the prescription is written by an optometrist or ophthalmologist, he or she can make your child's glasses so they have the proper correction.

Helping Your Child Adjust to Wearing Glasses

Parents are sometimes worried that young children will have difficulty keeping glasses on, or may lose or break them more frequently. This is possible, but, if the glasses help your child see, you may find that she adjusts fairly quickly to wearing them. If this does present a problem, your child's teacher of students with visual impairments will be able to help brainstorm some strategies to help you child. These may include:

- *Make sure that your child's glasses are comfortable and fit well.*
- *Analyze when it is that your child benefits from her glasses.* For example, are they meant primarily for reading or close work? Then you can make sure that she is wearing the glasses at appropriate times when she will benefit most from them.
- *Determine ways to reward your child for using her glasses appropriately.* It may be possible to combine the reward with an activity that will allow your child to use her glasses. For example, a trip to the zoo or circus is reinforcing and gives your child an opportunity to use her glasses in a fun activity.
- *Use commonly available devices (such as back straps and glasses cases) along with a routine of cleaning and caring for the glasses so that your child gradually begins to take more and more responsibility for the care and safety of her glasses.*

Your child's ophthalmologist might also discuss the possibility of using contact lenses. The use of contact lenses will be dependent on many factors, including your child's eye condition, the structure of her eye, her age, and other environmental factors.

∷ Conclusion

The importance of proper eye care for your child who is visually impaired cannot be overstated. Neither can the importance of your involvement in decisions related to your child's eye care. As the expert on how your child uses her vision on a daily basis, you play a crucial role in ensuring that she gets the medical treatment that will help her maximize her vision. Understanding your child's eye condition will help you find the best medical care for your child and will help you, along with your child's medical and educational team, make the best decisions for your child's future.

▪▪ Parent Statements

I will always be grateful to our ophthalmologist. When he told me that he suspected that Ryan was blind, he said that they would do everything that they could medically but that I needed to be strong and see that Ryan got the services he needed. Then he gave me the card of another parent of a blind child in our town. Some people might not have liked our doctor's abrupt style but he really started me out on the right foot.

❧❀❧

Once I drove for three hours to get to an ophthalmologist in another city. He was with my child for about ten minutes and seemed too busy to answer my questions. I've become much better at demanding attention, but it is still difficult.

❧❀❧

Soon after Alexis was born, I had a suspicion that there was something wrong with her eyes. Everyone kept telling me that I was wrong, but somehow I knew. Before we went to the doctor, I spent a lot of time watching her and trying to get her to look at things.

❧❀❧

My child's teacher of students with visual impairments goes to our eye appointments with us as often as possible. It helps me so much to have someone else thinking of questions. Sometimes she thinks of things I would never think about and she says the same thing about me.

❧❀❧

My daughter hates to go to the ophthalmologist's office. We need to go for checkups every four or five months and it is so difficult that I begin dreading the trip about a month in advance.

❧❀❧

I have noticed that if I bring my child's vision specialist with us to an eye exam, the doctor talks mostly to her, not to me. I feel like I become invisible.

❧❀❧

Because of her age, the doctors were unable to tell us how well Maggie could see.

❧❀❧

The doctor who gave us the diagnosis had horrible "people skills." When he was explaining Justin's visual impairment to us he was so matter-of-fact. The whole time I thought, "Our world is falling apart and this doctor doesn't even care!" He wasn't at all sensitive to our feelings. We switched to a kinder, more personable doctor as soon as we could.

❧❀❧

Dr. Wright, our ophthalmologist, is very funny. Hannah loves him! He has toys in his office and he is so kind when he talks to Hannah. He's also great with us, answering all our questions and not making us feel silly to ask anything. We are lucky that we found a doctor that we like and trust!

❧❀❧

I wish, more than anything else, that one of the three doctors we saw the first day we got the diagnosis, the specialist who performed the surgery to try and reattach Taylor's retinas, or **anyone** else had told us the name of a single agency or organization we could turn to for help and advice. It seems like such a simple idea, particularly for specialists, to have the name of an agency or a list of organizations they could give parents when they deliver the news that a child is blind or visually impaired. My husband and I both believe that there is a simple way for this information to be provided. We used to leave our names with doctors, letting them know they could give our number to other parents who learn of a visual disability. Few doctors have passed it on.

❧❀❧

Our son endured about six months of pain related to glaucoma and several other eye problems, so after consulting with three specialists and taking him for an exam under anesthesia, Nicholas underwent bi-lateral enucleation (eye removal). This was not a decision made without a great *deal of thought and tears. However, Nicholas only had light perception and both eyes were causing him such pain he had not been able to sleep more than four hours a night for months, so we were grateful knowing Nicholas would no longer be in pain.*

❧❀☙

Sometimes you've just gotten a grip on dealing with blindness or visual impairment, when you learn there are additional disabilities or your otherwise healthy child with a visual impairment becomes very sick. It seems almost too much to handle. You've got to keep at it, though—especially during these times.

❧❀☙

I really feel like our medical doctors are members of Bracey's team. Our ophthalmologist made it clear that he doesn't make educational decisions, but he will be happy to weigh in on any questions or concerns we have. He has always been a good listener!

❧❀☙

We have been connected with a low vision specialist who works in a clinic with an ophthalmologist and optometrist. This allows us to move from medical issues to issues related to low vision devices and we are confident that all of these professionals consult with each other about our daughter.

❧❀☙

At first I was worried that I would have difficulty understanding the medical part of Gracie's visual impairment, but Dr. Stratmoen relieved my fears as soon as I met her. She took our concerns seriously and never made us feel rushed during our appointment.

ADJUSTING TO YOUR CHILD'S VISUAL IMPAIRMENT

Erika Forster

Welcome To Holland
by Emily Perl Kingsley

I am often asked to describe the experience of raising a child with a disability—to try to help people who have not shared that unique experience to understand it, to imagine how it would feel. It's like this......

When you're going to have a baby, it's like planning a fabulous vacation trip—to Italy. You buy a bunch of guide books and make your wonderful plans. The Coliseum. The Michelangelo David. The gondolas in Venice. You may learn some handy phrases in Italian. It's all very exciting.

After months of eager anticipation, the day finally arrives. You pack your bags and off you go. Several hours later, the plane lands. The stewardess comes in and says, "Welcome to Holland."

"Holland?!?" you say. "What do you mean Holland?? I signed up for Italy! I'm supposed to be in Italy. All my life I've dreamed of going to Italy."

But there's been a change in the flight plan. They've landed in Holland and there you must stay.

The important thing is that they haven't taken you to a horrible, disgusting, filthy place, full of pestilence, famine, and disease. It's just a different place.

So you must go out and buy new guide books. And you must learn a whole new language. And you will meet a whole new group of people you would never have met.

It's just a different place. It's slower-paced than Italy, less flashy than Italy. But after you've been there for a while and you catch your breath, you look around.... and you begin to notice that Holland has windmills.... and Holland has tulips. Holland even has Rembrandts.

But everyone you know is busy coming and going from Italy... and they're all bragging about what a wonderful time they had there. And for the rest of your life, you will say "Yes, that's where I was supposed to go. That's what I had planned."

And the pain of that will never, ever, ever, ever go away... because the loss of that dream is a very very significant loss.

But ... if you spend your life mourning the fact that you didn't get to Italy, you may never be free to enjoy the very special, the very lovely things ... about Holland.

Most people enter parenthood with an awareness that raising a child will be filled with joys and challenges, and that there are no guarantees. As you prepared for the birth of your child, you probably had your own ideas about what your child would be like. You may have imagined a little girl with her mother's smile, or a little boy with his father's red hair. You probably did not consider the possibility of a visual impairment, but you probably did express a hope that your new baby would be healthy. For many parents, the once hypothetical fears for the health of their young child become a reality with the diagnosis of a visual impairment.

When your child was diagnosed with a visual impairment, whether at birth or at a later time, you undoubtedly experienced a variety of strong emotions. As in the vignette above, you probably felt emotionally disoriented. Since you hadn't planned on having a child with a visual impairment, it may have taken you some time to sort out exactly how you felt about this change. Some parents take their new situation in stride rather quickly, while others may experience deep grief or confusion.

Some parents are immediately able to make statements such as, "I'm sure we will learn what we need to know in order to make adjustments to this unexpected turn." Or, "I love this child totally; his visual impairment makes no difference." Other parents react differently to the news and may say things such as, "I'm devastated" or "This is horrible."

It is very important to understand that all of these emotions are valid and valuable and that it is not wrong to feel one way or another. At the same time, it is important to note that almost everyone who goes through this kind of experience reports that their emotions change frequently and that how they feel one day may be very different from how they feel the next.

The adjustment process is different for everyone and there is no "typical" or "correct" timeline. Still, there seem to be several factors that contribute to positive adjustment. These include:

- the amount and quality of support available,
- the availability of appropriate resources, and
- personal beliefs and values.

This chapter provides information about these factors, as well as other aspects of the adjustment process and provides some suggestions that may be helpful as you work your way through it.

◈ A NOTE ABOUT HELP

While this chapter is designed to provide a perspective and some support for dealing with the process of adjustment, it cannot replace support that you may find in your own community. In addition, your family's experience is unique, and the generic advice given in this chapter may not cover some of your pressing concerns. Many parents find that professional counseling or group support is helpful. There is some information at the end of this chapter about finding this kind of support.

◈ Getting the News

One of the common stories that parents tell is how they heard the news of their child's visual impairment. For some parents, their child's visual impairment is obvious at birth. In other situations, parents or family members may suspect a visual impairment before it is confirmed by a medical doctor. Sometimes, a visual impairment is not recognized until the child begins to participate in educational activities. Regardless of when you receive the news, you will probably remember it as an important event.

A formal diagnosis of a child's visual impairment can have a far-reaching and pervasive impact on parents and families. For some families, the diagnosis can come, at least initially, as a relief. This is likely if there was a lengthy and protracted time of uncertainty marked by a myriad of medical appointments. In these cases, parents may have begun to gather important information and resources before they receive official news. This gradual realization can be frustrating, but can also provide some time for parents to gather informal information without the pressure of an immediate need. Some parents do not suspect a visual impairment, and so the diagnosis comes as a shock to them. In any case, receiving news that your child has a visual impairment can be a traumatic event that may begin a long and sometimes difficult emotional process.

Perhaps you are aware of the much publicized emotional aspects or "stages" of grieving, including denial or shock, anxiety or anger, guilt, fear, bargaining, depression, and acceptance. These stages were initially identified to describe the process of dealing with death. However, they have been widely applied to the acceptance of many other kinds of loss. In this chapter, we will explore how these stages apply to the acceptance of your child's disabilities, and, perhaps, to the loss of some of your expectations for your child. Some people find this type of analysis helpful, while others do not. In fact, this chapter only uses the specific stages as an organizational tool for discussing many of the different emotions that parents often feel.

It is important to reiterate that no two people react to the news in the same way. The duration, intensity, order, and frequency of the feelings and experiences associated with the process of getting a handle on a child's visual impairment vary from individual to individual. Moreover, not everyone necessarily experiences each of these stages, and people from the same family may go through the emotional experience very differently. It may be reassuring, however, to realize that you are not alone in feeling a particular way after your child's diagnosis and that these feelings are part of a normal process of adjustment.

As a teacher of children with visual impairments (TVI), I have worked with many families who were in the process of adjusting to their children's visual impairments. These families came to the diagnosis with their own outlook on life, their own set of coping skills, and their own supports, and grappled with the diagnosis in their own ways. Some of them agreed to let me share parts of their stories in this chapter to show that, although coping can be rocky at times, ordinary families do successfully cope with the challenges. The following two family accounts will give you an idea of how two families received the news about their children's visual impairments and their experience during their child's early years.

Barbara and Darrell's Story

When Amy was three months old, my mother, a trained nurse, noticed that Amy's eyes "danced and flickered." She told me that this was not normal and that I should take her to a doctor. After seeing Amy, our family doctor told me that something was definitely wrong and arranged for us to be seen at Children's Hospital the next day. The fear of not knowing what was wrong was overwhelming. I felt scared, shocked, and upset with myself for fear that I had done something wrong during my pregnancy. I was so fearful for Amy and what her life would be like. How would this affect us all?

My husband and I both came to the hospital appointment. There the ophthalmologist confirmed "nystagmus" and suggested one or two other diagnoses. Achromatopsia was one possibility, he said. Achromatopsia is a rare condition that affects the cones in the retina at the back of the eye.

He suspected that she would have problems seeing color and that she would have a high sensitivity to light. Amy would need to wear glasses, not to correct her vision, but to block light and to correct astigmatism in her eyes. He said Amy had a visual acuity of approximately 20/1600 and that she couldn't see anything unless held directly in front of her eyes. This explained why she slept so much. He said she was "legally blind," which seemed devastating at the time. I remember feeling a lot of avoidance, denial, guilt, anger, and sadness. I also remember wondering what this would mean for her quality of life. I felt as if her diagnosis had turned life upside down for all of us.

While all this was happening, Amy's twin brother, David, was in the hospital because of complications related to his birth. David was in the hospital four times that year, and it seemed as if we were constantly running back and forth to the hospital. It was exhausting. And Catherine, our four-year-old daughter, was also being greatly affected by the birth of her twin siblings, the medical emergencies, and the resulting loss of parental attention.

The doctor said that it was imperative that Amy start using and focusing her eyes. We were told she was sleeping so much because she was not able to see anything. Given David's medical complications and extended hospital stays, we did not have as much time or knowledge as we would have liked to help Amy use her eyes. It was Catherine who took over much of the training. She would sit in front of Amy's swinging chair and hold toys in front of her and then pull them away so Amy would have to work to focus. It was gratifying to see how Catherine and Amy bonded over the toys and the process of helping Amy to pay attention to what she was seeing.

The doctor also said that it was very important that Amy receive specialized help from the early intervention consultants. Unfortunately, another department in the hospital was on strike and they were not allowed to visit us. Our direct contact with them was delayed for several months as a result. This was agonizing. The two consultants, however, kept in touch via phone, giving us moral support and advice on how to help Amy. We were treated very well, but waiting for the job action to conclude was very difficult.

Amy also endured some very difficult tests. One of the tests involved electrode testing and required Amy to have copper foil in her eyes. This electrode testing was to tell us how many of her rods and cones were working. It wouldn't make any difference to Amy's vision but it would hopefully give us some answers. Amy screamed when they were trying to attach the foil in her eyes. She was supposed to be asleep for the test. We had been told not to let her sleep prior—to keep her awake so she'd be tired—but it didn't work.

Very soon we just decided that this was the way life was going to be and that we needed to get on with it. We were in survival mode and we were determined to do our best for our daughter and our family. We would do whatever it took to make it work. Still, early on, it was very difficult to deal with all of the information we were given—especially the big binders of ophthalmology information. I had three young children clamoring for my attention. There was no way I could get through a three-inch binder of text. It was overwhelming just to look at. I preferred having conversations with people. I learned to choose these people very carefully.

In the beginning, we also had trouble dealing with others' reactions. Some people asked the most unnerving and uncomfortable questions. Strangers would ask us, "Isn't there something doctors can do for her eyes?" There were also many comments about a baby wearing sunglasses.

We ultimately chose not to put Amy into a specialized preschool education setting, although we continued receiving invaluable support from the early intervention consultants. We decided to keep her with her brother until junior kindergarten. David looked out for her and made it easier for her to be included, for instance, by helping Amy in those jungle play places where adults can't fit. We had to balance David's need for freedom and his level of maturity with the incredibly valuable and natural assistance that he could provide for Amy during activities, outings, etc. I guess we just naturally expected David to help look out for Amy, which he did without complaint.

In those early years, we took Amy everywhere and she basically did whatever we were doing. We didn't want her to think she couldn't. She was such a happy child all the time, which made the adjustment easier. We also had good support from our parents and other relatives and friends.

Amy and David are now seven and a half and Catherine is twelve. Amy attends an all girl's school, so is on her own and loving it. We are still determined to enable her to be independent—to let her try everything, knowing that not everything will be possible without adaptations, but to have fun trying. We do a tremendous amount as a family, and our schedules are filled to capacity with the children's many extracurricular activities and school events. The children are active in a whole range of activities from ballet, biking, and soccer, to horseback riding, swimming, and gymnastics. Coordinating these many activities is a full time job, as all busy parents can attest.

Given our hectic lives, it can sometimes be easy to temporarily forget that Amy has a significant visual impairment. Periodically, however, there are painful or uncomfortable occasions that remind us. Amy is wonderfully artistic and throws herself into ballet, gymnastics, and swimming with joyful abandon, yet when she starts a new activity or when there is a change in the nature of that activity, we must address any potential implications of her visual impairment—either those based on other people's fears or upon reality. But that is our life and we will do whatever it takes!

Tim and Michelle's Story

Soon after our son, Jason, was born, I (Michelle) noticed he wasn't tracking my finger with his eyes when I tried to engage him. We also thought that his pupils seemed a little hazy. Then again, he was our first child, so we didn't really know what we were looking at. In my gut, I kept feeling, "I think something is wrong" but I didn't want to find out what. When he was three and a half weeks old, I mentioned our concerns to the doctor at our regular infant check-up, at the end of the visit. She checked his eyes and couldn't find a "red reflux"—the reflection of light off the retina.

We were to wait until morning to see an ophthalmologist, but we couldn't. A dear friend who is an optometrist came to our house and had the hard, hard task of telling us he saw severe cataracts. At this point, we thought Jason would need glasses to do what his lenses weren't doing. First, though, he would need to have the cataracts surgically removed.

I was so worried about my tiny baby having this surgery. Then the surgeon came out of the operating room early and told us there was more difficulty behind the cataracts. Jason's retinas were malformed (dysplastic) and pulled off the back of the eye into the "stalk" that provides nourishment to the developing lens. This stalk re-absorbs into the vitreous (jelly inside the eye) in normal fetal development, but Jason's hadn't. Instant crisis. It was that "pit in the stomach" feeling. Jason had to go through a battery of tests. He had a CAT Scan, an ECG, blood tests, urine tests, etc. Eventually, ophthalmologists gave us our first diagnosis of bilateral Persistent Hyperplastic Primary Vitreous (PHPV). Jason had two vitrectomies (surgery through the sclera, the white of the eye) to remove his lenses, cut the "stalk," and check the state of his retinas. It was bad news after bad news.

The doctors always wanted to give us hope. I understand this need. They hope, too. But it was hard to hope and then have it dashed. I just remember sobbing and weeping and holding Jason. I remember going outside for a break at the hospital with Tim. It was a crisp fall day. I was so sad Jason would never see the fall colors, the sky, all that I see. People kept saying, "It won't be sad for him because he won't know any different." I hated this. It didn't relieve me of my grief. At that time I was so afraid for him. I thought, how can he grow up in this world? Kids are mean. People don't care for the differently-abled. Will he have friends? Will he ever get married? Who will take care of him when we die? I remember that first week going out for dinner and seeing a family with a baby who was sighted and just silently weeping because I couldn't stand it to know Jason would never see my face.

After the surgeries came genetic testing. The doctors all thought Jason had PHPV, which is usually not a genetic thing. They recommended genetic testing to completely rule out what they assumed they had ruled out by the way Jason's eyes looked. There was some red tape related to getting the testing done, and the upshot was that we had already decided to have another child by the time we got the results. When all was said and done, Jason's results arrived positive when I was two weeks pregnant with Matthew. Jason has a genetic condition called Norrie's disease. We had no family history of this. Was I a carrier? I did not want to risk Matthew by having fetal testing done. It would not have changed my mind about having him. I wondered the entire pregnancy, but tried not to worry. Surely it wouldn't happen again?

When Matthew was born, a pediatrician was there to assess him, but couldn't tell a thing about his vision. Once again, our good friend came to our house and once again he had to tell us our son's eyes were not formed properly. Matthew had been reacting to light in the hospital, so I had been feeling "It will be okay." It wasn't. The same road. The same surgeons, the same surgeries, but this time with an added test to determine if his retinas were responsive to light. In one eye, the retina was.

For the first two and a half years, Matthew had enough sight in one eye on the temporal side (toward the temple, not the nose) to be able to reach out and grab a juice cup, or see the white lines on the parking lot. A little bit of sight goes a long way for a child's mobility. Over that time, however, he struggled with glaucoma and endured three surgeries. He went for monthly EUA's (examinations under anesthesia). He remained on daily eye drops.

Two months ago, Matthew had surgery to remove a white mass in his lens cavity. The surgeons noticed he had some retinal detachment, so he had surgery to reattach it. One week later, I noticed his lens cavity was darkened with blood. I checked, fear in my soul. He couldn't see light from a flashlight. A rush visit to specialists and an ultrasound showed his retina floating in the middle of his eye. Our ophthalmologist, who has known us through our two sons, could only say how sorry he was. This meant a lot, because we know that he was grieving with us. We had all hoped so much. Our surgeon was unable to reattach the retina because of a huge build-up of scar tissue.

I find it hard to write this now, because my grief for Matthew losing the rest of his vision is so recent. I feel like I had a sighted child who just went blind. I had to watch him go from a child who would escape out the door to find the swings across the yard to a child who would take two steps and start crying because he was scared and didn't know where he was. He stopped eating properly. He was grieving, scared, and depressed. But slowly Matthew is learning to cope. He is gaining confidence around the house, mapping the rooms by trailing the walls. It will take him a long time to regain his confidence, but his exploratory nature asserts itself bit by bit as we try to give him tools to cope with his new situation.

As with many visual diagnoses, there can be accompanying concerns. With Norrie's disease, there is a good chance our sons will lose some or all of their hearing. As well, some kids with Norrie's disease have mental impairments. Matthew isn't talking yet. This weighs heavily on my mind, although we are thrilled that he is trying to communicate with some sounds.

Jason, while he didn't walk independently until twenty-six and a half months, is an active, almost five-year-old well on his way to being the class clown.

I have learned so many things over these last years. It's true, blindness isn't a loss or a tragedy to Jason. It won't be to Matthew two years from now. There will be struggles to help them deal with, realizing the ways they have to do things differently because of the blindness. We do this in little ways every day—encouraging them to do everything their peers are doing in a safe, secure, and nurturing environment.

At first I was overwhelmed trying to picture their whole lives. I very specifically said to myself, "No more. Only one day at a time." There are times I have to remind myself of this. I have also realized that my whole life vision for each of my babies failed to account for the fact that every baby is his own person. My job is to equip him to be skilled to make his own life decisions. Although my sons will always be my children, at some time they will be adults like I am now. A friend with a visually impaired child had her pediatrician gently remind her in her fear that, "He will be who he will be."

I used to always second guess myself. What if…? But there is no "what if." We do what we can with what we know at the time. We need to find the right people and resources to be as best informed as we can, but we can't beat ourselves up for retrospectives. They can eat us alive.

It is hard to deal with so much grief about your child. You deal with your own feelings of loss—you lose some of the dreams and visions you had for your child, your family, and yourself. It's hard not to try to find someone to blame—your doctor, for not noticing sooner; yourself—for not dealing with your "gut feeling"; your spouse—for discounting your concerns; God—for doing this or for allowing innocent children to suffer. A helpful picture for me has been God's arms surrounding me, surrounding Jason, and God crying with us. A loving God would never punish us like this, or hurt our child with intent.

When I was still raw in my grief, I was given the phone number of another mom who had a nine-year-old daughter blind from birth. This gracious lady and her daughter visited our home and let us ask her and her child anything. This went a long way in giving us a positive picture of a child with visual impairments. I would strongly recommend meeting other parents and their children.

My husband and I got a great deal of support and encouragement from our sons' therapists. Many of them have gone above and beyond their job descriptions in caring for our family. Our therapists encouraged me to put both boys in therapy playgroups with children with other disabilities.

This was a great experience for them and for me. I also joined a mom's support group for parents of children with disabilities. Talking with other parents in similar situations is essential. It can be hard to overcome the tendency towards isolation.

With family, it was important for us to be aware that our parents were just as concerned as we were. They needed information, too. They needed to know what was going on. They needed time to process their grief. It wasn't a time to withdraw, but to realize what a support network we could develop. When I couldn't read any more books, I passed them on to grandparents who were eager for them.

Our church also reached out to us. I have always been a private person. It has been hard to allow others to help when I felt like we needed to do it all ourselves. Allowing others to help us, however, has given me a new perspective on community. My advice is, when people ask, "How can we help?" tell them you can use some help with meals, with baby sitting your child while you go out (even on a date!), with funds—whatever you truly need. (Our church has set up a trust fund for the boys.) Allow others to be a blessing to you.

Another issue for me was the inevitable change in my public and social life. I remember feeling so angry that "now I won't ever be able to fade into the background. I will always stick out. I will always have the staring eyes and the hastily averted gazes to deal with." But you know, I don't. I make sure I have time to go out without the kids, so I can blend in. I don't have to be always "on" as the mom of the blind boys. Now when people say of Matthew, "He looks so tired." I just respond "Uh, huh." I spend time explaining things to the people in my life I see all the time. The others, I don't bother with. It takes too much energy to try and educate the world.

It can be difficult accepting the role of advocate for my children. I would just like to be a parent and focus on raising my child, but we have to fight (often tooth-and-nail) for services, funding, accessibility, and equal opportunity. I am glad that this new role has been only gradually thrust on me. When my kids were babies it was not the time to be on committees. We attended every event and seminar on visual impairments we could, as well as parent advocacy group events (family picnics). Now, four years later, I find myself on two committees. Every time advocacy is successful, I rejoice that our small part will have done so much to change things for the next child with disabilities who will come along. I will always remember telling one of our friends that Jason was blind and having him not react with concern. He had grown up with someone who was blind and was so matter of fact about it. Blindness wasn't a big deal to him. It was normal.

Blindness is no longer tragic for us. We just need to use different ways of interpreting information about life. For those of you who may be crying all the time, I want to assure you that there will come a time when the clouds will lift. You learn that life goes on and your child needs you to go on with him. Tummy time! Open up! Chin up! No pressing! Use the spoon, please! Use your words! On your tummy, feet first! Feet on the pedals, hands on the handlebars! Finger one, finger one on number one is the rule of the Brailler! Nose, belly button, toes, cane tip! Away we go!

▟ Your Emotions

As these two family stories illustrate, emotions do not always come individually, in tidy, isolated little packets that you can deal with one by one. Sometimes you may feel several emotions simultaneously or in rapid succession, making it difficult to pinpoint exactly how you are feeling. Still, for ease of discussion, the following section will go individually through each of the emotions often identified with the process of acceptance and provide an explanation of the "stage" that you might be in if you are feeling that emotion. But remember: Although some people do experience all these emotions in this exact order, it is also normal for people to experience different emotions or to have them in a different order. In addition, as Darrell and Barbara point out, sometimes an emotion that you thought you were through with will return to be dealt with again—often at transition points in your child's life. Although this chapter offers some suggestions for dealing with emotions, please remember that this chapter is no substitute for in-person support from family, friends, and professionals.

Shock and Denial

It is very common for parents to react with shock or denial when first faced with medical news. Phrases like "I can't believe it" or "It can't be true" reflect the types of emotions that parents feel during this time. Some parents describe this feeling as being completely numb and divorced from the events and people surrounding them, living in what feels like a surreal world. It is not unusual for parents to say that their child's diagnosis is the first thing they think about when they awake in the morning and that each day it comes as a surprise again. This can be a very stressful time for parents because shock makes it difficult to function normally in everyday life.

Denial is closely re-
lated to shock because it
reflects a parent's feeling
that something is not correct. Some parents may
find themselves denying
that the visual impairment
is permanent or minimiz-
ing its severity. While denial is often discussed as a
negative thing, in reality,
denial may buy parents
time to gain the personal
strength and external sup-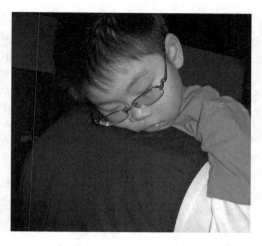
ports necessary to help them ultimately cope. In fact, it is often difficult
for parents, families, and the professionals with whom they work to have
a clear picture of what the child's life will be like at this early stage. As
much as we would like to have definite, long-term answers to the questions about what impact a visual impairment may have on a child's life,
it is not possible to have this definitive answer.

Many parents also report that denial had a significant impact on
their ability to cope with and interpret factual information that they
received, especially in the early stages. If you have only recently learned
of your child's disability, remember: Denial may cloud your understanding and ability to digest information, especially soon after learning of
your child's visual impairment. Just because someone, even an "expert,"
says something is true, does not mean their "fact" will hold true for your
child. Similarly, some information you hold to be true may not be realized in your child's situation. We know that denial is a common emotion
for people who are under this kind of stress, so when you have trouble
believing any of the factual information provided to you, consider that
the information may be true and you may yet be unwilling or unable to
cope with it at this point. At the same time, just because you disagree
with what is presented to you as "fact" doesn't mean that you are "in
denial" about the issue. You may be right! Here is an example:

*Scott and Judy are parents of Cody, a child who has been diagnosed
with a visual impairment. Scott and Judy have been talking with a teacher
who has watched Cody and has stated that in order for him to be included*

in her preschool class, he must be assigned a full-time paraprofessional for his own safety and to help him be included in the class. Scott and Judy think that Cody would be able to participate independently, given appropriate levels of support from a teacher of a student with visual impairments, and there has been quite a bit of conflict between them and the preschool.

At the most recent meeting, the director of the preschool told them that they were "in denial" about the difficulties that Cody will face as he enters preschool. Scott and Judy took some time to consider this statement. They took a step back and really looked objectively at why they believe that Cody would be successful, while seriously considering the concerns of the preschool director and teacher. In the end, they had a team meeting to discuss everyone's concerns. Scott and Judy suggested a trial period without a paraprofessional to see if Cody could be successful. This constructive solution satisfied everyone and changed the focus of the discussion from Scott's and Judy's possible "denial" to what everyone's realistic expectations for Cody should be.

In any case, you have the right to seek another opinion as you would when considering investments or an upcoming surgery. Maintain a realistic outlook, but by all means look around for other or new services, treatments, or devices that may benefit your child. You have the right to keep exploring possibilities. Doctors, teachers, and other service providers should not be threatened by your expertise and suggestions, especially when you present your case in a thoughtful, respectful manner. If you ultimately do not find a receptive audience, you may need to go to another service provider. By the same token, it is your prerogative to take a break or stop following up on suggestions from well-intentioned relatives, friends, or professionals.

Anxiety

Feelings of worry, fear, and anxiety are normal responses to learning of your child's visual impairment and they can be some of the most stressful human emotions. Parents frequently report feeling anxious about their child after a diagnosis of visual impairment. You may be worried about your child's medical condition or fearful about his future. Your feelings may be based on what you currently believe having a visual impairment is like and what impact you think it may have on your child's life. These feelings may eventually help you adjust your attitudes and may help mobilize you into action.

In the beginning, many parents attempt to allay their concerns by broadening their understanding of the medical diagnosis and its implications. Often they seek medical advice or investigate information on their own. Others alleviate their anxiety by seeking out other parents of children with visual impairments for support.

As time goes on, many parents are calmed and encouraged as they get to know their child and see how he is growing. Parents report that anxiety lessens as they begin to recognize and celebrate the progress their child achieves day by day.

Although a certain amount of anxiety is normal, it is best not to communicate your anxiety to your child. If he senses your anxiety, this may interfere with his motivation, confidence, and enjoyment of social events. Monitoring your own behavior and pinpointing anxiety triggers can help relieve feelings of anxiety and help your child gain confidence. Obtaining details or information regarding any area of concern is another useful strategy.

Carmen, a thirty-two-year-old mother of a toddler with a visual impairment, was extremely anxious about involving her daughter, Sara, in play-dates with her neighborhood peers. She desperately wanted the social contact for Sara and herself, however. Carmen confronted her anxieties head-on by identifying worrisome thoughts. ("Sara won't be able to find the other children as they move around the room." "Will she be safe with toys and children moving about?" "How will the other children react to Sara?"). She then got suggestions on including children with visual impairments from her local support group for parents of children with visual impairments, an early intervention specialist, and the Internet.

Carmen decided to start the process slowly, within her comfort level, by inviting two neighborhood moms and their children to her house for a play-date. By using her house as the venue, she was able to control the play environment and carefully select children she thought would respond best to Sara. During the play-date, she was relieved and encouraged to learn that she and the other moms shared many of the same parenting experiences and concerns. She was also pleased to see that each child needed some general prompting and guidance regarding how to play nicely with one another and that the moms welcomed her input regarding how to help Sara stay in the mix.

Anger or Resentment

Your feelings of anxiety can be closely linked with feelings of anger, especially if you are deeply distressed and disappointed by the diagnosis. You may experience anger toward yourself, God, medical professionals, your spouse, and even your son or daughter. Rightly or wrongly, you may feel angry at the thought that faulty medical care may have contributed to the visual impairment. It is natural to want to blame someone or something, especially as you begin to recognize the irreversibility of your child's visual impairment. Some parents are frightened by their feelings of anger, and may react by becoming aggressive or overprotective. You have the right to feel angry, but if you find yourself experiencing severe anger, you may want to seek professional help.

Feelings of resentment are closely associated with feelings of anxiety and anger. In fact, many parents report feeling resentful toward parents of children without visual impairments or in response to the increased burden of childcare and medical expenses that they experience. For example, it is common for at least one parent's career to suffer as a result of frequent and unpredictable medical appointments or emergencies. Often, one parent tends to take responsibility for most of the medical scheduling and this can lead to feelings of resentment towards the spouse or the child. Although anxiety, resentment, and anger are normal, whether justified or rational, these feelings will not minimize or undo your child's visual condition. Ultimately, you will likely come to realize that you can best recognize and address your child's concerns if you focus your feelings and energy on advocating for his needs.

Guilt

Parents also often tell of feeling guilty, sometimes thinking that they must be to blame in some way because their child has a disability. They may feel guilty because they fear they may have caused the disability in some way due to their genetics, for example, or that the disability is a kind of punishment for some past misdeed. Others feel angry with themselves because the visual impairment exists, and this self-blame can result in more generalized feelings of guilt. For example, mothers who are typically already tired and frustrated from arranging and attending medical appointments may now feel that something that they did or didn't do during pregnancy may have caused the visual impairment.

Some parents also feel guilty that they didn't notice signs of the visual impairment sooner and avail themselves of specialized treatment and intervention at an earlier stage.

At times, insensitive comments from strangers, or even trusted loved ones, may feel devastating, especially if you continue to make the mistake of blaming

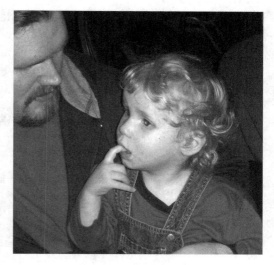

yourself. Some mothers report probing, tactless questions such as, "Did something go wrong during your pregnancy?"; "Shouldn't you get that visual problem corrected with surgery right away?"; or "Do visual problems run in your family?"

Usually, consultation with a trusted, sensitive, and knowledgeable medical professional will address your concerns and relieve your fears that you are somehow to blame. Even in the case of a visual impairment that has genetic links, you will in the end discover that being an effective parent has more to do with helping your child maximize his potential than worrying over something that you may or may not have been able to control. Feelings of guilt cannot typically be willed away, but diminish in time. Prolonged guilt can interfere with your relationships if you fear that others will "find you out" or that they consider you and your (imagined) guilt contemptible. If you feel persistently guilty, consider seeking professional counseling.

Grief

When the dream of having a totally healthy child is not realized, parents may feel sadness and depression. The sadness can be overwhelming and omnipresent. Some parents report feeling happy for the first few minutes upon waking in the morning, only to despair upon abruptly remembering about their child's visual impairment. The sadness can permeate everything. Sometimes only the passage of time and seeing evidence of what can still be wonderful helps.

Sadness is a difficult emotion to recognize and define. Sometimes this is because sadness can be complicated by other emotions. For example, you may feel guilty about your sadness because it may seem unnatural to be *sad* about the birth of your child. Similarly, your sadness may make you angry, or you may try to deny that you are sad at all. For some people, focusing on their own sadness is the first time they allow themselves to acknowledge the impact that this loss has on them. One parent I know stated, "I'm not sad. This isn't about *me*. I only want to focus on how this will have an impact on my baby."

If and when you experience sadness or grief, it can help to know that this is a natural reaction and that allowing yourself to recognize your feelings can help you get past them. There are many resources to help you deal with this and other emotions. Use your support system to help you and realize that there are also professional resources available to you.

Bargaining

Many mothers and fathers go through a period of bargaining during which they make "deals" to help them cope. John, a twenty-four-year-old student mechanic, was devastated by his daughter's diagnosis of optic nerve hypoplasia. He found himself bargaining with God. ("If the visual impairment clears up, I will always be kind to my child." "If you fix her eyes, God, I won't ever ask for anything else."). Later, he realized that this negotiation served as a kind of temporary relief from the pain he was experiencing.

Other parents bargain about the degree of their child's visual impairment. When Kate first learned of her son's visual impairment she found herself thinking, "OK, I'll accept that he may become totally blind only if he is the smartest and most athletic kid to ever have Leber's Congenital Amaurosis." Some of these types of parental expectations formed early on in a bargaining stage can continue to influence parenting. Some parents enroll their kids in a variety of sports, for example, in an effort to make their son or daughter the "best blind runner ever to step on a track." Usually, however, parents slowly move through this bargaining stage by taking pleasure in discovering the complexities and uniqueness of their children and in loving them for who they are.

Acceptance

Acceptance refers to the stage when the intensity of the grieving process lessens and parents are able to accept the diagnosis and their child for who he or she is. They then begin the gratifying, if at times seriously challenging, process of working toward finding supports and treatment that will help their child lead a fulfilling, enjoyable life.

Acceptance also marks the stage when you begin again to have hopes and dreams for your child. Parents sometimes state that the recognition of their child's visual impairment temporarily brought an end to hopes and dreams that they had for their child. Since most parents do not have previous experience with blindness or visual impairment, it takes some time for them to gather enough information to realize that their original hopes and dreams for their child may still be intact, or that they can be replaced by other hopes and dreams that are just as valuable and exciting.

In reality, almost all parents—whether or not their children have disabilities—go through this process of adjusting their dreams and expectations. For instance, a father may dream of his son becoming an Eagle Scout or playing basketball only to find out that his child's dreams for himself are different. The key for all parents is to provide opportunities for their children to reach their maximum potential in their specific, constantly changing dreams.

Parents of children with visual impairments often mention how much their child has brought to their lives. There are countless stories of families recognizing that working through the challenges posed by a visual impairment encourages creativity and family togetherness. Accepting your child doesn't mean that you have to be happy about his visual impairment or that you never again feel angry or resentful or frustrated. It is normal to periodically revisit one or more of these emotions as your child grows older. It is also normal to still need occasional (or frequent) support from others to help you deal with your emotions and some day-to-day practical matters related to the visual impairment. Most days, however, you will be able to spend large portions of the day thinking about things unrelated to visual impairments.

■■ How to Adjust

Lauren and Mark, both dentists, have an eight-month-old son, Luke, who was recently diagnosed with (bilateral) retinoblastoma, a cancer of the eye. These previously career-driven parents have seen their daily routines turned upside down since the birth of their son, and the disruption and resulting feelings of anxiety and anger are far beyond what their other friends with young children are going through.

Not only are Lauren and Mark worried about the health of their son, but Lauren has come to the conclusion that it would be in the family's best interest for her to quit her job indefinitely so she can take Luke to a myriad of appointments and attend to his other medical needs. While Lauren's first concern is the well-being of her son, she does, at times, resent having placed her career on hold for the foreseeable future. And, even given her medical background, she is exhausted by the need to advocate for her son to receive prompt and high quality medical attention, deal with breastfeed-ing issues, establish sleep schedules, and cope with the many other stresses confronting new parents.

In an effort to address her feelings of anger and resentment, Lauren and Mark have made a commitment to reevaluate the division of responsi-bilities in their household on a monthly basis. In the meantime, Mark has taken over responsibility for household chores that sap Lauren's energy such as grocery shopping, looking after the family dog, and paying the bills. Lauren has also contacted her local family support worker, plans to join a local group for parents of children with visual impairments, and has joined a retinoblastoma chat group on the Internet. In order to help meet her needs for up-to-date medical expertise, she signed up for an informa-tive newsletter from a retinoblastoma research group. And one evening a week Lauren and Mark make a point to do something fun or interesting as a family, a couple, or individuals with friends.

Although Mark and Lauren are still stressed out at times, they have actually begun implementing four of the most important strate-gies to adjusting to the diagnosis of a child's disability. These important strategies are:

1. Express your feelings;
2. Obtain additional information;
3. Get support;
4. Remember that neither you, your child, or your family are defined by the visual impairment.

Express Your Feelings

A key strategy for this couple was acknowledging their feelings to the best of their ability from moment to moment, since bottling them up had only caused them pain and frustration in the past. For example, once Mark knew that Lauren was feeling resentful, they could develop new ways to help improve the situation and their relationship.

Although you may believe that some of your feelings are inappropriate or "bad," they really are very natural. You can express your feelings in whatever way you are comfortable. Sometimes you may want to just "vent" your emotions without any expectation that someone will have a solution to make you feel better. If so, you may want to announce beforehand that that is what you are doing: "Do you mind if I vent for a little while?" If you are listening to another family member who is venting, it is important to let him say what is on his mind, without trying to talk him out of his emotions. Just because you do not feel depressed right now does not mean that your spouse shouldn't be allowed to feel that way. At another time, you could perhaps return to your spouse's emotion, however, and talk about why *you* feel there is reason for more optimism. Online listservs, bulletin boards, and email groups can be good places to vent your emotions if you have a computer. (Be aware, however, that some of these groups are open to the general public, so be careful to safeguard your family's privacy.)

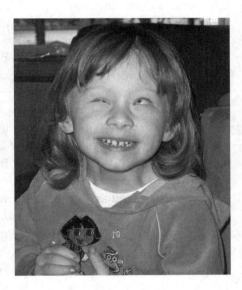

Other times, you may hope that once you express your emotions to a particular person, he or she will be able to help work out a solution. That is, you don't want to just vent; you want to problem solve. If you think your listener may be part of the problem, it is important not to express your feelings in an accusatory way. Often, counselors suggest that these types of feelings are best expressed using comments that begin with "I" rather than "you." For example, if you say to your spouse, "You always turn on the TV as soon as you come home from work without even asking me how my day went with Kayla" that is likely to make him feel defensive. On the other hand, if you say something like, "I feel so stressed out by the end of the day; I really wish we had some time to talk about how little progress I feel like I've been making with Kayla lately," your spouse is more likely to feel like working toward a solution with you.

Even though it can be extremely helpful to share your emotions, remember, you do not owe people an explanation. You are in control of your information. If you do not want to share your emotions with someone who asks, you do not have to. Many parents report how empowering it has been to reclaim their own information, following many emotionally invasive medical interviews, family "talks," and so on. If you don't really want to discuss your feelings, perhaps keeping a journal might work.

Obtain Additional Information

Obtaining additional, accurate information can help you along in your adjustment process and improve your ability to access the most appropriate early intervention services and supports available for your child. After the initial diagnosis, information about your son's or daughter's visual impairment may have been hard to digest, given the denial or sadness you may have experienced. Before long, however, you may realize that you need more information.

Take control of how much information you receive, and do not feel pressure to "read everything" regarding a particular visual impairment or any related issue. This is your experience and you are the expert on what additional information, if any, you require.

Parents are often prompted to investigate visual impairment further when they experience new issues or questions from relatives or friends about the child's educational or medical concerns. You may want to contact your ophthalmologist, pediatrician, local support group, books, or journals in an effort to learn more. Some parents rave about the benefits of joining listservs or researching issues through online databases like Medline. It may be hard to believe, but there are many parents who are addressing these same issues, and they have blazed a trail for others who need resources. There are many organizations dedicated to visual impairments. Be very cautious, however, about believing whatever you read on the Internet. Visit a reputable site and validate your new information with other parents and medical, educational, and legal professionals.

Many parents find that the right kind of information is empowering. Knowing more about your child's visual impairment may, for example, minimize your desire to overprotect your child, and instead allow him the chance to take appropriate risks and experience the joys of achievement. Likewise, finding out about educational rights and special education services can help you feel confident in advocating for the program that will help your child maximize his abilities.

The Reading List at the back of the book includes some good publications for you to refer to when you are ready for more information, and the Resource Guide lists organizations that can help answer your specific questions or point you to other sources of useful information.

Get Support

Parents have a dizzying array of often demanding roles and responsibilities. It can be argued that, at some point, all parents need the support of other parents, relatives, friends, their faith and church, community organizations and resources, or international groups. Given the particular needs of children with visual impairments, you may wish to include other parents with children who have visual impairments or other disabilities within your support network.

You may develop some strong ties with parents who can help you navigate through the sometimes complicated personal, physical, and emotional needs, as well as the financial stresses involved in meeting your child's needs. It is often validating and empowering to meet other honest, capable parents who are struggling with and, ultimately, succeeding in, dealing with issues similar to your own. You can't compare your family with any other family, but you can learn from other people and get strength from interacting with other parents who have had similar experiences.

There are many ways you can locate other parents. In this electronic age, perhaps the easiest place to "meet" parents of children with visual impairments is online. Some of the national organizations for people with visual impairments host bulletin boards or listservs where you can post questions or join in discussions about particular topics or "threads." If you don't feel up to introducing yourself or speaking up yet, you can also "observe" for a time—read other people's questions and comments without joining in the discussion yourself. Information about groups that have these kinds of resources can be found at the back of this book.

Local parent groups often set up convenient ways to meet other parents and their children face-to-face. Many communities sponsor picnics or family weekend camps that provide opportunities to learn from and socialize with other families who are facing the same questions you may

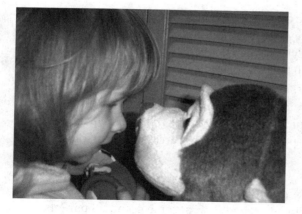

have. In the stories at the beginning of this chapter, the parents stated the importance of connecting with families who have experienced these challenges. The more connected you are to service providers in your community (local, state, or province), the better your chances of hearing about opportunities to connect with other families. Teachers of students with visual impairments in your communities, schools for the blind, agencies such as state division of blind services in the U.S. or the CNIB (formerly Canadian National Institute for the Blind) in Canada are all good sources of information to get you connected to other families in your area. Please refer to the Resource Guide at the back of the book for a starting point.

Other Sources of Help

Although other parents of children with visual impairments are priceless because they have been there too and can fully empathize with you, don't overlook other sources of support. If friends, neighbors, and extended family ask you how they can help, don't automatically turn them down. Probably many people would honestly like to support you and your family. Allowing them to be involved when you are ready will help to pave the way for your child's inclusion in your extended family, local schools, and in your community at large. Even though you may be feeling intensely private about your emotions and may fear the possibility of being pitied, most families in your social network have undergone at least one challenging situation and will come alongside you and your family in a supportive, nonjudgmental way in an effort to share the load of parenting. By accepting help, you are likely modeling this sense of connection with others for your family. You may also be opening yourself up to be a source of support for others, as you reciprocate for help you have received in the past.

Try not to overlook educational and medical professionals as a source of support. Many TVIs are very empathetic to families going through these difficult changes and can draw on many years of experience helping families make transitions with their children with visual impairments. At your request, ideally they can serve as a buffer between you and "the system," helping you to navigate more effectively through the educational system, make helpful links with the community, and access governmental support services (e.g., respite care). Many teachers are also parents, sometimes of children with disabilities, and we know firsthand how overwhelming parenting can be. We feel privileged when you share personal information with us, and we want to do our best to enhance your experience with the school system and your larger community. It is our job to be a support and a resource for you. We can often pass along tips and information that other parents have found helpful. Additionally, at your request we may be able to go with you to community events, school field trips, and medical appointments. Finally, we can be strong advocates for you and your child within the school system.

To maximize the quality of medical and educational care your child receives, make your needs known to the people who work with him. If you have a negative experience with a professional or other service provider, seek out another specialist. For example, if, even after you have clearly articulated your concerns and needs, a doctor or teacher continually rushes through your appointments, fails to answer your questions in a way that you can easily understand, or treats you in a condescending way, find another professional.

When you ask for help or when others offer help, give specific suggestions about what might be most helpful for you. Could your oldest child use a ride to soccer practice while you are taking your daughter who is visually impaired to early intervention? Would it help if you could just keep one designated person updated about your child's surgery and then let him or her pass the information along to other interested people? Could you use help gathering information on various treatment options?

Ray, a single parent of a young daughter with congenital glaucoma, asked friends and neighbors to make dinners for him and his daughter every Tuesday and Thursday immediately after his daughter returned from an extended stay in the hospital. This gave him the support he needed to accomplish other tasks without worrying about getting food for him and his daughter.

As hard as it is to believe, many, many parents have gone through situations that are similar to what you are now experiencing. These other parents have helped to pave the way for you, advocating for specialized services and programs that can help. Continue to ask around (at your community center, ophthalmologist's office, your doctor's office, etc.) until you find the support you need. The search can be draining, at least initially, but the rewards can be immeasurable.

■ Helping Other Family Members Adjust

At the same time you are coping with your child's diagnosis, everyone in your family and social circle is trying his or her best to adjust too. The timeline and nature of the process looks different for each person. It is important, as your energy permits, to provide support tailored to that person. Perhaps you can synthesize some of the medical information that you have learned into a few phrases that you can use to quickly and comfortably convey the main gist of the visual impairment and its implications. Sometimes these "scripts" can help you feel prepared to deal with potentially tricky social situations with relatives and friends—and maintain the degree of privacy you prefer.

Helping siblings, uncles and aunts, grandparents, and other relatives make a positive adjustment to your child's visual impairment will, in the long run, benefit your efforts to normalize family life. Your child is an important part of the family, but the family should not revolve around the implications of the visual impairment. By helping other family members as they go through a range of emotions that may be similar to those you experienced, you can have a positive effect on their ability to love and nurture your son or daughter appropriately. Your approach to these challenges should be dictated by what you think is most appropriate.

Your Child with Visual Impairments

You may not need to address this now, but at some point, your child with a visual impairment will realize that the way that he sees is different from the way that most people see. He may have questions about his visual impairment. The realization of visual impairment occurs gradually over months and years and the most important thing you can do is to be open for discussions whenever your child has questions or concerns.

Some people talk about a child's "acceptance" of his vision loss. If the child has had a visual impairment since birth, acceptance means something very different for him than it has meant for you. A child who grows up with parents who are creative problem solvers and who find alternative ways of accomplishing daily tasks will continue this process throughout his life, even when solutions are challenging to find. Chapter 7 provides some additional information about this topic.

As impossible as it might seem on some days following a difficult conversation with an ophthalmologist or a neighbor or while facing a mountain of housework and bills, try to consciously recognize and put words to your positive views of your child who has a visual impairment. If feeling positive seems to be an impossible task right now, there are many strategies that can help you develop a positive attitude and realistic hopes for your child. For example, focusing on the "little picture" instead of the "big picture" can help turn your attention to positive views. Pay attention to the small steps toward progress; keeping a journal or photograph album (or video diary) can help you see how far your child has come. Another strategy is to pay attention to your child's unique personality. Is he playful or giggly? Does he like bright colors or spicy food? Your child's personality will come through and delight you if you are paying attention!

You have the right to have "bad days" and to feel overly unenthusiastic at times, but try to focus on your child's strengths rather than on his current or anticipated limitations. You are his champion, cheerleader, and primary source of love and acceptance. Be realistic, yet lovingly positive. Excessive anxiety on your part will only worsen the situation, making it more difficult for you to respond well to meeting your child's needs. Your child's internal plan will dictate how he grows and develops, and having realistic goals is the key to avoiding disappointment and to noticing—and celebrating—the development and accomplishments that do happen. Try not to compare your child to other children in your family or in your neighborhood. Your child will thrive from your unconditional love. What he achieves shouldn't dictate how much he feels loved.

Your Other Children

Your other children will have many of the same needs that you do when adjusting to their brother's or sister's diagnosis of a visual impairment. That is, they will need opportunities and encouragement to express their feelings, information appropriate to their age level, and support. For example, the way that you approach telling your children about their brother's or sister's visual impairment will likely depend on their age. Very young children might not realize that there is something "unusual" about their sibling, and so you may be able to give them information on a "need to know" basis, or as they ask questions. Older children who have been aware of your concerns about their sibling need to be told something soon after you receive the diagnosis. Children are perceptive and will pick up on your anxiety. If they do not obtain information from you, they may imagine something that is even more concerning. Model the use of terminology such as "blind" in a comfortable way.

Overall, each sibling will have unique needs that can usually be met best with honest and simple answers. Reviewing and updating their knowledge, understanding, and feelings on a reasonably regular basis often minimizes fears, confusion, and frustrations. Answering their questions in an optimistic and upbeat manner is advisable, but be sure that your answers do not stretch the truth. For example, don't imply that your child's visual impairment will improve if this is not possible.

There are many good children's books that you can read to your children (or have your children read) that include characters with visual impairments. Your children may enjoy reading about strong, successful characters with visual impairment, and you will probably enjoy them too!

Other Relatives and Friends

Paradoxically, members of your extended family can be a huge support for you and your child, but also may need huge amounts of your support, at least initially. Especially if they were not aware that there was any concern about your child's vision, they may be even more shocked than you were to hear the diagnosis. In addition, grandparents in particular often feel a double dose of grief at the news—one for your child, and one for you, their child (or son- or daughter-in-law).

Occasionally, grandparents or other relatives may have reactions that are less than helpful. Some grandparents may suggest "cures" for the child's visual impairment or spoil the youngster. Other grandparents may avoid visiting the grandchild. Sometimes the problem is that grandparents have outdated attitudes, because in their day people with disabilities were much less likely to be included in normal community activities. However, most relatives, in time, will take their cues from you and learn to treat your child with a visual impairment just like any other child.

Including extended family members in your search for information can help both them and you. Consider suggesting that other family members gather information for you on the Internet or accompany you to parent conferences focusing 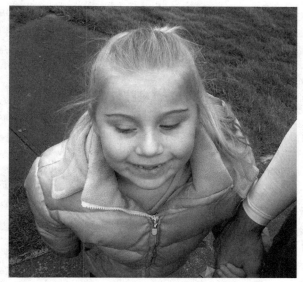 on visual impairments. This can provide invaluable support for you and open doors for increased awareness and acceptance on the part of your child's extended family members.

Having a child with a visual impairment will usually have an impact on your relationships with adult friends. At some stage, you may feel lonely and overwhelmed and may need to withdraw from old friendships. Alternatively, you may develop new friendships with people who can give you the kind of support that you need now. Eventually, you may find that as you move through the adjustment phase, you feel compelled to reactivate those past friendships. Strive to recognize your own personal needs as these evolve, and take care of yourself.

▋▋ Conclusion

Over the past ten years as a teacher of students with visual impairments, I have had the privilege of working with a wide variety of families of children with visual impairments. Although many of the parents struggled with their emotions during the early stages of our work together, virtually all of them were able to put their children's disability in perspective and see the visual impairment as just one aspect of their children's lives. Drawing on their love for their children, they were able to focus on all the wonderful things that their children could do. Perhaps it's hard for you now to imagine that one day your child's visual impairment will cease seeming so huge, but these parents' experiences have shown me that this is not only possible, but highly probable. I have seen it happen time and again.

⠿ Parent Statements

Joining a support group either on the Internet or through a local or national agency is a great way to get a handle on blindness issues. Everything seems so different when you first become aware of your child's vision problems. We were relieved when we found an Internet group for parents because questions will crop up almost daily when your child is very young. The web group offered an immediate forum for posting questions and getting many different responses.

⠿

We have found that you have to be very careful about listening to other people. When the ophthalmologist told us that David was blind, he said that we would want to put him in an "institution." Who says something like this these days? It became clear pretty quickly that we needed another doctor!

⠿

I'm a single parent and my daughter, Brianna, is three years old. I really am on my own, I have no family in the area, and Brianna's father is not in the picture. Sometimes that makes me sad, but other times, I'm glad just to be able to take care of things by myself.

⠿

We found out that Emma was blind when we were still in the hospital after her birth. I was so glad that my mother was there when I heard the news. She has always been Emma's biggest fan!

⠿

While I was still in the hospital after Tony was born, the pediatrician told me that he was blind, but it didn't sink in. I really believed that all I had to do was get him home and then he would be okay.

⠿

I really didn't have much trouble with the initial news that John Henry has a visual impairment. I know he can see some things so it really didn't have a big impact on me that he would have trouble in other areas. But the thing that really got to me was seeing him in his first pair of glasses. He was so tiny and the glasses seemed so big. I started to cry. Thank heavens the doctor stepped in and gave my son some encouragement while I composed myself.

⊰⊱

After a few tries of going to the store or to church, I just stopped. I couldn't stand how people looked at my baby (or at me). For a period of time, I only saw my parents, my husband's parents, and every once in a while a neighbor. It's a lot less stressful that way. But recently, I've tried to venture out more because I know I need to do that for me and for my daughter. I'm just taking it one step at a time but already it's getting a little easier.

⊰⊱

Hearing about Franny's blindness was the worst moment of my life. I never thought this would happen to me. I know probably everyone feels that way. I trust other people who tell me that things will get better, so I'm just holding on until that time happens.

⊰⊱

I get so annoyed at the strangers who ask what's wrong with my baby's eyes. Sometimes I just say she's sleeping and try to be polite. At other times I growl something and walk off. What's wrong with people anyway?

⊰⊱

After my son was born, I kept on going back over the events of my pregnancy, wondering if there was something I could have done differently to prevent this from happening. I felt very guilty.

⊰⊱

This probably sounds strange, but I spent several days when Amy was about six months old worrying about whether or not she would go to her senior prom.

⊰⊱

We have had to be patient and go at David's pace.

⊰⊱

Some people just want to feel sorry for Brian but I don't want that. If I can't have an influence on how other people feel, I think I can at least make sure that Brian doesn't feel sorry for himself.

❧

My biggest pet peeve is people who stare. Don't just stare at my child. Come and talk to me. I am proud of him and I can talk about him all day long.

❧

My wife and I have difficulty communicating with each other about our child. She is probably farther along in the coping process than I am so I always feel guilty about what I am thinking.

❧

I don't think my husband and I have been on the same wavelength since our daughter was born. It seems like one of us is always up, while the other is down. Sometimes I think he is being unrealistically optimistic or pessimistic, and sometimes he thinks the same of me.

❧

I think my husband and I have gotten a lot better at communicating with each other since Amelia was born. Nothing is off limits. Often at night when we're lying in bed, we talk for an hour about what's on our minds. Sometimes it's just trivial things, like what kind of spoon seems to work best for feeding Amelia, but other times it's real big-picture things, like our hopes and concerns about her future. It's like we're partners on this complicated but important journey now, and honest communication is essential to us staying on track to achieve our goals.

❧

At first, It was really hard telling everyone at work about Joshua's diagnosis. Everyone had been so happy for me when they heard I was having a baby, and I felt somehow as if I was letting them down by having to tell them about this serious medical problem right off the bat. But they have all been extremely supportive right from the start. My boss asked me if I wanted to do some of my work at home before the thought even crossed my mind to ask for that!

❧

Right now I just try to treat Jessica as normally as possible. I try not to make too many exceptions for her. I especially try to make sure that Jessica knows I expect the same things from her that I expect from her sister.

❧

I hate it when people say "I know exactly how you feel." I know they are just trying to be nice but I don't think anybody understands unless they've been through this.

❧

I think I've started to trust my instincts more. I'm beginning to believe that what I know about my child is correct even if other people don't see it.

❧

At support groups, you may not necessarily find parents with whom you have much in common besides your child's vision loss. It is important to try out a variety of sources of support to find the one that matches your needs and your personality.

❧

I would recommend that parents who have just received the diagnosis create their own support group. Find specific people who can meet your needs. Ask questions. Control the amount of information that is coming at you, if it is overwhelming. Ask for help and guidance. Do not try to deal with it entirely on your own. The most important thing, though, is to just love your child and try not to automatically put up barriers. See what he or she can do first.

4

YOUR CHILD'S DEVELOPMENT

Kay Alicyn Ferrell, Ph.D.

Most childcare books include lists or charts of the skills that children are learning and doing at particular ages. You have probably scanned these charts, wondering where your child fits in. Perhaps you have been concerned that your child seems to be lagging behind in certain skills. Or you may have been puzzled because she has picked up some of the older skills without first learning the younger skills. These types of reactions are common among parents of children with visual impairments. Although all children with visual impairments grow and learn, or *develop,* the pattern and rate of their development is often different from other children's.

Unfortunately, health and education professionals have not studied the development of children with visual impairments as thoroughly as that of children without disabilities. In fact, we know very little about the development of children with visual impairments. To make predictions about development even more difficult, every child with a visual impairment is a unique individual, born with her own unique traits into a unique environment. Some are precocious and seem to be older and more advanced than their friends without disabilities. Others make much slower progress, and every new behavior learned becomes a cause for celebration.

The point is, even the experts do not know what makes the difference among children with visual impairments—why some sail through life effortlessly, while others seem to take one step backward before taking two steps forward. We think we know where some of the problems occur, and why. We think we can help parents work around these problems. But we don't have all the answers.

This chapter will look at what is known and unknown about the development of children with visual impairments. You will find some things that are true for your child, and some things that are not. Hopefully, this chapter will help you to enjoy your child as an individual, to recognize what she does best and where she needs your help, and how to make the most of her educational opportunities.

▪▪ What Is Development?

When educators talk about development, they mean the process by which children grow physically and mentally and learn increasingly complex skills. It includes mastery of skills such as making sense of the environment, communicating with others, making purposeful movements, caring for oneself, reading and doing math, and figuring out a bus schedule. It is, in short, the process that enables a child to change from a tiny, helpless newborn to an adult who is capable of looking after her own needs.

There is tremendous variability in human development. Some children make faster than expected progress in all areas of learning, and others make slower progress. Some develop quickly in some areas, but have more difficulty in others. Usually, however, most children acquire skills in the same sequence at about the same age. For example, children without disabilities usually learn to roll over by the time they are about three or four months of age, and then learn to sit up at about six to eight months. They begin to babble at about six to eight months, and then learn to say "mama" sometime around twelve to fourteen months of age.

Developmental Areas

During the course of development, children learn many different types of skills and behaviors. Child development experts usually group related skills into six general areas (or domains) of growth: cognitive, communication, motor, self-help, sensory, and social. In each of these areas, there are certain important skills, or *milestones,* that children are expected to acquire as they develop into more capable individuals.

For example, standing alone is a milestone in motor development and smiling is a milestone in social development.

The domains are interrelated. That is, growth in one area usually affects growth in other areas. For example, a child who has learned to take turns with others when communicating will also develop social skills such as sharing and working with other children in play. In spite of this, there are many children with really good abilities in one domain and poor abilities in another, as well as children whose progress in one developmental area seems to hamper their progress in another area, at least temporarily. A child who is having difficulty with motor skills, for example, would have more difficulty working on self-help skills such as dressing or eating by herself. Development is a dynamic, constantly changing process.

Understanding how skills are categorized into developmental areas is important if your child will be receiving early intervention or special education services. Before beginning school, your child will probably be evaluated in each of these developmental areas, since these areas help us to organize our thinking about how children grow and learn. Developmental areas also help us to identify strengths that can be used when children need help. For instance, a child who is especially good at social interactions might benefit from being placed in a play situation to work on motor skills or cognitive skills. The child's strengths in social interaction would help her develop abilities in her weaker areas (motor and cognitive skills).

Cognitive Development

Cognitive development involves acquiring the ability to think, reason, and problem solve. Babies learn the building blocks for these more advanced skills by manipulating toys and other things in their environment. For example, babies learn such concepts as *object permanence*—that things continue to exist even when they can no longer be seen, heard, or touched. They also learn *object constancy*—that objects that look different can still be the

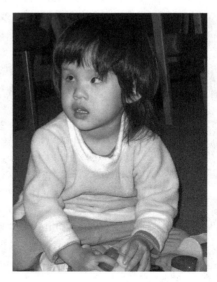

same thing. (An egg is an egg whether it is fried or boiled; the kitchen chair is the same chair whether you sit on it or someone else does.) In addition, they learn that their own actions can make something happen (*cause and effect*); and that objects can be organized according to characteristics such as color, size, how they're used, and what they do (*categorization*). These concepts lead to memorization and abstract thinking and help the young child understand how the world works and how her own actions can influence what happens.

Communication Development

Communication development enables the child to understand what is being communicated to her by others (*receptive language* skills), and also to make others understand her wants or needs (*expressive language* skills). Communication does not just involve speech, but also gestures, body language, reading and writing, crying, even whining. In addition, it can include the use of communication boards (laptop devices containing pictures or words that the user points to) or sophisticated electronic equipment that produces synthesized speech.

Motor Development

Motor development allows the child to move around in, and act upon, her world by controlling the muscles of her body. Motor skills are usually divided into two basic types: gross motor skills and fine motor skills. Gross motor skills involve large muscles such as those in the arms, legs, and abdomen. Examples of these skills include crawling, walking, and sitting up. Fine motor skills involve small muscles such as those in the hands and face. Examples of fine motor skills include grasping a crayon, fastening buttons, smiling, and moving the eyes.

Motor development follows four general principles:

1. It moves from head to toe, so that you expect a baby to be able to hold her head steady before you expect her to sit, and you expect the baby to sit before she can walk.

2. Control over large muscles occurs before control over small muscles, so that you expect a baby to play patty-cake before you expect her to tie shoes or print her name.

3. Muscle control moves from inner body to outer body (from the child's trunk to her fingertips; from the center to the extremities) so that babies will use their abdominal

muscles to sit upright before they are able to use their fingers to pick up tiny objects.

4. Motor development moves from simple movement to complex movement, so babies first swipe and pat objects before they are able to manipulate, poke, push, and pull objects.

The development of all children—with or without disabilities—follows these same four basic principles.

Self-help Development

Self-help development involves learning skills that enable a child to take care of herself and gradually become less and less dependent on adults for meeting her needs. For young children, this means learning to eat, dress, bathe, and use the toilet. While self-help skills may seem relatively unimportant compared to walking and talking, they are especially critical because they help children develop self-confidence and an understanding of their own abilities.

Sensory Development

Sensory development involves learning to recognize and use the information that is being gathered by our senses of touch, vision, hearing, smell, and taste. Sensory development is not always viewed as a separate developmental domain. It is usually considered part of cognitive development. This is because we typically measure how our senses have developed by the way that we use the information received through them, which is a part of our thinking and reasoning process. But however you look at sensory development, learning to make the most of *all* the senses is extremely important. As explained in the section called "Developmental Hurdles," when a sense such as vision does not develop properly, a child's entire course of development can be altered.

Social Development

Social development occurs as children learn to interact with their parents, family members, other adults, and other children. Babies begin life as very self-centered little beings; gradually they learn to build relationships, to seek out others, and to care about how others feel. During the preschool years, your child will learn some critical early social skills, such as taking turns and sharing with others. Social development is an important prerequisite for entering school.

❚❚ Differences in Your Child's Development

Much of the research on children with visual impairments compares them to children without disabilities. In such comparisons, children with visual impairments almost invariably seem behind their peers. But why shouldn't they? Think about how much babies use their vision. It is a constant source of information and sensory input. Research suggests that infants use their vision to enhance their understanding of the world long before they can demonstrate what they are thinking. Some studies, for example, have shown that five-month-olds, when shown pictures of various people, recognize their mothers not only from a black-and-white photograph, but even from a black line drawing! To do this, they must make the transition from real experience (from real moms in real color, who touch and talk and smell), to abstract concepts (to two-dimensional *representations* of moms, in black and white, who don't *do* anything). Those babies have so many visual experiences of their mothers stored in their memories that they can make the connection to a visual experience that is unlike the real thing—and at five months of age!

Now think about what that experience is like for infants with visual impairments. First of all, depending on the degree of impairment, their visual images of their parents might not be constant—they might only be able to see Mom's or Dad's face when it is a few inches away. Or, the image they see at six inches away might be much clearer than when Mom or Dad is three feet away. Their visual image of Mom and Dad is changing constantly, depending on where their parents are and how much light is in the room. Instead of storing *one* image in memory, they have to store *several*. Eventually their brains will merge these images, and they will understand that these images belong to Mom or Dad. But it is certainly a much slower process.

It would be nice if the other senses could substitute for vision—if they could provide the same type of information that helps babies to learn and form concepts about their world and if they could do so as frequently as vision. Unfortunately, they do not. What they do is provide a different set of experiences, which may or may not be confirmed by visual experiences. When a baby with typical vision plays with a squeeze toy, for example, she primarily uses vision, even though hearing and touch also provide sensory information. A baby who has a visual impairment, however, primarily uses hearing and touch, and only secondarily (if at all) uses vision. The difference occurs when that squeeze toy is held by someone else. The infant with typical vision can see the toy and recognize it as what she was playing with before; her vision helps to connect new experiences to what has occurred in the past. The infant with visual impairment cannot make such easy connections. The toy doesn't look the same, because it is further away; the toy is not being held by the baby, so memory is not triggered by what the object feels like; and the sound may be similar, but not quite the same (softer) because the toy is not as close as it was before.

Children with visual impairments do learn how to put all of these bits of sensory information together, but the process takes longer without reliable sensory input. The brain learns by repetition, but infants with visual impairments don't have the repetition opportunities when every time they contact an object or a concept, it looks, feels, or smells different.

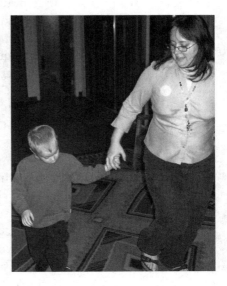

Another way visual impairments can slow development is by making it harder for children to learn incidentally, without their parents doing anything out of the ordinary to teach them. You cannot assume that incidental learning occurs for children with visual impairments, because whatever is happening has to occur in such a way that they *know* it's happening. For example, one popular game to play with infants is "So Big," where an adult says the words, and then raises his arms and hands up into the air. The baby responds by smiling and raising her own arms in the air in imitation. The adult then smiles, too, and both are enchanted with each other. The blind baby, however, doesn't know what's expected or how to do it, *unless* the adult shows her how to raise her arms. There are many things that happen in the course of the day that occur outside of the blind infant's direct experience.

Another example of this issue is the family pet. Children with typical vision see a cat's mouth open when it meows or spits, so they can connect the sound to the cat. When they pet the kitty, they feel the soft fur and see the cat's entire body simultaneously. When Dad tells the cat to stop scratching the couch, they look at Dad, see that he is looking at the cat, and follow his gaze over to where the cat is pawing at the couch.

The experience is different for children with visual impairments. They have no way of knowing what that meow, growl, or purr is. They may be able to pinpoint *where* the sound is coming from, but they cannot see *what* it is coming from. When the cat remains still long enough, they can feel its soft fur, but they can only feel one part of the cat at a time. They can't see that the cat has a head with ears, a body, four legs, four paws with claws, and a tail. When Dad yells at the cat, they cannot be sure what he is yelling at, or why. And if they get scratched, the paw comes out of nowhere and quickly disappears. Of course, children with visual impairments still learn the concept of cat, but if they rely on incidental learning, it will take quite a while to put this jumble of discrete, unrelated experiences together.

One teacher talks about the Good Fairy Syndrome—how, for children with visual impairments, objects and people seem to come out of and disappear into a secret world. Children need to learn the totality of actions: that clothes come out of a chest of drawers, or that toys do not get back into the toy chest by themselves, or that a banana has to be peeled to get to the edible part. Again, this is something that children with visual impairments can and do learn, but unlike other children, they need deliberate teaching to do so.

Because learning *is* more difficult without the clues provided by sight, it makes sense that children with visual impairments do not develop either at the same rate or in the same sequence as children without disabilities. They have much more to learn. For these reasons, comparisons to normal development are not really relevant for children with visual impairments. In other words, what is considered a delay for other children may not be a delay for your child—it may, in fact, be normal.

∷ Developmental Milestones

Even though your child's development may differ somewhat from the norm, this does not mean that you shouldn't have expectations for her development. If you do not expect your child to be able to do something, the chances are good that you will not try to teach her *how* to do it. If you do not teach her, then she has no chance to learn. Or if you teach your child but do not give her a chance to practice it, she may not learn it correctly. What this means is that your expectations—your belief in your child's abilities, or your ideas of what people who have visual impairments can and cannot do—have a lot to do with your child's development.

To help you set reasonable expectations, Table 1 (on the next two pages) suggests some developmental milestones that are important for your child's development. This list may look different from other developmental checklists you have seen. It includes skills that are important to children with visual impairments, but not necessarily important to children without disabilities. The age ranges are estimates, since we do not know exactly when children with visual impairments learn these behaviors. Your child may do certain skills earlier and others later. This table should help you understand what you and your child are working toward.

▪▪ Developmental Hurdles

Although we still have a lot to learn about developmental ages and sequences, we can identify some areas that seem to be more difficult for children with visual impairments. These areas are described in the sections below. Bear in mind, however, that visual impairment has a very individualized impact on a child's development. Your child may have relatively few problems in some of these areas, or she may have a great deal of difficulty in most. For strategies to help your child over these hurdles, see the section on "Helping Your Child's Development" at the end of this chapter.

Cognitive Hurdles

As Chapter 12 explains, some children with visual impairments have mental retardation and therefore encounter more difficulties than usual in learning. Visual impairments, however, do not cause mental retardation. As in the general population, most children with visual impairments have at least average intelligence, while some are intellectually gifted. A visual impairment in and of itself does not affect *what* a child is able to learn cognitively. It does, however, affect *how* children learn, as the section on "Differences in Your Child's Development" discusses. As a result, children with visual impairments often have trouble with several areas of cognitive development, including parts to whole learning, object permanence, and categorization.

:: TABLE 1—DEVELOPMENTAL MILESTONES FOR INFANTS

Developmental Area	Birth – 12 months
Cognitive	Imitates sounds, gestures, or actions Shows displeasure at loss of toy or object Demonstrates object permanence Begins to demonstrate cause and effect or means-end behaviors
Communication	Smiles Makes eye or face contact Babbles Laughs Says first word Understands "no" Responds to own name
Gross Motor (large muscles)	Controls head (holds upright when being held or when lying on tummy) Rolls over Sits Crawls
Fine Motor (small muscles)	Brings hands together Grasps objects Reaches for toys (either visually or auditorially) Searches for a dropped toy Explores objects (pats, pokes, hits together)
Self-Help	Eats with spoon Holds and drinks from bottle Eats some finger foods
Sensory	Focuses on and follows objects Turns to sound Explores objects by touch
Social	Makes eye or face contact Smiles Recognizes parents and family members Reaches for familiar person Cries when parent leaves

WITH VISUAL IMPAIRMENTS

13-24 months	25-36 months
Imitates use of toy Points to body parts Demonstrates memory (e.g., sings a song) Uses objects as tools Uses trial and error	Matches objects Remembers past events Begins to sort objects by size, color, texture, and shape Tells use of objects
Uses gestures (points, waves) Uses 2-word sentences Follows simple directions Names familiar objects and people	Uses first person pronouns (I, me) Asks questions Understands some prepositions (on, next to, on top of) Begins to use imagination
Pulls to stand Walks Climbs into adult-size chairs Rolls, then throws balls	Walks up and down stairs Begins to run Begins to jump Balances on one foot
Releases objects on purpose Uses pincer grasp (thumb and index finger) Scribbles Puts objects inside containers Completes simple form board puzzles Turns pages of books Uses wrist rotation (turns doorknobs, jar lids, etc.)	Stacks objects Copies geometric figures (either tactually or visually) Strings beads Sorts objects by size and texture
Drinks from cup Removes some clothing independently Indicates toilet needs Anticipates some daily routines	Puts on some clothing independently Puts toys away Partially or fully toilet trained
Identifies hot and cold Identifies familiar sounds Identifies familiar odors Recognizes objects by touch Explores objects or surfaces with feet	Recognizes places or activities by odors or sounds "Tracks" braille (follows along in book or on label) Identifies textures
Plays interactive games with adults Hugs Repeats actions that others laugh at Imitates household activities (feeding baby, sweeping, etc.); fantasy play Plays independently	Plays interactively with peers Shows signs of ownership Asks for help Pretends

Parts to Whole Learning

While most people see the whole object first, and then explore the little parts, children with visual impairments are limited to what they can see or feel at any one time. They have to construct a whole image or idea for something they will never experience as whole. It is like putting a puzzle together without seeing the photograph on the box. This may not seem like much of a problem, given the size of infant toys, but as your child grows, she will begin to explore toys and objects that are larger and more complex. And what about that pet kitty? Since your child can only feel one body part at a time, the image of the kitty in your child's mind could be entirely different from yours. This does not mean that learning is impossible—only that it needs to be structured, so that you are sure that your child is getting all the information, and getting it in the right order.

Imagine that you want to show your child her brother's new wagon. You might first let her sit in the wagon and explore the bottom and sides with her hands and feet. As soon as you feel that she is comfortable with the inside of the wagon, you will want to encourage her to feel the outside of the wagon and the wheels. You can do this first while she is sitting in the wagon and then you'll want to take her out of the wagon to continue exploring the outside. As you do this, place her hand on the inside (or seat) of the wagon to remind her that she was sitting inside the wagon just minutes before. Finally, show her the handle and demonstrate that as you walk with the handle in your hand, the wagon follows you. Now you're ready to go! Help your child place a favorite toy or stuffed animal in the wagon and then let her pull it a short distance and check to make sure the toy has "followed her" in the wagon.

Your child will also enjoy sitting in the wagon and being pulled by you. As you pull her, talk to her, so that she can feel the movement of the wagon and hear your voice in front of her. A word of caution: as you are about to begin to pull her in the wagon, make sure you warn her and tell her to hold on. While her brother may see you prepare to pull the wagon and grasp the sides of the wagon, your child with a visual impairment will not have the visual cues to prepare herself.

Object Permanence

Object permanence is the concept that something continues to exist even when you can no longer see, hear, touch, or otherwise perceive it with your senses. For example, a teddy bear still exists when it is stashed out of sight in the toy box; the vacuum cleaner still exists when it is turned off and put in the closet. If a child does not understand object permanence, everything is new to her each time it is presented; there is no continuity from time to time or object to object. Mastering this concept is a little more difficult for children with visual impairments, because they cannot rely on their vision to inform them about what happens to things. Even the toys they throw disappear, from their perspective. When they drop something, the only way they know it still exists is if they are able to touch or hear it. Yet babies with visual impairments seem to develop "people permanence" fairly easily. They know Mommy and Daddy, and they know that their parents will return even if they "disappear" momentarily. You can help your child develop object permanence by helping her feel around for dropped objects and by using the same words for objects consistently.

Categorization

Categorization is a way of ordering or sorting people and objects that most children begin doing actively around age three. Children begin by sorting objects by physical attributes, such as color and shape. Later they sort by group ("foods"), function ("things that you eat with"), and association ("things you need for a trip"). By categorizing things, we begin to organize our thinking so that we can be successful in learning new things and building on existing concepts and knowledge. This cognitive skill is difficult for children with visual impairments because they may not be able to see the similarities and differences among the objects in their environment. You can help your child learn to categorize by verbally pointing out similarities and differences and showing her the tactual qualities as well. For example, the first time your child encounters a motorcycle, point out that it has two wheels and a seat like a bicycle but it has a key to start it and it sounds more like a car.

Social Hurdles

Social development is important for all children, including children with visual impairments. Just as with children without disabilities, some children with visual impairments have an easier time picking up social skills than others. Some children are just naturally more outgoing and at ease in social situations. There are, however, some common problems encountered by children with visual impairments. For example, preschoolers with visual impairments often have a hard time initiating interactions with other children, choosing social activities, and playing alongside peers. You can help your child by arranging opportunities for her to play and interact with other children on a regular basis.

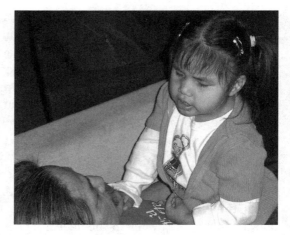

Attachment

Attachment is the process by which infants and parents learn to care for and love one another and form a human bond. It is important because it provides security and assists in emotional development. This process can be slower in babies with visual impairments, primarily because they often do not seem to cuddle like other babies. In fact, they may respond to being picked up by stiffening their bodies, arching their backs, and crying. Their message seems to be that they want to be left alone. In reality, however, they may merely have been surprised when they were picked up, and therefore responded in fear. Remember: babies with visual impairments are not always able to watch people approaching them, and you can't be sure they can hear or understand the sound of approaching footsteps.

Babies with visual impairments do attach to their parents, and they do cuddle. But they need some preparation before sudden moves. Try touching and talking to your baby first, giving her time to adjust, before wrenching her from the comfort and security of her crib or infant seat. Although your baby may give different signals, with patience and understanding you can learn to read them and to respond to them with love. Eventually, your baby will learn your signals and respond with just as much love.

Communication Hurdles

Vocal and verbal imitation are usually not problems for children with visual impairments—they very quickly learn verbal play like repetitive nursery rhymes and songs and it becomes a source of pleasure for them and their parents. There are, however, other aspects of communication that children with visual impairments typically have trouble with.

First, communication can be difficult when there is little visual feedback. Children with visual impairments may not make eye contact, so it is hard to tell whether they are paying attention to what someone is doing or saying, and it is hard for them to know if someone is paying attention to them. Without the cues from others' facial expressions (the raised eyebrow or the smile), children with visual impairments may also have trouble understanding when it is their turn to speak. You can help by practicing turn-taking with your baby, even in early infancy—imitate your baby's sounds, then wait and give her a chance to respond, then repeat your imitation again.

Another aspect of communication that may be difficult for your child is nonverbal gestures such as waving, pointing, or nodding. If your child cannot observe these gestures being used by others, she will not automatically learn how to make them. Teach your baby about these simple, but meaningful gestures that will add to everyone's understanding. It will be most effective if you use naturally occurring events to teach your child about nonverbal gestures. For example, when you are playing with your child and she smiles, you might tell her that you like it when she smiles and that it lets you know that she is happy or pleased.

Motor Hurdles

Although a visual impairment does not affect a child's ability to use her muscles, it does affect the way she learns to use them. One reason is that many of the motor skills children learn are acquired by watching someone else do things, imitating them, and then repeating them over and over again. This means your child will not automatically pick up skills such as crawling, walking, skipping, and jumping the way other children do.

Another reason visual impairments can affect the development of motor skills is that if a child can't see an attractive toy or mobile, she won't be as motivated to try to touch or grasp it. In addition, children who can't see where they're moving may be reluctant to explore their environment.

Fine Motor Skills

You would think that babies with visual impairments would just naturally use their hands, because so much information is available

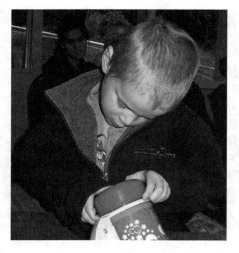

that way. But remember that they have not had the same visual experiences—they may not be able to watch their hands, or see their hands contact and manipulate objects, or watch what other people do with their hands. You can show your child what to do—whether it's eating or stacking or scribbling—by using a hand-over-hand technique. Some children will like your hand on top of theirs, while others will like their hand on top of yours—but in either case, the purpose of a hand-over-hand technique is to show the child what to do until she can do it herself.

Your child's fine motor skills may also be delayed if she does not like lying on her tummy or crawling, as is the case with some babies with visual impairments. This is because a baby's hand grasp tends to become more mature when she bears weight on her hands and shifts weight from one hand to the other. If your child does not get these experiences, she will probably have difficulties in eating finger foods and playing with objects. Other than showing your baby how to do these things with her hands, the next best thing is to make sure she gets lots of gross motor activity. Good activities for encouraging movement include: playing with a variety of toys that require your child to use her hands in different ways; patty cake; ball play; rolling a wheelbarrow; and making obstacles courses that encourage climbing and scooting.

Locomotion

Moving independently from place to place *(locomotion)* seems to be one of the most difficult skills for children with visual impairments. For children without visual impairments, the motivation to move comes, first, from watching others move, and then from seeing something desirable that is just out of reach. Children with visual impairments do not have these experiences. Consequently, they can be delayed in skills such as crawling and walking. You can show your child how to move, even if it means you have to get down on the floor! You can also use other sensory cues (your voice, the sound of a favorite toy) to help your child understand that something is "out there" and worth going after. See Chapter 11 for more suggestions about helping your child with locomotion.

Sensory Hurdles

According to some researchers, vision is involved in 90 percent of the learning that takes place in early childhood. But the way your child learns about the world will be different. To a greater or lesser degree, your child will have to rely instead on her senses of smell, touch, hearing, and taste for information. As mentioned earlier, this will make it harder for your child to learn because she cannot watch and imitate what others are doing, and may make her less motivated to learn if she cannot see enticing objects in her environment. It will also make it harder for her to learn about objects and people in her environment through intersensory coordination.

Intersensory Coordination

Intersensory coordination is the process of taking information learned through one sensory system and using it in another. It involves figuring out how the information obtained through one sense is related to the information obtained through another sense. For example, a young child might hear a siren and figure out that the noise goes with the big red fire engine that just sped by. Vision plays an important role in intersensory coordination, because it seems to blend the other senses automatically. Vision, because it is always present, can take all the separate pieces of sensory information and pull them together into a whole.

In the absence of vision, this process is more difficult, because the other pieces of sensory information occur intermittently. Toys sometimes make sounds, but they may sound different across the room than they do close up, and may stop making sounds if batteries or wind-up mechanisms run down. Toys can be touched and smelled, but only if they are within reach. Babies with visual impairments do eventually develop intersensory coordination, but until they do, it is probably a good idea not to overload them with sensory stimuli. Give your child one sensory input at a time—let her touch an object before squeezing it to make noise, and let her touch food before you give her a taste of it. At the same time you are presenting a new object to your child, be sure to explain what you're showing her: "Feel the fuzzy bear. Listen to the pretty music the bear makes. . . ." As mentioned in the section on Object Permanence, be sure to use the same words in describing objects at first, so that your child does not become confused. For example, at the beginning don't alternate using "bear" and "teddy"; use the same word each time.

▪▪ Helping Your Child's Development

One of the best ways you can help your child's development is to get some help yourself. As Chapter 8 explains, there are laws that entitle your family to early intervention and special education services. These services are intended to help maximize your child's development.

Be sure that the services you receive are what you want—they should never feel burdensome or intrusive. And because children with visual impairments send different signals and experience the world differently, insist that your services include a professional who is knowl-

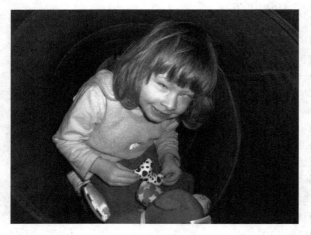

edgeable about blindness and visual impairments (a teacher of children with visual impairments and/ or an orientation and mobility instructor). These professionals have been trained to understand the experiences of children with visual impairments and to help them learn. Perhaps most importantly, they have also been trained to see the possibilities for people with visual impairments and not the limitations—just as you will see the possibilities, as you watch your child grow and learn.

Besides getting professional help for your child's developmental problems, there are also ways you can help her learn. Some general principles include:

- *Experience the world from your child's point of view.* This might mean getting down on the floor and learning to crawl all over again, or it might mean closing your eyes before you try to hold and drink from a cup. The point is that you want to get an idea of what you are asking your child to do before you ask her to do it. It might not be as easy as it seems!

- *Create opportunities when the opportunities do not create themselves.* Although we are still learning about how babies with visual impairments develop, one thing is certain: They will not learn what they have not experienced. Since you cannot rely on incidental learning, you have to *make* opportunities for learning. If you drop an egg on the floor, your toddler can help clean it up, while you talk about eggs and compare *this* egg to the eggs she had for breakfast. Seize the time!

- *Make your child a do-er instead of a done-to-er.* Help your child to learn on her own, instead of always doing things for her. By allowing her to accomplish things on her own, you are sending a clear message to her that you not only *expect* her to do things on her own, but you also trust her to accomplish them correctly. While your child is very young, it will be important for her to experience success often as she tries new things. As she grows, however, it will be just as important for you to know that some of the things she tries to do will be difficult. You must encourage her to work through her frustration. It will be well worth it as she grows into an independent and capable young adult.

- *Give enough time.* Give enough time for your child to learn a skill, and then give enough time to practice it. This may mean you have to change your schedule a bit, but it will help make your child a do-er.

- *Help make connections.* It is difficult to apply what you have learned in the past to a new experience (*generalize*) if you are unable to see the similarities in the situations. You help make connections when you relate the broken egg on the floor to breakfast. You help make connections, too, when you point out that the wheels on the car are circles, and serve your child mashed, baked, scalloped, and diced potatoes instead of only French fries.

- *Use co-active movements.* Hand-*over*-hand and hand-*under*-hand are *co-active* movements that are great for showing your child what your expectations are, especially when introducing a new skill.

- *Use concrete (real) objects and experiences.* It will be easier for your child to understand the concept of the *real* object before asking her to understand a representation of that object. The family cat is a better learning tool than a stuffed animal toy.

- *Beware the fairy godmother.* Help your child to understand the totality of actions, instead of thinking that things just happen. Make sure that she knows that the apple juice doesn't just "appear" in her cup at breakfast—that *you* open the refrigerator door, pick up the juice bottle, pour the juice into her cup, and set the cup on the table. It will be helpful to talk to your child about what you are doing as you do it.

- *Use touch.* Your touch means a lot to your child. Sometimes a touch on the shoulder can be just the reassurance your child needs to plow ahead!

- *Use language that is rich in description.* You do not have to talk *at* your child all day long, but when you do talk, try to be as informative as possible. Explain what is going on, or why everyone is laughing. Tell her about colors and textures and the weather.

- *Be consistent in the names you use.* It can be confusing if you talk about your baby's overalls one minute, and then refer to them as pants the next minute. Try to use the same words for objects and events until your baby is old enough that you can point out similarities and differences and can help her make connections for what seems obvious to you.

- *Use your child's name.* A child with a visual impairment cannot see the facial expressions or body language that tell her she is the one being spoken to. Especially if there are other adults or children in the room, speak to your child (and everyone else) by name.

- *Point out visual features.* If your child has some vision, it may help her sort out what she is seeing if you draw her attention to various visual characteristics of objects. Point out that her toy is bright yellow or that her patent leather shoes are shiny. "See" and "look" are appropriate terms to use, even if your child is totally blind.

- *Point out the sensory qualities of people, objects, and events.* If you walk past a bakery, comment on the wonderful smells coming through the door. Your baby will smell it, too, but will not necessarily know what it means unless you tell her. Point out that Aunt Sara always smells like flowers and Uncle Dan has hairy arms. Show her that grass feels and smells different from carpeting.
- *Make no assumptions.* You can never be sure your child has witnessed events that you have, and you can never be sure that she understands them in quite the same way. Do not assume that learning has occurred—check it out, probe, ask questions. Exposure does not mean absorption.
- *Encourage interactions with people and places.* It can be difficult for children with visual impairments to take risks in social situations because they do not have the same clues available. For example, they cannot read body language to tell if they would be welcomed into a group. Help your child to feel comfortable with adult family members, and, if necessary, show her how to play with her peers. In new places, help your child explore the surroundings and feel comfortable in them.
- *Encourage socially appropriate behaviors.* Children with visual impairments may not be able to make eye contact, but they can turn their head toward someone who is speaking to them. "Please" and "thank you" are appreciated in any youngster. As your child grows older, you may also have to explain which habits are appropriate in public (scratching your head) and which are not (picking your nose).
- *Remember that eye function can vary.* Children with visual impairments are affected by different lighting conditions, different times of day, and even different weather patterns. Their behavior may not be consistent, and they may have legitimate reasons for this inconsistency because of what's going on around them. Be patient if your child comfortably completes visual tasks one day and seems frustrated by them the next.
- *Use your voice to convey meaning.* The volume and tone of your voice can tell your child a lot about your current state of mind—whether you are angry, sad, happy, exasperated,

or thrilled. This will be another clue that your child can use in social situations.

- *Relate directions to body parts.* Whenever possible, give directions by referring to positions in relation to your child's body parts. Instead of saying, "You dropped your rattle on the floor," say "Your rattle is on the floor next to your foot." As your child grows, her orientation to the world will occur in terms of her body—in back, in front, next to, on the side, left, and right.

- *Challenge your child.* No one knows what makes the differences among children, and with today's technology, no one knows what the possibilities are for your child's future. Try to create experiences that will help your child make connections, reach a better understanding of the world, and seek out her own opportunities for learning.

■■ Conclusion

As a parent, you have probably already realized how fascinating it is to watch your child as she learns new things. Day by day, week by week, you watch as she develops her own strengths and discovers her unique likes and dislikes. Still, you likely have some concerns about your child's development. This is only natural—all parents do.

Your child with visual impairments may need your help to discover the many opportunities for exploring the world. These experiences will help her develop skills and understanding in the cognitive, communication, motor, self-help, sensory, and social domains. By encouraging this development when your child is young, you are helping her establish a firm foundation for learning later in life.

■■ Parent Statements

We were fortunate we didn't have to take Brandon to a daycare, so my wife was able to work with him every day. She began with simple movement—pushing one hip, then the other, to show him how his hips would propel his very first rolling movements. Then, it was on to arms and legs, and eventually to sitting up, and eventually, to crawling. He showed us early on that he would let us know when he'd had enough. He would start to fuss when he was tired.

❧

We worried about how John would clean himself properly when using the restroom; how he'd never play baseball or ride a bike. There are so many things sighted people just presume cannot be done if one cannot see. Happily, our desire to raise a happy, confident young man super-seded our misconceptions. Our son is eight, now, and although he hasn't yet gotten interested in bikes, he did enjoy playing tee-ball for two years, has taken gymnastics, and is planning on taking karate at some point. He also loves swimming, jumping on trampolines, flying on zip lines, explor-ing, and digging for treasure!

❧

Try to ensure that your day includes unstructured time. It is easy to fall into the habit of spending most of your time together doing physical therapy exercises, visual development games, and other helpful, yet time-consum-ing activities. Your family needs time to laugh and just hang around too.

❧

I know Jason has delays—I just keep expecting them to go away. I figure if we work on things step-by-step and Jason continues to progress, then he is continuing to learn. It doesn't matter to me if it takes him longer to learn than other kids.

❧

I always thought I would be the expert on my own child. Now I have to rely on all these outsiders—teachers, therapists, psychologists—the list goes on and on. I should be the boss—not them.

❧

Don't feel sorry for my child. Just be proud of her accomplishments.

❧

My friend's baby is the same age as Josh, and she's way ahead of him. When I'm depressed, I don't want to visit them. But then I look at how far Josh has come and I know that is what is important!

❧

I talk to Katie a lot—I try to explain everything I'm doing, even though I know she doesn't really understand yet. Some day she will.

❧

The early intervention team told us that Marty's motor development might be delayed because she doesn't reach out for things since she can't see them. We bought all kinds of toys that make noises so that she will have something to reach out for, but she is really interested in people and will be more likely to reach out to someone she loves than to a toy.

❧

I get very defensive when people point out what Carrie isn't doing yet.

❧

It frustrated me that my baby never does as well when his development is being assessed as he does when he's with me at home. But I guess what matters in the long run is that he is making progress, even if he doesn't demonstrate that progress to his therapists and teachers.

❧

The therapists in the early intervention program have really helped me understand the areas in which my daughter excels, as well as the areas in which she is lagging behind.

DAILY
LIFE

Beth Langley, M.S.

When your child has a visual impairment, day-to-day activities still go on. Family members need to sleep, prepare and eat meals, dress appropriately for the events of the day, do chores, run errands, and take time to relax and have fun. In the beginning, your child will need a great deal of help to participate in these activities, just as any child would. As he grows older, however, you can expect him to learn self-help, social, and other skills that will enable him to become more and more independent.

Ideally, by the time your child reaches kindergarten, he will be well on his way to having the basic social and self-care skills that will enable him to get along fairly independently at school and in the community. Imagining how your child will accomplish so many skills by kindergarten age may be overwhelming, but from the first few weeks of his life, your child must be held to the same expectations and standards as his seeing peers. Even if your child has other disabilities in addition to his visual impairment, he should be expected to participate in the same activities of daily life that other children do. While your child's visual impairment may dictate that he learn through a slightly different process and timeline, unless he has a significant physical and/or mental challenge, he will learn basic life skills in a manner that closely parallels his peers'. However, how effectively and quickly your child masters daily living skills will largely depend on you, at least in the beginning.

To help you anticipate and cope with the demands of encouraging your child's independence, this chapter suggests hints, tips, and strategies accumulated from personal experience, well-accepted techniques that have proven effective for children with visual impairments, and clever ideas shared by other parents and professionals. You will find that your child will often discover his own compensation and that the ideas in this chapter serve only as a catalyst for igniting your own fires of ingenuity. If you have older children, you may find that the suggestions included in this chapter sound very familiar because you may have used these or similar strategies to help them become independent. This chapter includes discussions about some issues that may not be relevant to you and your child, while other suggestions may be helpful for you.

:: Your Role as a Parent

One of the most important things that children learn is independence. Being independent includes managing your personal needs, safely navigating your environment, knowing the expectations and rules associated with a variety of home, school, and community settings, and having the confidence to seek out information critical to dealing with new situations and advocating for your needs and dreams. In no other area will you be such a powerful influence in your child's life. You will need to set the tone for expectation, opportunity, patience, motivation, and persistence.

Because you are a parent, your first instincts are to protect your child and to provide for his needs. When your child has a visual impairment, the emotional part of you may want to wrap him in an eggshell and do everything for him to alleviate the stress and inconvenience of him trying to do things for himself. The intellectual side of you will need to take over and do the exact opposite (within reason relative to his age)! Your child will never be too young for you to begin to encourage independence if your goal is for him to be a competent adult. Here are some strategies that must become second nature to you if you want to promote the development of an independent and well-adjusted child:

- Depending on the severity of your child's visual impairment, you will need to think and perceive for two people (avoid that shopping cart coming at him, cue him about that upcoming curb, alert him about the sprinklers headed your way!).

- Because so much of learning to do for yourself is typically achieved by imitating others around you, you will have to offer appropriate opportunities at the appropriate readiness level and physically and verbally guide your child through activities that other children learn through visual imitation. Figuring out all of the nuances associated with eating, dressing, toileting, and chores may take your child longer to master since vision is the great integrator of other senses.

- Help your child discriminate whether his behavior is the same as his peers', and encourage him to learn skills in functional and meaningful settings and consistent routines. This helps with *generalization*—that is, being able to use a skill learned in one context or setting in a different context or setting. You need to think about where and when other children typically acquire a skill and then be consistent about ensuring the opportunity is available. It will be important to both your child's development and your sanity that skills be taught within existing household and family routines.

- As with other children, your child will have his own unique learning style and preferences and you must honor and follow his lead when introducing compensatory strategies for achieving independence. The extent of his visual impairment and the presence of other disabilities may govern the nature of adaptations and compensations needed. However, what your child enjoys, avoids, and rejects may provide more insight into how best to help him learn skills.

- Ingenuity in arranging, designing, and adapting experiences and then providing for practice, practice, practice should be the shared responsibility between you, your family, your community, and your child's interventionists.

- Finally, you and all the members of your family will need to become ambassadors and role models by demonstrating what to expect of your child, how to respond to those around him who lack your expertise, and by setting the tone for a sense of humor, grace, and dignity when the inevitable potentially embarrassing moment ensues. My son's grandmother continues to be alarmed that the light in his room or the bathroom is not on but she now easily laughs at herself when someone mentions we save a lot on the electric bill because of his visual impairment!

:: The Compensatory Role of Other Senses

Development of self-care and other independence skills is dependent on appropriate and timely opportunities, the quality and extent of the child's posture and movement patterns, and his ability to use his other senses. Even a small perception of light is valuable to your child in helping him orient and localize to participate in tasks of daily living. If your child has other disabilities in addition to vision loss, you will need to be creative in finding ways to engage him actively in caring for his own needs. If he lacks efficient balance, coordination, and fluid control of his muscles, additional strategies and different approaches may be needed to give him a sense of control over his life. In addition to your child's teacher of students with visual impairments, an occupational therapist and/or physical therapist can assist you with alternative techniques and equipment as well as activities that will help him make progress in sensory development and motor control.

All children learn to adapt to their world through their senses. Sufficient and appropriate sensory information guides a child to make the right response to a given situation, whether it is to push his arm the rest of the way through a sleeve, to turn left to go into his room, or to step quickly across hot cement. The sense of vision plays an enormous role in integrating information from the other senses, sometimes alerting the child that something needs to happen and at other times confirming for him that he did hear the ice cream truck or that it was the family dog that just brushed by him. Without vision, the responsibility of alerting and confirming falls to the other senses. Your child will learn to use and trust his hearing to recognize the voices of friends and relatives, his sense of smell to know that Mom is cooking his favorite dinner, and his sense of touch to avoid the spinach and search for the applesauce!

While you may be tempted to bombard your child with multiple sensory experiences to make sure he learns as much as possible as quickly as possible, this can be a mistake. Overloading your child with sights, sounds, textures, and smells can be just as damaging as a complete lack of sensory information. For example, while driving down a country lane, you might think it is a good idea to keep a running commentary going: "We're driving down a little gravel road. We're passing a barn and a farmhouse and some cows. Can you hear that I am rolling down your window? Can you feel the wind and smell the fresh-cut grass?" As you can see, it would be difficult to keep such a commentary going and so much information may be overwhelming and potentially meaningless.

Sensory information will be more meaningful to your child when emphasized within a natural context or routine so that what he hears, feels, tastes, and smells has relevance. When sensory input is an integral part of the activity, your child is more likely to accept it, process it, and use the information functionally.

Most of us readily apply information gathered from multiple sensory experiences without difficulty and even tune out sensory input if it is not immediately important to us. This process is referred to as *sensory integration.* That's why you may have been somewhere numerous times and never have noticed a particular feature until someone directly pointed it out to you. If your child was premature or has additional disabilities, his sensory systems may be immature and he may display behaviors that indicate he has a difficult time making sense of sound, touch, smell, and taste.

Chapter 4 presented information on how children use their senses. The five basic senses are vision, hearing, touch, taste, and olfactory or smell. You may hear about two other sensory systems that play a very important role in your child's ability to integrate sensory information, coordinate, and plan movement, and to know where his body is in space. They are the vestibular and proprioceptive systems. If your child has cerebral palsy or other neuromuscular impairments that result in too much or too little muscle tone, his vestibular (sense of movement) and proprioceptive (unconscious awareness of where he is in space) systems may also be impaired. This, in turn, presents additional challenges in eating, playing, dressing, moving safely and independently, and adapting successfully to a variety of different environments. The vestibular system provides a framework for all of our experiences and paces the functioning of the entire central nervous system, preparing it for other sensory input. When your child's brain cannot sufficiently register information received from the vestibular system, he may react defensively (by pulling away or crying) to touch, sound, and movement, especially if he has had limited opportunities to adapt to feedback from these sensations in a variety of settings.

▪▪ Why All This Discussion about Sensory Processes?

Since your child will need to rely so much on other sensory systems to learn and adapt to his world, it is important that you understand why many children with visual impairments may have difficulty with daily life activities that depend on responding effectively to movement, touch, taste, and hearing. Researchers have found that sensation is influenced by the context and the demands of the moment as well as the child's prior sensory experiences, current state of alertness, and emotional state (Williamson, Anzalone, and Hanft, 2001). This helps explain why an only child may respond negatively to the noise of a busy birthday party or a mall while a child reared in a home full of busy children is not fazed by noise and may even be happiest in the midst of chaos and activity.

▪▪ The Function of Sensory Information

While well-meaning friends, neighbors, and interventionists may suggest specific "sensory experiences" for you to try, consider first whether the recommended activity will give your child a more functional (real-life) way to control or adjust to his environment. "Stimulating" should not take the form of "doing to the child," but of allowing him to actively explore, control, and make accommodations in a naturally occurring setting or play opportunity. Rather than devise isolated ways to "stimulate" sensory development, look for ways to involve your child in sensory experiences that occur naturally and that match his level of readiness. For example, exposing your toddler to different textures such as a feather duster, a wire whisk, and strips of velvet, corduroy, and sandpaper in the absence of a meaningful context may result in tantrums or boredom. However, he may be much more accepting of his bath towel, the plastic of his highchair tray, the graininess of his Cheerios, and the rubbery feel of Dad's sunglasses because he has explored them in the comfort and security of pleasurable situations and familiar routines.

The bottom line is this: your child needs to learn to use sensory information (sights, sounds, smells, surface changes, textures, and taste) for:

- anticipating what is happening or about to happen;
- being alert to dangerous situations;
- calming and organizing;
- helping make appropriate choices or decisions;
- controlling the environment;
- orienting in time and space; and
- moving safely in the environment.

If a sensory experience does not meet one of the above functions, it may serve no useful purpose and, in fact, may be disorganizing. The smell of powder may cue your child that he is about to have his diaper changed; soap bubbles signify it is bath time; and the smell of toast means breakfast is finally ready. Calling your child's attention to the oven buzzer or microwave beep helps him orient to and navigate his way into the kitchen for mealtime and alerts him to prepare for eating. When your child can anticipate what is about to happen, he will gradually begin to initiate control and independence. Table 1 on the next page provides examples of natural sensory cues and potential meanings associated with each cue.

A Word about the Tactile System

You will need to be proactive about providing your child appropriate touch experiences during the first months of life to encourage the development of a normal touch system. This, in turn, will enable him to use his hands for exploring, processing, and adapting to self-care routines; and, possibly, reading braille.

When children with visual impairments are hesitant to touch and explore different types of textures, they are frequently labeled "tactilely defensive." Often, however, this label is misapplied. If your child is reluctant to experience touch sensations, it is more likely because his sensory system is trying to protect him from dangerous or unpleasant experiences. To some degree, everybody's sensory system does this. Most people are hesitant to touch unknown objects as well as substances that are associated with unpleasant events and experiences. This is a survival technique intended to help the touch system recognize danger and regulate sensory input that is too intense. All babies and young children are more likely to have these primitive, protective responses to touch and other sensations because their sensory system is immature.

Immature touch systems respond best to pressure, weight bearing, and hard, firm textures, and resist light touch at all costs. Providing sensory input from soft materials such as fur, silk, or velvet, or from light stroking may not only disorganize a child's behavior, but cause a great deal of emotional stress. Offering your infant playful deep pressure into his palm with your thumb, providing a variety of firm, hard toys, and guiding his hands to firmly contact your face are only a few ways of helping your child develop his protective touch system.

:: TABLE 1—NATURAL ENVIRONMENTAL CUES

Natural Cue	Associated Event/Location
Mom's perfume/Dad's shaving lotion	Informs child who is approaching
Music from clock radio	Time to get up
Bib on/off	I'm going to eat/I'm finished
Bath water running	Time for bath
Smell of powder	Time for diaper change
Sound of battery-operated toothbrush	Time to have teeth brushed
Banister	I'm going up/down stairs
Tile/rug	I'm in the kitchen/family room
Sound of radio/TV	My toys are near
Blender	Time to eat
Keys	Time to go for a ride
Book	I get to sit with Dad
Toilet flushing	That's the bathroom
Coffee, meals cooking	That's the kitchen
Warmth from sunshine	That's a window
Pulling on outerwear	Time to go outside/playground
Sound of bike horn	I'm going to ride my bike
Sliding doors opening	I'm at the grocery store
Moisture, splashing water, sounds of voices, smell of chlorine, swim ring	Time to go swimming
Leather shoes	Time to go to church
Crinkly paper	I'm at the doctor's

It is all right for your child to be somewhat tentative when touching something for the first time. He also has a right to refuse to touch particular textures or to engage in specific tactile experiences. For example, he should not be forced to play with Play Doh, finger paint, or glue if he finds these substances unpleasant. Children with visual impairments learn most efficiently when they have some control over the amount of incoming sensory information. Offer your child encouragement, choices, and frequent opportunities to participate, without imposed judgment or expectations. Once he knows what to expect and can trust that an experience is predictable, he will often accept new objects, textures, and substances and incorporate them into his play and sensory repertoire.

Occasionally, tactile defensiveness can be so severe that it interferes significantly with everyday routines or contributes to delays in development. If you suspect that your child has tactile dysfunction, seek assistance from a pediatric occupational therapist with sensory integration training and/or certification. See Chapter 8 for more information on occupational therapy.

■■ Mealtimes

Mealtime can be the most frustrating time for both your child and your family. Mealtime can be hurried, noisy, and messy. What should be a relaxing time for families to get together and review their day often turns into a stressful situation if a child resists eating, is highly selective in what he eats, lacks the motor skills to eat age-appropriate foods, or has sensory issues that cause him to reject specific temperatures and/or textures of food.

Many children with visual impairments master eating skills with little difficulty, while others may be quite delayed in learning to eat independently and have significant feeding problems. How your child reacts to eating will depend on how well he perceives sensation in and around his mouth, his posture, his general temperament, whether specific eating experiences and textures are introduced at the right time, and, most importantly, your attitudes, emotions, and consistency in feeding your child.

Early Eating Experiences

Babies with visual impairments follow the same developmental feeding milestones as sighted babies. You should therefore follow general feeding guidelines when selecting and offering different textures of foods.

Children with visual impairments usually manage pureed foods as well as sighted infants do unless they have poor oral motor skills due to prematurity. Most feeding difficulties coincide with the introduction of cereals and foods with more consistency and texture. Often premature babies, especially those with visual impairments, do not spend time exploring a broad array of textures with their mouths. Low tone around the face and difficulties coordinating arm movements at midline may impede early hand-to-mouth behaviors, including bringing toys to the mouth to explore. Without these early oral exploratory experiences, your child may be resistant to having something grainy or coarse in his mouth. You can help your child by gently guiding him to place his hands in his mouth and by helping him explore a variety of different textured teething toys. Later, giving him foods such as zwieback toast, teething biscuits, hard pretzels, strips of hard cheeses, frozen vegetables, and graham crackers may help him accept different textures.

Children with visual impairments who have low muscle tone may also have poor sensation within their mouths and have a difficult time managing soft and gooey foods. Often firmer, "regular" foods provide more sensory input and are easier for the child to manage. Other reasons to avoid feeding your child pureed foods for too long include the following concerns (Orelove and Sobsey, 1996):

- lack of development of more advanced eating skills;
- risk for aspiration pneumonia;
- constipation, dental cavities, and vitamin deficiencies; and
- increased likelihood of developing weakened and deformed structures in and around the mouth.

The most difficult textures for children with visual impairments are those without a definite consistency, such as jello, and those with mixed textures, such as casseroles, soups with several items, and beef stew. You may wish to consult books such as the *M.O.R.E.* book (*M.O.R.E.: Integrating the Mouth with Sensory and Postural Functions* by Sheila Frick, Patricia Oetter, and Eileen Richter) for suggestions about how to help prepare your child for different textures inside his mouth (see *Reading List*).

When you introduce your baby to unfamiliar foods, he may react by coughing, sputtering, gagging, and spitting. These are typical reactions from all infants. If you have not experienced these reactions with other children, however, you may be alarmed and think that your child is struggling because of his visual impairment. As with other babies, you should calmly alternate bites of preferred foods and cautiously present the offending food for another try. Your child may require a longer period of time to adjust to new foods, but he will most likely get used to the new textures with experience and warm encouragement.

For age-appropriate guidelines for offering your child different types and textures of foods and addressing feeding issues typically seen in children with visual impairment and other disabilities, you may wish to consult the book *Let's Eat: Feeding a Child with a Visual Impairment* by Jill Brody and Lynn Webber. See the Reading List at the end of the book. Some suggestions for helping your child learn to eat independently include:

- Let your child actively participate in the feeding process as soon as possible.
- Guide him to assist with holding his bottle, which encourages the integration of touch and cause and effect understanding, and builds hand skills.
- Look for utensils that will give your child tactile feedback. For instance, there are textured bottle holders that offer tactile feedback as well as visual input if your child can appreciate bright colors and bold patterns. There are also many wonderfully textured utensils for little hands when your child is ready. Many of these are arched and curved to help him get food to his mouth more easily. Explore the infant/toddler section of your favorite drug, discount, grocery, or department store to find feeding tools that are appropriate for your child.
- Devise signals to let your child know what is going on at mealtime. For example, some children like to hold onto a spoon of their own throughout the feeding process. This can be a signal to them that food is approaching. Other signals can include a consistent phrase such as "Ready for a bite?" or encouraging him to put his hand on your wrist before you offer him a spoonful of food.

Sometimes children with visual impairments have significant oral motor problems and just cannot seem to adapt to new food. If this occurs, consult a pediatric occupational therapist or speech therapist with specialization in treating oral motor difficulties and feeding problems. Even if your child has feeding difficulties, always encourage him to stay with your family during mealtime, even if only to play in his highchair or infant or booster seat while the family eats. Your child needs to learn that, regardless of his behavior, you still expect him to participate as a family member during family events.

Poor Appetite

Poor appetite can be another obstacle to overcome with children with visual impairments. While every child is different, poor appetite is often due to the oral motor problems discussed in the previous section. Other common causes include too little physical activity and meals served too closely together. One mother was surprised when her child brought a note home after the first day of school asking her to send snacks for her child, as she was still hungry after lunch. Typically, this child refused to eat more than a few bites at any meal. The mother admitted, however, that her daughter spent most of her days at home listening to music or lying on the sofa and listening to television with her siblings. Another child ate heartily at lunch once his class switched to the last lunch period, allowing more time between meals.

If your child has a fairly inactive daily life, offering several "little meals" throughout the day, rather than the traditional breakfast, lunch, and dinner, may entice him to eat. Also consider whether your child finds his meals tasty enough to eat. Although each child has his own preferences, children with visual impairments often prefer spicy foods over sweet ones. Many children have highly developed taste cells and acquire a preference for specific types and brands of foods, refusing the same food of another brand. One deaf-blind child had such refined taste buds that she would eat French fries only from McDonald's, Mrs. Baird's bread, Oreo cookies, and Birdseye orange juice.

If your child is not getting sufficient calories, either because he is a "picky" eater or because his metabolism is high, ask your pediatrician to refer you to a certified pediatric nutritionist or dietitian. The dietitian can recommend simple ways of providing more calories, including adding Instant Breakfast to your child's milk or cereal, offering fruit and yogurt milkshakes, and blending peanut butter, wheat germ, mayonnaise, butter, or oil into foods your child will eat.

Finger Feeding

As mentioned above, many children with visual impairments are hesitant to touch and handle unfamiliar objects, including foods. This hesitancy often delays finger feeding, a critical step in the acquisition of self-feeding skills. Finger feeding aids in the development of fine motor skills and reinforces scanning techniques as the child searches for food on a tray or plate.

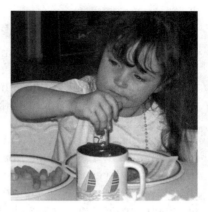

Even though tactile sensitivities may delay finger feeding, you should still introduce your child to finger feeding at the usual age (about six months). To help him make the transition to finger feeding, try letting him hold his hand over yours while you place bites in his mouth. Some children may require most of the food to be fed to them and then can be encouraged to feed themselves the last couple of bites. Also try offering a small taste to entice him to grasp and self-feed the remaining portion. If you can identify one favorite food that lends itself to finger feeding, it may help to allow your child to perfect his skills with that food before moving on to others.

One parent decided that if her child was motivated to open his mouth when his favorite food was offered, he should be motivated to hold it and feed himself. After only two short sessions in which his parents placed the cookie in his hand and quickly guided it to his mouth, the boy began to hold a broader variety of finger foods.

Whatever your child's age, remember that most individuals have a few foods that they would rather not eat. When your child rejects only certain foods, his "message" should be honored. However, from the very beginning, it is critical for you to be consistent in your approach to feeding your child. Children learn quickly how to get what they want. If you allow your child to have juice boxes and chips when he won't eat the family meal, he will "hold out" for those items.

Although it is extremely frustrating and worrisome when your child won't eat, most children eventually eat when they are hungry, especially if they know there is nothing more preferable coming before the next meal. A word of caution, however, some children with significant neurological involvement truly may not have the hunger sensation. Only a qualified feeding therapist and your physician(s) can determine this with your help. These children require a different therapeutic regimen and approach to mealtime.

Independent Feeding Skills

Although most children with a severe visual impairment learn to feed themselves as well as sighted children do through patience and gentle guidance, some children have difficulty learning the process. Certainly the inability to imitate others when they are eating contributes heavily to difficulties. Cognitively, children need to understand the process of taking objects from containers so that taking food from the plate follows naturally. Additionally, many children with visual impairments have not developed wrist control or sufficient supination of the forearm (turning the arm so that the palm of the hand faces up). Sighted children automatically develop these skills as they turn over toys to visually explore all surfaces. Finally, if your child is tactilely defensive, he may be less motivated to seek out and discriminate foods on his plate.

Scooping

Your child can begin building the motor skills he needs to manage utensils as he plays with toys requiring a variety of hand, wrist, and finger movements. Toys that make a funny sound when they are rotated (such as rain sticks) are excellent for building the action needed for scooping. Being able to bring his hand to his mouth, orally explore a toy he is holding, and maintain grasp while playing with a toy are fine motor precursors to feeding himself with a utensil. Working from behind your child rather than in front of him helps develop movements needed to scoop and bring the food to his mouth in a more natural way. First attempts with scooping are most successful with foods that tend to stick to the bowl of the spoon—for example, macaroni and cheese, oatmeal, and pudding.

To help your child learn to use a spoon, you can use a technique called *fading*. At first, allow your child as much support as he needs but quickly reduce (fade) the amount of assistance as he gains control. The best way to help your child learn the scooping action is to stabilize the handle of the spoon against his palm with your index finger (your right index finger if he is eating with his right hand). Your thumb should rest gently on top of your child's hand. With this approach, your child has more contact with the spoon, your hand is less distracting, and you can turn your child's hand as needed with minimal control.

Before guiding your child to scoop, allow him time to tactually explore his bowl or plate and to take his fingers to his mouth for a taste of what is to come. Securing the bowl to the surface with suction cups, Dycem™ or Rubbermaid™ rubber matting, or a vinyl placemat will eliminate the need for your child to chase his bowl as it slides away from him. Additionally, a plate with high sides, divided sections, and/or curved edges will provide boundaries that let your child know where to place his spoon and give him a stability point and cue as to when to lift his spoon.

Initially, guide your child hand over hand to approach the plate with the bowl of the spoon at a 90-degree angle (perpendicular with the plate) and firmly contact the surface. The feedback from the contact of the spoon with the plate cues him to rotate his hand and to scoop. This downward approach also tells his large muscles what they are supposed to do and provides a cue as to exactly where his plate is on the surface. Once your child understands this initial step, he can be guided to approach the bowl or plate from a more natural angle. As you guide him, make sure that the elbow of his feeding hand is angled away from his body and slightly higher than his hand as he brings the spoon toward his mouth. This motion helps your child hold the bowl of the spoon level to prevent food from slipping off.

As your child's arm and hand skills improve, encourage him to hold the spoon against his curved fingers with his thumb and with the palm of his hand facing toward him (the more conventional way). This position makes it easier to scoop and requires less arm motion and effort. Show your child how to use his other hand to check that the spoon is loaded. A transitional step that may help your child learn to scoop is for him to pick up appropriate foods with his fingers and place them on the spoon or the fork.

Locating Food on the Plate

To help your child learn what is on his plate and where to locate it, teach him to explore his plate with his nondominant hand (the one he does not use to hold utensils). Learning to use a fork when you can't see what you are spearing is tricky! Teach your child to use the fingers of his nondominant hand to locate and stabilize the food and serve as a reference point as to where to aim. Give him a small cracker, piece of roll, or bread to use as a guide when scooping. Your child can place the cracker on the plate, behind the food to be scooped and the spoon can be pushed against it. Many children are more willing to use their fingers during eating if a wet cloth or towel is immediately available for them to clean food from their fingers. When your child is older, you can teach him to look for foods based on the positions of a clock. For example, his peas are at two o'clock and his meat is at six o'clock.

Drinking from a Cup

When your child is learning to drink from a cup, always encourage him to search for and pick up his cup from the surface so that he knows where it comes from and the location in which to return it. One mother found that guiding her child at his forearm to firmly return the cup to the surface with a "bang" motivated him to independently position the cup in an upright position, as he was rewarded with the sensory information to his hand and he loved the sound it made.

Use small open cups rather than sippy cups so that your child will understand exactly how far he can tip the cup to control the liquid. Initially this will be a very messy process but will make the transition easier in the long run than moving from the bottle to a sippy cup. You may also want to make your own "nosey cup" by cutting a lip-sized half-circle from one of the edges of the cup. Your child drinks from the cup so that the cut-out space is on the side opposite his mouth. The cut-out space prevents the cup from covering your child's nose as he drinks and he may be more willing to try to do it himself.

To eliminate messy clean-up, purchase an inexpensive plastic film or drop cloth from a hardware store and place it under your child's chair. At first, fill his cup with only an ounce or so to encourage him to tilt the cup effectively without drowning in spillage! Your child may find drinking more motivating if you find a cup that plays music once empty or that activates music when lifted from the surface. A word of caution: as early as possible, offer your child a variety of cups, spoons, and forks to prevent him from becoming "stuck" on one particular cup that you may not be able to replace later on!

Once your child is proficient with drinking from a cup, teach him to pour his own liquids. Show him how to secure his cup with his thumb and fingers while placing his index finger inside his cup. As he pours, he will know when to stop when the liquid reaches the tip of his index finger. To begin with, use small containers with only an ounce or so of liquid. When there is less liquid in the container, your child will have to really rotate the container to bring the liquid to the surface. Gradually fill the container with more liquid as your child learns to perfect his pouring motion.

Selection and Design of Eating Utensils

Utensils that are designed for use by any child are often more appropriate than utensils designed especially for children with disabilities. Even musical plates and spoons/forks are commercially available. These can add to your child's motivation and help him locate his utensils. Remember, whenever possible, your child should use items that do not set him apart from other children his age. One utensil, however—the Steady Spoon® from Sammons—is an exception. The Steady Spoon's bowl stays level regardless of the angle or direction in which the child holds the spoon. In addition, the spoon can be Velcroed to the child's hand to help him hold the spoon, if necessary because of a physical disability. The one disadvantage of this spoon is that it does not do well with thickened or heavy foods that offer resistance. It works well, however, for cereal, oatmeal, pudding, and ice cream!

Creativity and ingenuity, as well as brainstorming, may be necessary to construct or modify utensils for your child's needs and still be aesthetically pleasing. The need for adapted eating utensils must be continually reevaluated. You should consider new eating utensils as your child grows and either becomes more independent or continues to need assistance of some nature. An occupational therapist can help modify utensils and help your child with any problems he might have holding them.

Mealtime Preparation

Even very young children should have experience helping in the kitchen. Being in the kitchen during mealtime preparation affords your child a myriad of sensory experiences. Supporting him in a highchair or a small box and allowing him to play with measuring spoons, plastic containers and lids, and even bits of food you are preparing, helps your child associate sounds, smells, and textures with relevant activities. Additionally, these experiences build language, memory, spatial, and motor skills and facilitate social interaction.

Helping with meal preparation can be both educational and enjoyable for your older preschooler. It gives him opportunities to make choices, assume responsibility, and interact with family and friends, and exposes him to many concepts, textures, and cognitive and motor experiences. For example, your child practices memory and classification skills as he recalls the location of the milk, the napkins, and the silverware. As he helps set the table, an older preschooler builds directionality and spatial orientation skills and learns about one-to-one correspondence (each family member gets one knife, one fork, one spoon). A younger child can fill glasses with ice from a container strategically placed to avoid a mess if a few cubes are dropped, or can help remove lids from the milk or plastic containers. Throwing away empty cans and boxes provides practice in orientation and mobility skills. "Guessing" what is being prepared or which food was in each empty container builds inferential reasoning abilities and promotes language development. Finally, helping in the preparation of the family meal may motivate your child to try different foods and to view mealtimes as a fun part of the day. Of course, you will want to spend some time "childproofing" your kitchen and watching your child carefully to make sure he is safe.

▪▪ Dressing

As with all aspects of daily living, your child should be an active participant in dressing as soon as possible. Many children with visual impairments tend to be passive learners and to wait for things to happen. Following your child's lead and permitting him to make choices reinforces that he has control over what happens to him. Always talk with him using short phrases about what is happening to cue him to anticipate, and, hopefully, initiate the next move! For instance, if you always dress and undress your baby in the same place (perhaps on a terrycloth changing pad), he can begin to anticipate that he will have his clothes changed. When children know what to expect, they are more cooperative with the process. Many infants become fearful when having items removed over their heads; this process may be even more frightening for a child with a visual impairment. If your child has postural insecurities because of his visual impairment and/or poor postural control, dressing can be not only scary but frustrating.

The first rule of dressing an infant or young child with a visual impairment is to ensure that he is physically stable. This may mean that you place or support your child in a variety of different postures for dressing and undressing, all governed by his postural control. For example, it may be easier to take a T-shirt off a small child who has minimal trunk control by laying him on his belly over your lap with his arms extended. A child who doesn't have good trunk or standing balance can lie on his back to pull on his pants. Have him bend his knees so that his feet are flat on the surface and then push his bottom up to pull his pants over his hips. There's no right or wrong way; only what works for your child to be as independent as possible.

Instructional Strategies for Dressing

You can lay the groundwork for teaching your child to dress or undress himself when he is quite young by consistently naming clothing items and relating them to body parts as you engage him in participating. Body parts are more likely to have meaning if they are connected to a functional activity. For example, better to encourage him to: "Give Daddy your foot; pull on your shoe" than to rehearse out of context: "Show me your foot."

One way to teach clothing labels is to be consistent in the order that you take off and put on clothing. Consistency will also help your child learn to anticipate and assist with the next step. Even a toddler can begin to help by lifting his bottom during a diaper change if he knows what is coming next. To help your child anticipate actions, always give him a cue by tugging gently on the clothing article prior to its removal and then pause to see whether your child will lift his arms or hold out his foot.

Once your child has the motor skills to begin learning to take off or put on clothing articles on his own, there are several points to keep in mind. First, be sure that he has a stable sitting base, either on the floor or on a sturdy chair, low to the floor, and with support to the back or sides. Second, dress and undress your child from in front of him. Although dressing him from behind may teach him more normal movements, he may feel more secure with you in front of him and you will be better able to communicate with him.

There is no one best procedure or order for what to teach when. Removing unlaced or opened shoes and socks from the tips of his toes are often the first skills mastered. Some children more readily learn how to pull down their underpants by grasping the leg openings and pulling. As long as you are there to encourage, allow your child to do as much as he can without becoming stressed. Sometimes a child learns more easily from mistakes than from your explanation. For example, at one time or another, your child may accidentally put both legs in one pant leg. Once he realizes he can't move, he will pull one leg out of the pants opening and direct it to the opposite leg opening.

Regardless of what you teach first, be sure that your child's efforts are rewarded with success. To ensure success in removing socks, be sure they fit very loosely and have stretchy cuffs. Cross your child's leg over his other leg to bring the foot closer to his hands. First, let your child simply pull his sock from his toes once you have pulled it over his heel. Gradually increase the number of steps your child must do. When he is ready, show him how to hook his thumb into the cuff of his sock to pull it off. Similarly, when you are teaching him to remove a pull-off shirt, begin with the last step first. Once the shirt is over his face, have him pull it the remaining way. Later, teach your child to grab the back of his shirt near his shoulders and pull it over his head.

Watch your child for preferences in getting dressed and undressed. For example, it is easier for some blind children to first push their arms into the shirt sleeves of a pull-over shirt, raise them, and then tug the shirt over the head. Be patient and systematic. A word of advice to working mothers and fathers: Teaching your child to dress and undress is best done at bedtime, when the pressures of time do not exist! If you are in a hurry, it is better to help your child than to frustrate him and risk confusion and error.

Dressing: Clothing Selection

Clothing selection involves two phases: 1) selecting and purchasing appropriate clothing for your child to wear, and 2) choosing (or asking your child to make choices when he is able) appropriate clothing to wear on any given day.

Clearly, if your child is to succeed in choosing clothing to wear, his wardrobe must first be stocked with clothes that he can match himself and easily put on and take off. When buying clothing for your child, consider his age, level of vision, tactile and motor skills, as well as your family's and child's preferences. In general, however, there are several considerations to keep in mind. For young children just beginning to dress and undress themselves, and for children with poor motor control, buy clothing that fits loosely but still looks appropriate. The looser the clothing, the easier and less stressful it will be for you and your child to pull it on, up, and over. In particular, the neck openings should always be sufficiently loose or flexible to allow your child's head through easily and smoothly. If a tight shirt becomes "stuck" while you are pulling it over your child's face, he may become fearful and protest about all pull-over shirts in the future.

Clothing with Velcro closures or magnetic snaps may be a good choice at first, since they are easier than zippers or buttons for young children. But remember that you want your child to be able to wear all types of clothes, so buttons and zippers will eventually be important to learn about.

Clothing in the bright fluorescent colors so popular among children today can be a good choice for children with some vision because they can more easily distinguish the clothing item from its surroundings. It is also easier for children to distinguish their clothing from other family members' if it is brightly colored, especially when made with puffy, shiny, or sequined textures. When teaching fronts and backs of clothing, a textured item on the front of the shirt can be a natural cue as to what is front and back. Most preschoolers are capable of feeling for tags in clothing and know they typically signal the back of the item. However, if a label irritates your child, removing it will prevent protests and refusals to wear an otherwise good shirt or pair of pants.

When your child is ready to match his own clothing, there are several strategies you can try. Buying clothing items that he can discriminate by touch, such as clothing decorated with puff or slick paints (available at most craft stores), rhinestones, critters, or other textures is one strategy. You can then teach your child that the shirt with the bugs matches his long, soft pants. You can also buy clothing in colors or patterns that can be mixed and matched so your child can put together an outfit acceptable to the most conservative person. For instance, you might want to buy pants only in solid colors so they will not clash with any patterned shirt he might choose.

When your child is ready to take his shoes off and on, look for those that fasten with a zipper or Velcro or else substitute brightly colored, fluorescent shoelaces for the more typical cotton laces to encourage use of vision as well as independence. One helpful technique for children with low vision who are beginning to lace their own shoes is to coat one half of the shoelace with one color of puff paint or fluorescent, colored glue and the other half with a different color. Using matching colors of paint to encircle the shoe eyelets will help your child discriminate the eyelet and to correctly lace his shoes by matching the lace to the same colored eyelet. If your child has no vision, try using a slick paint on one side and a textured paint on the other instead of different colors. Elastic shoelaces may also be used so the shoes can be simply pulled on and off.

Presenting a Neat Appearance

It will be just as important, if not more so, for your child to have clothes that match, zippers zipped, and tags tucked in as it is for any child. However, your child may not realize this on his own because he cannot see that other people have clothes that match, zippers that are

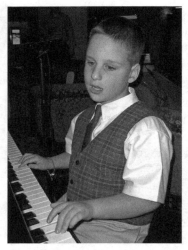

zipped, and tags that are tucked in. The best way to teach your child about the importance of these things is to mention them to him over and over as you work with him on daily routines and offer him choices.

Don't hesitate to use color names with your child. As with any child, associating a color with a specific piece of clothing is just another way of describing the item and your child will encounter color words in the natural environment. Some children with visual impairments want to know about colors and can learn that reds are "warm" colors and blues are "cool" colors, etc. Children learn to make their own associations from experiences and good memories. One child told me yellow was "bright like the sun" and green was "slimy like her pet frog!"

Your child will hear others talk about color and, in some situations, identifying his things by color may come in handy such as when someone naturally asks "whose swimsuit is the black one with zig zags?" When you are helping him dress in the morning, you might say, "You chose to wear your blue shorts today with the cool zippers on the pockets. Do you want to wear the blue striped shirt or the tan shirt with the zipper?"

Letting your child help as you pack a small suitcase with clothes for an overnight stay at grandmother's house can be a fun time to talk about matching clothes and to do some problem solving about the types of clothes he may need while there. Letting your child organize clothing and hygiene items in the suitcase also encourages spatial planning and problem solving. Your child will benefit from multiple opportunities to learn to plan what, when, why, and where to choose specific clothing items and to pull them on and off efficiently.

:: Grooming and Hygiene

Bath Time

Some children with visual impairments are initially afraid to sit inside the tub. If your child is afraid of the "unknown," it may help to allow him to sit on the side of the tub with just his feet inside or to sit next to the tub and splash or play with toys in the bath water. Slowly and gently, but firmly, you should encourage him to put more of his body in the water. Depending on your child, this process may take one bath time, or it may take weeks or months. Simply providing him with a secure surrounding may also help eliminate his fear of the "wide open spaces" of the bathtub. An infant can be eased into the tub in a plastic infant seat. A toddler can be "grounded" in any of the bath frames commercially available. For a larger toddler or a preschooler, plastic laundry baskets are an inexpensive solution for holding the child while he plays in the tub. Another strategy is to let your toddler participate in bathing a favorite doll or stuffed animal or choosing which toy he will play with in the tub today.

To make the tub a safe environment, consider using one of the many different faucet covers, especially if your child likes to "swim" in the bathtub. These covers, which are available in a variety of shapes, colors, and themes, help protect little heads from being scraped during play and the child from being burned. (Eventually you will point out that hot and cold are controlled by different knobs or come from different faucets.) You may also want to use adhesive stickers on the bottom of the tub to prevent slipping. If you use bar soap, be sure to select a brightly colored bar or one that contrasts well with the surrounding tile and surface areas in the bathroom. You may also want to purchase the commercially available cloth pockets that contain bars of soap. The child just applies the cloth directly to his hands or body and doesn't have to worry about it slipping from his hand.

Most children love bath time, so it is a natural time to foster independence and teach a variety of skills. Encouraging your child to splash, reach or search for toys in the water, and play with cause and effect water toys or an empty squirt bottle builds motor, cognitive, and tactile integration abilities. Letting your child wear a sponge or terry cloth bath mitt in the shape of an animal or favorite character is an enticing way to get him to cooperate with bathing. Talking to your child about body parts he is "washing" is a natural way to increase body awareness and function: "John, you are washing your feet; they help you run." Gently trickling water over your child's head with a strainer or a sprinkling water toy or guiding him to do the same will help prepare him for having his hair washed and rinsed. Purchase towels with appliqués of your child's favorite animals or cartoon figures or with a brightly colored pattern or stripe if he has some vision so that he can locate his own. Consider sewing a pocket onto your child's towel in which he can store his washcloth or bath mitt.

Brushing Teeth

While many children with visual impairments enjoy the sensation of having their teeth brushed, just as many find it an unpleasant activity. In particular, children who are sensitive to other types of touch are extremely hypersensitive to brushing their teeth. Often, however, these children will accept deep pressure inside their mouths. Consequently, they may not mind having their teeth "brushed" with a warm washcloth rubbed over their gums and teeth. Gradually, they may tolerate the firm rubber surface of a Nuk™ or Sassy™ toothbrush. Next, you can try a small finger brush placed on your finger. Simply using an electric or battery operated toothbrush may also persuade your child to cooperate, especially if you get one in the shape of your child's favorite character or other preferred items such as robots, racecars, and rockets. Some children more readily accept brushing their teeth in conjunction with a song (e.g., "This is the way we brush our teeth," etc.).

As soon as your child can accept the different textures inside his mouth, encourage him to hold the brush on his own. To entice your child to brush his teeth on his own, you might try a toothbrush with a musical handle. Older children can be motivated to brush their teeth with toothbrush bases with popular characters who say familiar phrases and encourage the child to brush while they talk. Reach™ toothbrush company makes a toothbrush that glows in the dark, which can be a great source of motivation for both brushing teeth and using residual vision.

As with other self-care skills, you may want to help your child initiate the process by first guiding him hand over hand and then moving your support back to his elbow. Even if your child only holds the brush a few seconds and then drops it, he has succeeded. Simply pick up the brush and calmly state, "My turn," and brush his teeth for a few seconds before returning it, verbalizing, "Your turn." Making a game will encourage cooperation and the phrase will signal him that you expect him to try again.

As your child becomes more capable, help him learn to place the toothpaste on his brush. Letting him help select his own toothpaste is the first step in the process. A flavored toothpaste may make him more eager to brush. Be sure your child has the motor abilities to handle the applicator he selects. Many pump-type dispensers are too complicated for a young child to manipulate with one hand. The flip top lids on many toothpaste tubes eliminate the need for more refined motor skills and the search for a lost cap. Show your child how to extend his index finger, third finger, or thumb on the bristles so he can tell where to place the toothpaste and know when he has applied enough paste.

Toilet Training

Toilet training can be another area of difficulty for children with visual impairments. Still, how you go about training your child will be very similar to toilet training any child. Signs of readiness for toilet training are the same for children with visual impairments as they are for other children:

- Your child is aware of being wet or soiled.
- He perceives an urge to go and signals that in some way.
- He follows simple directions.
- He stays dry throughout a nap or waits at least one and a half hours between elimination times.
- He sits (even with support) in a chair for five minutes.

Once your toddler seems ready, you can begin by reading one or more of the many good children's story books designed to prepare a child for toilet training. In addition, give your child repeated supervised opportunities to explore all components of the toilet, including flushing, and the toileting process. Your child will need to understand what that splashing in the toilet is all about.

In their book, *Steps to Independence: A Skills Training Guide for Parents and Teachers of Children with Special Needs,* Bruce Baker and Alan Brightman and their co-authors have proposed a very functional and systematic approach to toilet training. While many steps are involved in teaching your child to use the toilet, these authors suggest that your initial goal is simply to get him to eliminate on the toilet. Your first task is to define the range of time when your child is most likely to wet or soil his pants. Baker and Brightman recommend starting the toileting process only after you have two weeks of data and specify the following steps to take during these two weeks:

1. Check your child when he first gets up the morning and note whether he is wet or soiled.

2. Check him again one hour later and continue to check him every hour until bedtime.
3. Each time, record whether he is dry, has urinated, or has had a bowel movement.
4. Change him when he is soiled when you check him.

Some children are more readily bowel than bladder trained, as bowel movements tend to occur more regularly. Once you can tell the general time range when your child is most likely to void or defecate, take him to the bathroom approximately fifteen minutes prior to the usual elimination time. Repeat the process for each timeframe you have noted that he is wet or soiled, depending on the schedule noted for either urinating or having a bowel movement. Baker and Brightman suggest sticking tightly to your schedule, using the same phrases, always training your child in the bathroom, removing distracting toys and people, and refraining from irrelevant talk (e.g., songs, rhymes, talk about what the dog is doing, etc.). Some experts suggest having the child wear regular underwear once he remains dry for a period of two hours so that he can readily distinguish when he is wet.

It is very important that your child feel safe and secure during early toilet training. A small potty chair may ensure that he has a stable base of support and will not cause any gravitational insecurities as the large toilet might. Some professionals, however, propose sitting him on the regular toilet from the beginning to avoid difficulties later when transitioning from the small to the regular toilet. You can purchase child adaptations for the regular toilet in most discount or large toy stores. Regardless of your choice, your child's feet must always be supported so that he has a stable base.

Let your child sit on the potty while Mom and Dad carry out grooming routines in the bathroom so he can become accustomed to his potty. Later, gently encourage him to sit, even for a few seconds, at regular intervals throughout the day, and then reward him with hugs and praise for at least trying. You may want to help your child understand that there is an end to the process by setting a timer to go off after several minutes, after which you let him get up, regardless of success, and reward him with hugs for sitting and trying.

Your little boy should be shown how to raise the lid against the back of the toilet and to hang onto it or to the outside of the toilet base to center himself since he may not be able to see where to aim. Or you may want to show your son how to position his knees on either side of the narrow front of the toilet (if sufficiently narrow) and lean forward, placing his hands on the wall behind the toilet (Simmons, 1993). He will quickly understand that his aim is not accurate if he is not rewarded with the sound cue of urine splashing in the toilet bowl. Provide a small stepping stool or bench to ensure that he is able to urinate into the bowl.

Some children benefit from singing a "transition" song about toileting as they move toward the bathroom which alerts and helps him anticipate the activity. Other children enjoy "training" a favorite doll or stuffed animal. Often the best method is simply to be consistent in offering encouragement and opportunities without pressure over time. If your child is successful, let him help dispose of the waste and flush the toilet, if he seems to enjoy it. Even if your child has already had an accident, take him to the bathroom to sit or stand briefly and to change his clothes to reinforce where this process should take place.

During the toilet training process, dress your child in loosely fitting clothing that he can manage with very little help to encourage him to do as much as possible for himself during this time. Make sure that the toilet paper is always in the same place and use the same techniques for tearing the appropriate amount and placing in the toilet each time your child goes to the bathroom.

One word of caution: never leave your child on the potty for longer than five or ten minutes and always supervise him in the beginning. He needs to know that you are there to support him. Also, if left with too much idle time, your child may engage in eye-poking or other types of "mannerisms." (See below.)

Bedtime Routines

Many children with significant visual impairments have sleep difficulties due to confusion between day and night. There are several theories as to why this might be. Some children may have no light-dark contrast to signal time of day. Other children may be passive the majority of the day and may not be tired and ready for sleep at bedtime. They stay awake most of the evening and then sleep during the day to compensate for lack of sleep. At night, they are not tired and the cycle repeats itself.

The most practical solution to sleep pattern difficulties is to establish a consistent daily routine. An essential part of this routine is to keep your child active during the day. It is also helpful to develop an evening bedtime routine and stick to it, regardless of the setting. There will always be times when your child sleeps away from home such as when he is at the babysitter's, in hotels or motels, in the hospital, and at relatives' homes. Thus, the actual activities and physical actions included in your child's routine are more important than the bed or room. Your child's nighttime routine will necessarily vary as he grows older, to match his chronological as well as developmental needs. When your child is an infant, simply rocking and singing a specific song, sung at no other time except when putting him down for the evening (for the first or last time!), may be all that is needed.

As your child grows older, you can allow him to sleep with a stuffed animal which plays a brief song. Some toys are specifically

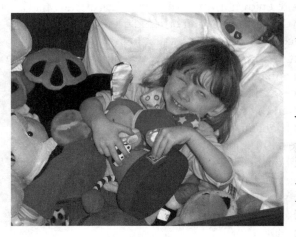

designed with a light that dims gradually, which your child may enjoy if he has some vision. Older children often enjoy a favorite nighttime poem, story, or phrase. One child loved Dr. Seuss's *One Fish, Two Fish, Red Fish, Blue Fish.* When his mother began to read the last page, which began "Today is done; today was fun," he would turn over and hug his pillow, ready to settle for the night as Mom finished the story. To cue him that it was bedtime in other settings, Mom simply recited "Today is done..." and that was sufficient to signal bedtime.

When your child balks at going to bed, even after his routine, it is critical that both parents react the same way to ensure that your child remains in bed, or at least in his room. Make sure that toys or other items that might invite play are not available.

When your child becomes sleepy during the day and wants to rest because he did not get enough sleep the previous night, try not to let him to do so. If sleep is allowed, do not permit more than ten to fifteen minutes of rest within a two-hour framework. Walking your child, playing with him, or offering a healthy snack may distract him. Coping with a cranky, miserable, screaming child is a very difficult task. It will, however, be well worth the misery and effort to ensure a peaceful night of sleep in the long run. While some children have a will of iron, most get the message within at least one to two weeks.

One clever mother initiated her own plan of attack when her deaf-blind youngster refused to sleep at night, playing into the early morning hours. When he began to curl up on his favorite chair in the middle of the day, his mother commented on his need for sleep. She led him into his room to change into his pajamas, then into the bathroom to brush his teeth, the same sequence followed prior to putting him to bed for the evening. Brushing teeth was definitely a nonpreferred activity for this youngster, and subsequently, a natural negative reinforcer. He quickly learned that sleeping in the daytime was not worth the work or aggravation of having his clothes changed and teeth brushed. After being awake all day, he was too tired to play at bedtime and began to sleep most of the evening. Over a two-week period, his sleep patterns became more appropriate.

∷ Household Responsibilities

Your child with a visual impairment can and should reap the same benefits from doing chores as any other child. He can gain self-esteem from being a useful, participating member of the family, build cognitive, motor, and sensory skills, and become increasingly independent. By pitching in and doing his share, he can also contribute to family harmony. After all, if he is excused from chores and his siblings are not, there are bound to be cries of "That's not fair!"

A good place to start with any child is to give him responsibility for his own items and room. For example, he can take his dirty clothes to the laundry hamper. He can also help identify and put away his own laundry by searching for specific sizes or for easily identifiable features such as puffy paint textures, loops on pants, metal clips on the end of suspenders on painter's pants, or bows or lace on socks. To provide cues as to where clothing items belong, you might stick a sample of that clothing on the outside of a drawer (for example, put a small piece of denim on his jeans drawer). You could also suspend one sample of an item from the shelf above the place where similar items should be hung in the closet.

As your child grows older, you should expect him to participate in household chores with the same expectations as you have for your other children. For example, filling the dog's water dish, pouring dry pet food, transferring silverware from the dishwasher to the utensil drawer, emptying his own trash can, or taking dirty dishes to the sink are all activities that may be suitable for a preschooler. Provide a specific basket or container for toys in each room in which your child plays so

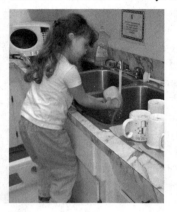

that he learns where to return and find toys, building memory and classification as well as spatial understanding and orientation and mobility skills.

Recycling is a great activity for involving your child in both home and community responsibilities, and an excellent means for teaching and reinforcing concepts, motor skills, tactile skills, and classification. Having your child help separate paper, cans, bottles, and glass into the appropriate containers offers opportunities to reinforce memory skills, discrimination, and concepts such as heavy, light, smooth, rough, big, little, empty, full, in, out, over, beside, right, left, etc. Auditory localization skills (being able to listen to something and locate it) can be integrated with classification as your child sorts plastic, glass, and aluminum containers.

With practice, you will learn how to take advantage of readily available and natural situations to enhance your child's development. In time, helping your child develop sensory, motor, and social skills will become spontaneous and routine. You may also wish to refer to a curriculum called *Preschool Attainment Through Typical Everyday Routines (Patter),* which was designed for preschool children with visual impairments. It focuses on building critical thinking, language, independence, and motor skills through involving children in typical household activities, including doing the wash, setting the table, and washing the family car. You will find *Patter* listed in the Reading List under Lewis.

▪▪ Do's and Don'ts of Daily Care

The suggestions about daily care in the sections above are intended to be just that—suggestions. The way that you deal with daily care routines will depend largely on your own family's schedule, routine, and priorities. Below are some general strategies that may help you in figuring out how best to manage daily care routines.

- *Be patient and persistent.* Sometimes you may feel as if teaching your child to feed himself, dress himself, etc. is too difficult. He won't achieve independence in self-care, however, unless you insist that he try.

- *Feel free to get advice from friends, relatives, and professionals.* However, you also need to learn to trust yourself and your instincts since you will be the major influence on your child's success in learning self-care routines.

- *Talk to your child about what you are doing whenever you are working on daily care routines.* When he is very young, you might say, "Let's take off your T-shirt now." As he gets older, this becomes, "It's time to take off your T-shirt. Why don't you help me by holding up your arms?" Still later, you might say, "Go ahead and take off that dirty T-shirt. Let me know if you need help."

- *Don't assume that your child can't do something just because you don't think you could do it if you had a visual impairment.* Go ahead and try difficult tasks; your child will probably surprise you.

- *Don't be too quick to rescue your child in difficult situations.* Working through the situation will probably help him become a better problem solver. When he does need help, try to provide the least amount of assistance possible; for instance, start him out, but let him finish the task. Look for naturally reinforcing times for him to be independent. If your child loves to swim, require that he take off his own shoes or shirt before he can get into the water.

- *Make sure that your child has success with some aspect of every task.* Provide lots of hugs and praise for the tasks he does accomplish.

- *Anticipate potential accidents, and, when possible, teach your child how to address them.* For example, every child will eventually knock over a glass of milk. Show your child how to gently scan his place to know where things are. If he spills, use this opportunity to help him remedy the situation, get a paper towel, wipe the area, and request more drink, etc.

▪▪ Behavior Management

Some parents are reluctant to discipline their child who is visually impaired. They may feel that the vision loss is to blame for their child's misbehavior or fear what others will say about being too hard on a young child with disabilities. However, your child needs to be held to the same behavior standards as any child. Failing to discipline him may mean that he will grow up without rules or limits and that he may consequently be unpleasant to be around.

Consistency is the key to behavior management with all children. Make sure that your child knows the rules, as well as the rewards for following the rules and the consequences for not following them. The same techniques for disciplining any child should work with your child. Make sure, however, that the rewards you use are truly reinforcing to your child. For example, stars or smiley faces on a chart may be meaningless to your child if he can't see them, but he may find "scratch and sniff" stickers quite rewarding. The American Printing House for the Blind produces tactile stickers (including smiley faces and words like "wow" and "super") that can be used to reward positive behavior or hard work.

Remember that your child may miss many of the social cues other children perceive since he cannot see. He may therefore need more specific clarification and guidance to understand why he is not permitted to behave a certain way. However, when he is a toddler, he may not have sufficient language to understand danger and safety issues. You will have to guide him through experiences that help him understand about safety and social rules. Use very simple language to explain why he can't reach into the drawer and play with knives, or hold him at the curb to "listen" for the cars and reinforce that he must "wait." The lack of vision will interfere with his ability to integrate information about danger from simply being told about cars and busy streets. If your child throws toys, he should be led to touch the injured child and the same toy should be gently touched to his own leg or shoulder to help him understand he hurt a friend and that toys belong either in his hands or the toy box.

Always direct your child toward positive behavior so that he understands what to do rather than confuse him with what he shouldn't do. Saying, "we touch our friend gently" or "finished toys go in the box" is better than stating "don't hit" or "don't throw." When you tell your child what to do, he has information about what is expected.

Mannerisms

Mannerisms, sometimes called blindisms, are behaviors parents are often concerned about and interested in changing. Mannerisms consist of repetitive, seemingly purposeless, body movements. Mannerisms often seen in children with severe visual impairment include head weaving, flicking fingers before the eyes, flipping objects against the fingers, rocking, flapping the arms in space, light-gazing, and eye poking or rubbing. Although not considered a mannerism, the characteristic head drop associated with severely limited vision can be just as frustrating for parents.

There are a number of reasons mannerisms should be discouraged or prevented. Most obviously is that these behaviors are not socially acceptable. Mannerisms may make your child appear even more different from typical children. The more mannerisms your child has or the more frequently he engages in them, the less he can interact with and learn from his environment. This translates into decreased attention to what is going on around him and fewer meaningful experiences. Another reason for preventing mannerisms is the physical damage that behaviors such as eye rubbing or poking can cause.

The degree, frequency, and intensity of mannerisms are often influenced by stress, cognitive abilities, cause of the visual impairment, and amount of residual vision. Mannerisms are more common in children who are under stress, who cannot make sense of incoming sensory information, and in children with mental retardation. Mannerisms in general may be more common in children who are passive and who enjoy little physical activity.

Understanding why a child engages in a mannerism is critical so that both the origin of the behavior and the behavior itself may be addressed. Researchers Gordon Williamson, Marie Anzalone, and Barbara Hanft explain that these types of behaviors serve different functions, based on the child's current sensory threshold. For example, they note that a child who is easily over-aroused may use hand-flapping to help focus and screen out confusing visual information. Another child may hand flap to release tension. These authors encourage teachers and parents to analyze the underlying cause of a child's particular mannerism or ritual and respond accordingly to help him adapt more appropriately.

Some mannerisms may evolve out of a need for vestibular, proprioceptive, or visual input. For example, eye poking is most prevalent among children with retinal disorders. The poking creates phosphenes, chemically triggered constellations of light, which provide some form of visual sensation even for blind children. Other children who eye-poke enjoy the pressure and proprioceptive feedback they receive from doing so.

Often, simply providing your child consistent verbal feedback at the first hint of the behavior may help reduce it. A simple verbal cue such as "You are flapping" or "You are head weaving" may help your child realize what he is doing. If an occasional mannerism surfaces when your child is particularly stressed or excited, a gentle touch cue may be all that is necessary to redirect him. (After all, we all engage in some "mannerism" such as chewing pencils, clicking retractable pens, or twirling hair at various times in our lives!) Sometimes, calling too much attention to the behavior only strengthens it, particularly in very willful children. If your child tends to eye-poke, you might consider getting nonprescription lenses for him to wear for a short time while he learns to pay attention to this behavior. The glasses may make it more difficult for him to engage in the behavior and serve as a reminder to keep his hands away from his eyes.

Physical therapy designed to strengthen the neck and back muscles can help to minimize head drop and mannerisms such as head weaving and rocking that are vestibular based. You can learn to incorporate the specific techniques used by the physical therapist in everyday handling and play routines.

Another strategy that may reduce the frequency and intensity of mannerisms is to figure out what sensory information (visual, vestibular, proprioceptive) your child craves. Then, offer him this sensory information through alternative, more acceptable means. For example, a child who likes to rock or spin may enjoy opportunities to swing, spin in tire swings, rock on equipment designed for that purpose, or play on Sit N' Spins™. Giving your child toys, especially manipulatives, that provide him with the same type of sensory input as his mannerism does is often a good solution. For example, textured wrist bands, "funky" textured jewelry, and wrist-worn video game watches can be effective in reducing inappropriate movements of fingers and hands.

Even children with no useful vision may enjoy the noises made by hand-held video games or watches. Other toys that can provide socially acceptable alternatives to mannerisms include small party favors such as "crickets" or holiday noisemakers that are intended to be "flicked" and plastic toys designed to be twisted into various shapes or knocked together. When giving your child one of these alternatives, quietly point out the mannerism, as described above, and suggest that, alternatively, he play with the toy.

As your child becomes older and social acceptance is more important to him, he will probably begin to control his mannerisms on his own. Research also suggests that as your child's ability to interact with his environment improves, he will rely less on stereotypical behaviors or routines. If not, your child's TVI, orientation and mobility instructor, or occupational therapist can help devise a plan for addressing the behaviors and their underlying cause.

∷ Your Child in the Community

Daily life does not just go on in the home: your family and your child also have a life in the community. It will be very important for your child to accompany you on trips to the grocery store and to the post office as well as to the playground, zoo, and on walks around the block or through the woods. To an adult, a trip to the grocery store or the dry cleaner's is just another errand to complete as quickly as possible. To your child, however, that same chore is a wonderful opportunity to exercise his independence and learn about the world around him.

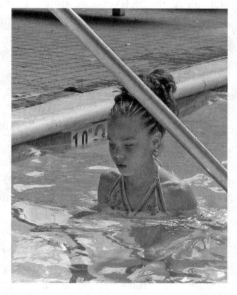

Your child needs to experience active participation in the community and to enjoy and learn from community activities as does any other child. Unlike other children, however, your child will be more reliant on you to bring aspects of the community to him and to help him explore features other children can perceive through their sight. Initially, it may be overwhelming to try to teach him all the things other children learn incidentally through watching. You will quickly learn to take advantage of a few learning opportunities at a time based on what you know about your child and his readiness to absorb information.

If you think about the routine things you do, you will realize the myriad of opportunities you have to reinforce many of the same concepts across settings. You want to expose your child, but not overload him with more than he can handle. Pick a few things to emphasize each time you do a particular activity and review and reinforce one or two things from previous visits. Think about or simply watch what other children your child's age are doing with their parents while in the same situation. Let your child participate as much as he can. For example, below are some ideas for turning a visit to the grocery store into a learning experience:

Hand your toddler a frozen juice can or vegetable bag or box and simply say, "Juice is cold!" Or give him a peach or banana and comment, "Peach is fuzzy; mmm, smells good, etc." The older mobile child can help pull a can of fruit or a box of macaroni and cheese from the shelf and put it in the basket. Simply allowing your child to reach into the refrigerated section at the grocery store and lift out the milk or pull his choice of cereal from the shelf tells your child (and the observing public) that he is just as capable as any child. Letting your child decide which of two frozen vegetables or which flavor of ice cream to buy tells him that you value his judgment. It also offers him the opportunity to have some control over the situation.

The grocery store also provides numerous opportunities to teach and reinforce concepts critical to mobility and orientation, as well as pre-braille, and other preschool learning activities. Involving your child in selecting and handling grocery items helps with motor skill development, language acquisition, classification and reasoning skills, math, and concept development.

You can teach concepts by asking your child to reach up, find something on the bottom shelf, select the bigger bottle or the smaller box, use two hands to carry the milk, get "one more" apple, and by commenting that an item is "cold" or "heavy." Your child's classification abilities are enhanced as he builds a repertoire of associations with specific smells and temperatures when he passes through the household cleaning aids, pet foods, seafood, florist, bakery, and frozen food sections at the grocery store. At the checkout counter, you can further encourage your child to classify by asking for his help in putting all the cans on the conveyor belt, or all the boxed items, all the cold items, all the beverages, all the fruits, or all the vegetables.

Be sure to let him help put away items once at home so he can learn that some things are kept in the refrigerator while others are kept in the pantry. Let your child help open the box, peel the banana, or slice the peach so that the experience comes full cycle.

Whenever you are in the community with your child, call attention to important sounds, smells, or textures or other tactile inputs (wind) that help define a context. Leaving a store, you may comment "Ooh! Feel the cool breeze? It feels good to be outside!" Entering a tire store, you can draw your child's attention to the smell of the rubber and let him feel the tires, etc. At the post office, let him hand the letters or package to the clerk, put money in the stamp machine and retrieve the stamps, open the mailbox and drop in the letters, etc.

Family life may also entail accompanying Mom and Dad to older siblings' sports or dance activities. Let your child help you gather several items that are associated with the sibling's specific activity, such as a soccer ball, old ballet slippers, an old rosin bag, a whistle, a hat or feathers from an old ballet skirt, etc. Pack these items in a backpack that accompanies your child when he attends siblings' practice times or activities. The objects help him understand what is happening far away; gives him something to do and to talk about; and provides an opportunity to build vocabulary, memory, and a means of sharing his siblings' experiences with others. Over time, your child will anticipate where you are going and what happens there and will initiate helping or asking to help with tasks associated with where you are going. You will not only be teaching your child, you will also be demonstrating for others your child's capabilities and modeling expectations!

As a parent, you do not have much control over how community members react to your child. You do have control over how you deal with others' reactions and how you teach your child to deal with them. In fact, how you choose to react to the attitudes and reactions of others will determine the extent and opportunities for acceptance and integration into the community. Additionally, parents are typically the first and only individuals in whom children have total trust for quite a while. Therefore, you are in the best position to help him understand how to behave in the community.

Handling Questions, Comments, and Stares

Almost everyone's attention is attracted to the unusual. Without realizing what we are doing, we focus on differences out of curiosity.

Then, just as quickly, we decide how to react to the novel information. Children of all ages are naturally curious about a child who is different. Many factors influence how a nondisabled child reacts to a child with a disability. These include the chronological age of the child and how much previous experience he has had with children with disabilities. Reactions from children range from a child who watches intently but without judgment to a child who forthrightly asks, "Can he see?" to a child who is so totally overwhelmed that he sees only the disability and none of the child. It is also not unusual to see parents of the sighted child cringe in embarrassment or even become angry with their child if he asks about your child or points and stares.

If you can respond to all of these situations in the most positive way possible, you can demonstrate appropriate ways to interact with your child and promote acceptance and understanding. The most important lessons you can teach are that your child is competent and independent; the vision problem just happens to create a need for doing things a different way. Respond positively to these opportunities for education based on a quick analysis of how much information you think the questioning individual will appreciate.

People who ask direct questions are generally truly interested in your child and want to know the most appropriate way to interact. For example, a Sunday School teacher who asks if your child can see bright colors may actually be asking the question in order to determine how to best plan your child's involvement in next week's lesson. You might say, "Yes, he can see some bright colors and he sees them best when there is lots of light in the room." People who give the impression that they are awed by your child and have no means of establishing contact simply need an example to sensitize them to your child's needs and competence. Cueing your child to say hello, extend his hand, or help with some simple task such as taking groceries from the cart or holding the door open demonstrates that your child is competent and can be expected to behave and respond as other children his age. My favorite approach to young children is to move to their level and compliment them on their perceptiveness, stating, "You are so clever to notice that Eric can't see." "I bet you figured that out because he held my arm as we walk."

Occasionally, you will run into people who are truly embarrassed or say things that are really hurtful. These people need more education than you can provide in a brief encounter. Your main concern is your child. The best thing to do is define your child's response or behavior that attracted the attention and calmly and briefly inform the individual, "Eric is blind. He touched your arm because he was searching for me. I hope he didn't startle you." If capable, your child might offer a simple explanation about his visual impairment or why he uses specific compensations, such as "Excuse me, since I can't see, my fingers help me know what is on my plate."

Trying to change attitudes may be one of the more difficult jobs you will undertake. Among your goals are to help people be realistic and open-minded and to change harmful stereotypes. You may have the experience of having someone offer to "heal" your child while you stand in line at a restaurant as I have (as well as in churches other than ours, on playgrounds, and even at the dollar store!). These well-meaning people need to be assured that everything possible is being done for your child and that "healing" takes many forms. For example, let them know that your child is learning important adaptive skills that will enable him to be independent and productive. You should feel comfortable expressing your wishes relative to the offer for healing. Some people may not take your "hint." Eric and I were in a dollar store one day when I politely declined an offer from a gentleman to heal Eric then and there. I turned my attention to a set of party favors when suddenly this gentleman began to chant and raise his arms and voice "in prayer." I quickly extended my arm to Eric and we fled the store!

Feel free to share your experiences and frustration with your child's teacher of students with visual impairments and with sympathetic family and friends. You will receive not only support but useful suggestions for handling embarrassing or uncomfortable situations in the future. Generally, you should openly and frankly model how you want others to address and interact with your child. The key is to encourage his independence and competence in everything you do or say. By showing others your standards and expectations, you are providing the most direct avenue for integration and acceptance. In addition, you are modeling for your child ways to respond to a variety of people, situations, and contexts. As he grows, you will want to show him how to refuse help politely and to express his independence assertively.

Social Acceptance

To dispel the general public's notion that being blind "must be awful!" your child will need to demonstrate his competence in all situations. When others perceive your child as competent, they will also interact with him as they would any other child, which will further motivate your child to take risks and, eventually to be his own best advocate.

Regardless of your child's age or abilities, the one variable that most obviously affects how others perceive him is his behavior. A ten-year-old child who is allowed to rock and bounce an eggplant in a vegetable basket during church is perceived as a severely limited child even though he may be quite capable of reasoning and decision making. In contrast, a child who participates appropriately in church activities such as making an offering or shaking hands is perceived as being alert and competent, even though his cognitive abilities may be far more impaired than the other child's. One child may be pitied, the other admired because of the choices the parents have made about how to manage their child in public. This underscores the importance of making sure your child understands developmentally appropriate expectations and of your developing creative ways for him to comply with societal "rules" associated with the context.

Health Care Settings

Behaving appropriately in a grocery store, restaurant, post office, library, or laundromat is one thing. Maintaining appropriate behavior when you are frightened or confused is something else again. Even adults become anxious when they are not sure what to expect in a medical setting. When you cannot visually monitor what is happening, the unexpected is even worse!

To make visits to therapists, the doctor, dentist, or other medically related appointments as bearable as possible, prepare both your child and the health care professionals. Inform everyone who will be interacting with your child about the functional nature of his vision, such as whether he is able to see light or has some perception of objects and the environment. Just as importantly, explain that they should tell your child before they touch him and let him explore any equipment before they use it with him. If your child needs to sit or lie on an examining table, let him first feel the table and its height. Otherwise, he may be frightened if he is suddenly lifted into the air and placed on the table or the chair suddenly is reclined.

If your child is old enough to be concerned about being in medical facilities, it may help to let him explore the office and equipment before any painful or frightening procedures may be necessary. You can often arrange a visit to establish a friendly rapport with the doctor and staff at a time when your child is not ill or in need of critical care. Even making brief but frequent visits prior to the actual appointment may alleviate fears and promote comfort and cooperation.

Sometimes it is possible to help prepare your child at home for upcoming medical or dental procedures. For example, many blind children are easily terrorized by a blood pressure cuff. To desensitize and prepare your child, you might give him many opportunities to wear inflatable arm floats (swim fluegals) when he plays or swims in the pool or to wear a small radio that can be strapped to his arm. While the pressure is not the same, children are not as panicked if they have had some simulation of the experience and know they will be okay afterwards. An older child may engage in taking the blood pressure of a doll or stuffed animal. Similarly, using an electric or battery operated toothbrush is often helpful in preparing your child for his first visit with the dentist.

When medical professionals do not respect your child's needs, you as his parent have the right to discontinue the visit and seek other care. How your child is treated may have lasting effects, and health care and management will be a lifelong process. Positive experiences early in life will make future medical appointments much more palatable.

▪▪ Conclusion

Enhancing your child's independence may be one of the most time-consuming but rewarding tasks of parenthood. When your child has a visual impairment, you will initially need to help him access information that others take for granted and to become accustomed to day-to-day demands through his other senses and systematic and varied experiences. Providing a variety of meaningful and repetitive opportunities to learn expectations and to practice relevant and appropriate behaviors will provide your child with the tools he needs to take on age-appropriate responsibilities. With planning, consistency, and creativity, you can foster independence in addition to self-esteem, acceptance, and competence in all aspects of your child's life.

▪▪ References

Baker, B.L., & Brightman, A.J. (1989). *Steps to independence: A skills training guide for parents and teachers of children with special needs.* Second edition. Baltimore, MD: Paul H. Brookes Publishing Co.

Bambring, M. (2001). Integration of children with visual impairment in regular preschools. *Child: Care, Health, and Development, 27* (5), pp. 425-438.

Brody, J., & Webber, L. (1994). *Let's eat: Feeding a child with a visual impairment.* Los Angeles, CA: Blind Children's Center.

Chen, D. (1995). Guiding principles for instruction and program development. In D. Chen and J. Dote-Kwan (Eds.) *Starting points: Instructional practices for young children whose multiple disabilities include visual impairment,* pp. 15-28. Los Angeles, CA: Blind Children's Center.

Kastein, S., Spaulding, I., & Scharf, B. (1980). *Raising the young blind child: A guide for parents and educators.* New York, NY: Human Sciences Press.

Lewis, S., Slay, S, and Pace, E. (1999a). *Preschool attainment through typical everyday routines: Assessment tool.* [videotape]. Tallahassee, FL: Author. (lewis@coe.fsu.ed or 850-644.8409.)

Lewis, S., Slay, S, and Pace, E. (1999b). *Preschool attainment through typical everyday routines: Curriculum guide.* [videotape]. Tallahassee, FL: Author. (lewis@coe.fsu.ed or 850-644.8409.)

Lewis, S., Slay, S., & Pace, E. (1999c, December). *PATTER: Preschool attainment through everyday routines: Study Guide.* Tallahassee, FL: Author. (lewis@coe.fsu.ed or 850-644-8409.)

Murdoch, H (n.d.). Repetitive behaviours in children with sensory impairments and multiple disabilities. http://www.deafblindinternational.org/review.

Oetter, P., Richter, E.W., & Frick, S.M. (1993). *M.O.R.E. Integrating the mouth with sensory and postural functions.* Hugo, MN: PDP Press, Inc.

Orelove, F.P. & Sobsey, D. (1996). Mealtime skills. *Educating children with multiple disabilities: A transdisciplinary approach.* 3rd edition. Baltimore, MD: Paul H. Brookes Co.

Scott, E., Jan, J.E., & Freeman, R.D. (1994) *Can't your child see?* 3rd edition. Austin, TX: Pro-Ed.

Simmons, S. (1993). Self-help skills. *First steps: A handbook for teaching young children who are visually impaired,* pp.139-150. Los Angeles, CA: Blind Children's Center.

Williamson, G.G., Anzalone, M.E., and Hanft, B.E. (2001). Assessment of sensory processing, praxis, and motor performance. *CDL clinical practice guidelines: Redefining the standards of care.* Bethesda, MD: The Interdisciplinary Council on Developmental & Learning Disorders.

▪▪ Parent Statements

I know that I should let Molly do more for herself and every morning I wake up telling myself that this will be the day I will back off a little bit. But it is so hard—we are always in a hurry to get somewhere or I watch her struggling to put on her socks and I just give in. Most of the time it is just easier to do it myself.

❧

We live in a small town and have had wonderful support from everyone. One day I was in the grocery store with Amelia and she started explaining the difference between an apple and an orange to the clerk in the produce section. We were all so proud of her. We were proud of her knowledge but even more thrilled at her initiative to "teach" someone else what she had learned!

❧

For a long time, Eric would only eat two things—macaroni and cheese and oatmeal. I tried and tried to get him to eat something else but he would just scream and spit it out. I worked with his preschool teachers to overcome this problem. Eric is still a picky eater, but he eats much better now.

❧

Ashley has trouble with anything different. She won't play with play dough and doesn't like to touch anything that feels different. She doesn't even like soft fabrics like velvet. It makes it very difficult to do anything new.

❧

I try to tell Andy I am going to pick him up before I do. I talk to him as I am walking up to him. I don't want him to be scared.

❧

We are a happy family. I don't think there is anything better than working together for a common cause. We have three children, and our middle child is blind. We have worked hard to make sure that all of our children feel valued and all feel responsible for each other.

❧

Sometimes you have to make choices. You can't do everything.

❧

Our son has loved spinning since he was about four months old. We would put him in a bouncer attached to the header in a doorway. He would stay in it for a couple of hours at a time, bouncing and spinning happily. As he grew, he enjoyed spinning in his swing and on our tire swing in the back yard. He is seven years old now and he still loves to spin in his room—or anywhere else for that matter! We tell him his other friends don't do that and that they might think he's odd if he does it at school. I don't think he does it as much at school, but I do know social stigma plays a big role in curtailing many of the quirky things all children do.

❦

I try so hard not to get angry when people stare at Tucker. My wife handles it much better than I do. Sometimes I just want to scream, "Where are your manners"? but I know that wouldn't help the situation. I've heard lots of advice about what I "should" say but nothing feels right. I just wish I didn't feel so angry!

❦

We are committed to making sure that we have high standards for Kiki. We expect her to behave appropriately, we expect her to be independent, and we expect her to contribute to our family by doing chores. It isn't always easy, but we will do everything that we can to make sure she can be successful.

6

FAMILY
LIFE

Leslie & Eric Ligon

When parents first learn that their child has a visual impairment, their chief concern is often: "How will this disability affect my child?" Sooner or later, however, parents realize that their child's visual impairment will also touch the lives of everyone in the family. Then their question becomes: "How will this disability affect my family?" There are many issues related to this question, including: "How can we balance the needs of all family members while still keeping a keen eye on the needs of our child who is visually impaired?" "Will our family have a 'normal' family life?" "Can we plan family activities without worrying that there will be difficulties related to our child's visual impairment?"

The answers to these questions depend largely on you, the parents. If you are determined that your family have the most "normal" life possible, then you will probably develop the coping skills and attitudes needed to meet the challenges that face you. All members of your family will learn effective methods of working through the issues related to your child's visual impairment by following your example.

Of course, you won't learn how to cope with your child's differences overnight. And en route to learning how to handle them, your family is bound to run into stresses and strains that other families don't have to address. Also, every family is different and will have different ways of coping with challenges and joys. This chapter describes issues related to family life from one family's perspective. You will be able to take this information and use it as it best fits your own situation.

We have written this chapter from our perspectives as a married couple raising two children. Our older son has a visual impairment, while our younger son does not. We realize that today's families are quite diverse and your situation may be very different from ours. We have tried to incorporate ideas and suggestions from many other parents with whom we have talked. Regardless of whether you are reading this as a part of a traditional or nontraditional family—with or without extended family support—it is likely that you will have the same questions and concerns. We encourage you to gather information from a variety of sources and trust your own ability to apply this information to your own situation. You will be the best judge about what will be valuable to you.

▪▪ Focusing on the Child First

When we were first learning about our son's visual impairment, like most parents, our overriding concerns were for our child. At Ethan's eight-week, well-baby exam, we were laughing one minute about how much weight he'd gained and stunned the next when the pediatrician said, "Brace yourselves; Ethan can't see."

Looking back, there were vague signs that something was not quite right with our baby's eyes, but we were dealing with and learning about so many other things with our first child, we didn't really jump to any worried conclusions. A couple of times I remember that Ethan's eyes seemed to roll way up and back. We had read about babies not seeing well at distances in the first two to three months, so we just thought it was probably a muscle spasm which would go away with age. Our pediatrician later said she'd seen no previous signs, either; she was as shocked as we were. At two prior check-ups, she'd checked his eyes and had gotten a good retinal reflection.

We were fortunate that our pediatrician knew an excellent pediatric ophthalmologist who agreed to meet with us a couple of hours later. We went on to an appointment with a daycare center, and then to try and eat lunch, before meeting with the pediatric ophthalmologist. I remember feeling like the woman in the kidnapping scene in the movie, *Fargo*. It was as if someone had pulled a sack down over my head, thrown me into the back of a car and sped away. I felt completely out of control.

The pediatric ophthalmologist told us Ethan's corneas were fine, but that his retinas looked detached. He was surprised when we told him Ethan had not been premature and had actually been two weeks late. He suggested we go on to a nearby retinal specialist. We spent nearly five hours at that doctor's office. I remember looking at the fish tank filled with beautifully colored tropical fish and thinking Ethan would possibly never see them. It seemed like nothing would ever matter again.

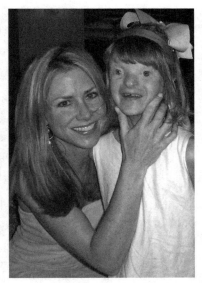

When we finally met with the specialist, he examined Ethan and did a sonogram on his eyes. That test showed his retinas were severely detached—floating toward the front of his eyes. He talked to us about all our concerns and put his arm around my shoulder and reassured me. He was a compassionate, caring physician, which I appreciated.

We ultimately spent the entire, long day in shock, waiting to see first one doctor, then another. We felt fortunate, though, to have at least gotten all of our information in one day, rather than waiting a week or more for subsequent appointments, as some parents have to do.

One week later, we traveled to Memphis, Tennessee, for an attempt to use cryosurgery to reattach Ethan's retinas. Afterwards, the surgeon told us there was hope that the retinas would stay attached and that Ethan would have a little residual vision. Unfortunately, when we returned for Ethan's check-up a month later, we got the news that Ethan's retinas were completely detached. I believed then that our little boy would never see our faces. I did, however, know that there are many ways of seeing, and that is what carried us through the first couple of years, which were often difficult.

▪▪ Shifting Focus

As the reality of your child's visual impairment sinks in, other realities will probably also become apparent. Perhaps little by little, or perhaps all in a rush, you will grasp that it is not just the future you imagined for your child that has changed. You and your spouse, as well as any other children you may have, are all facing a new future. For some families, these changes may ultimately contribute to the parents' divorce. Other families may emerge from the experience stronger than ever. Since how you and your spouse get along will greatly affect the family as a whole, it may be helpful for you to understand some of the ways a child with a disability may affect a marriage as well as family life.

We often talk about how important it is to focus on our marriage. We recognize that parenting a child with a disability carries with it potential problems for maintaining a strong marriage, but we also believe that both of our children are far better off if we work together, using each of our talents to strengthen our family.

As we began to think about ways that Ethan's visual impairment might change our lives, we worried about everything! For instance, when Ethan was about six months old, we had a conversation about having other children. We thought we'd need to have another child so there would always be someone for Ethan to rely on. (Of course, it didn't take long to learn that would *not* be necessary! Ethan can take care of himself!) We also thought that we'd need to buy lots of really expensive equipment and worried about how much it would cost. The reality is, the equipment does not have to be expensive—especially in the early years—nor does it have to fill the house! We found that Ethan loved to play with basic, everyday things we had around the house like pots and pans and plastic containers. Just like other children, Ethan enjoyed doing real-life activities and interacting with us more than he would have enjoyed playing with the newest electronic toy.

■■ Effects on Your Marriage

We discovered that there are several specific issues that parents should be aware of as they move forward. You will find that some of these issues are more important to your family than others, and you may be facing issues that we have not identified. We have briefly described these issues below.

Demands on Time and Money

All parents have the same basic responsibilities. They must see that their families are provided with food, shelter, health care, clothing, education, and love. This is a tall order for any parent. But when you have a child with a visual impairment, looking after these basic needs can sometimes seem incredibly challenging. To begin with, money may be tight because meeting the everyday and special needs of a child with a visual impairment is expensive. Two costs that add up very quickly for some families are loss of income from missed days of work, and health insurance co-payments and deductibles. This is especially true if your child has other disabilities or health issues in addition to a visual impairment. And health insurance often does not even pay for eyeglasses, vision aids, and assistive technology such as computers, reading machines, and closed circuit televisions. As your child grows, adapted equipment such as interactive toys, descriptive videotapes, and audiocassette tapes can also take a toll on the checkbook. In addition, childcare may be more costly if your child requires additional staffing and monitoring. The list of potential expenses goes on and on.

In our family we decided that I (Leslie) would reorder my life so that I could stay home with Ethan and later with his brother. We spent some time examining what was really important to us and made some sacrifices so that I could stop working outside the home. Eventually, I found that my creative talents and my love of making jewelry could combine with my developing interest in braille, and I created a company to make and sell braille jewelry.

As we mentioned before, it will be very important to approach these decisions as a couple or as a family, discussing and problem-solving together. We found that the more we talked about issues related to money and time, the more we could support each other in making the changes necessary to continue to do what we wanted to do. We found that this was actually an opportunity to simplify our lives and to concentrate on each other and our children.

One major time drain was gathering information and figuring out how to best use it to support Ethan and other family members. Sometimes it felt like we were spinning our wheels, although we were sure that other parents had traveled this road before us. We have increasingly used the Internet to help in our search for information and for connecting us with other parents. The Resource Guide at the end of this book should help start your search for information. We have also felt a keen responsibility to pass on what we have learned to other parents who have children younger than Ethan.

Sometimes, even in the best of times, we found that we felt overwhelmed. It is a little bit comforting to hear our friends with children who do not have disabilities echo our feelings of tiredness and irritability and sleep deprivation. While we have been careful to find time to spend together, we also benefit from time alone, so we try to "spell" each other from time to time. One day I may take the boys to the park and Eric gets to relax by himself or enjoy a special project on his own, while another day Eric has a play date with the boys and I can take off for an afternoon with a friend.

Challenges to Your Role as a Parent

Parents of children with visual impairments may sometimes encounter real or perceived challenges to their parenting abilities. This can lead to conflicts if parents don't agree about who is the "expert" on this or that issue, or if one parent begins to feel undervalued. Challenges may come from early intervention or school personnel, as well as from people in the community or family members.

All parents may feel as if others are second-guessing their parenting abilities at times, but these experiences can be especially upsetting when you know the individual judging you is clueless about visual impairments. We often felt we were under the microscope when Ethan began using his first white cane just after his second birthday. Texas summers are hot, so in an effort to help Ethan to learn to use his cane and not burn up in the Texas sun, we went to a local shopping mall to walk. Our little parades must have been quite a sight: a fairly frenzied-looking mother, a newborn in a stroller, and a cute little boy carrying a 24-inch white cane! People stopped dead in their tracks and simply stared. Completely forgetting all the manners they had been taught, they stood open-mouthed, ignorant of us and our feelings, only seeing this beautiful little boy who was blind and carrying a tiny white cane. In their defense, we both realized that we had never knowingly seen a blind child either before we had Ethan. Nevertheless, it was unnerving, and we handled it better on some days than on others.

We tried hard to reassure people that Ethan was all right, just blind, but very smart and happy. Many people recovered nicely, smiled, and went on their way (usually sneaking another glance over their shoulders as they left). Others, though, would swarm around in an instant when Ethan dropped his cane and it rolled a little. We would just put our foot on the cane and wait for Ethan to find it, saying, "Well, unless you plan to have him come live with you when he's eighteen, he needs to learn to find it on his own!" We were sure people thought we were horrible parents, making our "poor little blind child" crawl on the floor in public looking for things he'd dropped.

Changes/Challenges to Your Other Roles

Becoming a parent changes your life. Some of the changes are predictable, others are not; some are wonderful, others are not! We believe that the challenges that we faced as new parents of a child with a visual impairment are very similar to the challenges all parents face. However, we recognize that the addition of a visual impairment into the equation is not a small one, and, at times, ordinary challenges may seem magnified.

One of the most common complaints of new parents relates to the change in identity from individual and couple to mother or father and parents. One mother told me of going to her parents' house and waiting twenty minutes for someone to finally say hello to *her*; everyone was paying so much attention to her new baby it felt like she was invisible. The interesting thing was that she said this with both pride and longing in her voice. You may feel the same way sometimes. It will help if you make some time to continue to focus on activities that interest you outside of your parenting role. If you were in a book club before your child was born, try to continue after her birth. Maybe your club will come to your house more often to make it convenient for you. If you like to keep up with the local sports team, make sure you continue to do so and talk with others who have a similar interest.

Differences in Coping

Parenting a child with a visual impairment can arouse many strong emotions. These emotions are not just limited to the time when you are finding out your child's diagnosis and initially grappling with the implications. They can also besiege you when you are dealing with medical issues, vision testing, and decisions about early intervention and school. These emotions are not, by any means, all negative. Sometimes you may be excited by the new information you are finding or energized by the progress you see your child making. Sometimes, it will seem like a bit of a roller coaster.

Some parents report that it can be difficult if you and your spouse are not "on the same page"—for instance, if one of you is worried while the other one is excited by new information. In addition, friction may arise if one of you has a different way of coping than the other and tries to force the other to cope in the same way.

We decided pretty early on that if we were going to be on this journey, we were going to be on it creatively. We jumped in with both feet, talking to everyone we could, attending local and national conferences of both families and professionals, and imagining how we could use the information we gathered to enrich our lives. We decided that we would be upfront with information and with our emotions—we would cry when we wanted to cry and laugh when we wanted to laugh. We wanted to incorporate our compassion and our sense of humor; handling situations with both humor and respect.

We've found that there is a fine line between appropriate and inappropriate humor, and we try very hard to find funny aspects of our lives without resorting to sarcasm, which can be difficult for young children to understand. For instance, we thought it was funny when Ethan dressed up as a pirate for Halloween and wore two eye patches, but we bristled when, after Ethan won a board game, someone sarcastically said, "You played that game pretty well, for a blind kid!" We wanted Ethan to feel that his win was not qualified and feared that this sarcasm, while said in jest, would give him the impression that he was not an equal player in the game.

Even in harmonious homes, differences in coping and emotion can take a toll. And some families find that there is little harmony. We have heard our share of stories about how differences in coping can cause real stress. It can be very frustrating when you are experiencing emotions that your spouse or partner does not feel or understand. For instance, at a conference we met a woman who said that her husband gets angry when she expresses sadness. He feels that if she is sad about their daughter's blindness, then she must not love her. She said that not being able to discuss her sadness with her husband made her feel guilty and her isolation from her husband on this matter made her lonely. Stories like this abound. Even if you and your spouse experience the same emotions, you may not experience them at the same time and this disconnect can have an impact on your relationship.

If you and your partner have this type of emotional disconnect, it would probably be best to discuss your difficulties when you are not in the middle of a crisis. Just knowing that this can be a problem and a source of stress can help you recognize it when it happens. Coming up with a pre-agreed-upon strategy might help you get through temporary rough patches. (For example, you could agree to talk things out with a neutral third party or try to use nonjudgmental comments such as "I'm sure that must be difficult for you" when one of you is struggling.) However, if the discord is intense or ongoing you may need to get outside help from someone who will be able to give you strategies geared to your individual needs and family style. It seems unlikely that ignoring these differences will make them go away. Instead, it may lead to anger, isolation, and resentment, which can sometimes lead to permanent damage to a relationship.

:: Strategies to Keep Your Marriage Strong

There are many books written about keys to successful marriages, and just as many opinions about how to achieve a successful marriage as there are mothers-in-law. But really, you probably already know what you and your spouse need and what works for you. We have included some strategies to start your discussion, but feel free to find help from other sources and to trust your instincts about what you need to do to keep your marriage strong. The most important piece of advice that we have to offer on this topic is to pay attention to the need for keeping your relationship strong from the very beginning. It is much easier to work on your relationship along the way than to repair damage caused by neglect.

Share Your Emotions

If you or your partner are grieving or grappling with other strong emotions, you may have difficulty making decisions together. For example, you may not be able to agree about surgeries, educational or medical recommendations, having a care provider in your home, or any number of important issues. This sort of impasse can affect every aspect of your family life. How your relationship is affected depends a great deal on your ability to be open about your feelings with one another.

Sometimes one spouse (often the husband) feels he must be "strong" for the sake of the other. This is a mistake. First, the "strong" partner must publicly deny his real feelings, and therefore may not work through his emotions as quickly as he would otherwise—or at all. Second, the grieving spouse may mistakenly conclude that his or her spouse doesn't really care about what has happened to their child, or doesn't grasp the seriousness of the diagnosis. This can lead to feelings of loneliness and resentment.

You may need to give Dad special permission not to have to feel strong. It is OK not to be the "provider" and not to be able to "fix" this problem. Sometimes it helps to refocus the "fixing" to address the environment rather than the blindness. While you may not be able to "fix" the blindness, you can help figure out how to get the help you need and how you can be involved in the team! Our society has traditionally encouraged men to feel like they shouldn't say "I don't know." In these situations it is especially important to pay attention to this pressure and try to reduce it as much as possible.

If you share your emotions, you will often find that you and your spouse have or have had the very same worries. At the least, this discovery can help dispel some of your concerns; at best, the two of you may jointly be able to come up with some solutions.

In discussing your feelings, sometimes one or both of you may find that things are just too much for you to handle alone. That's when it's time to get some outside help from a friend, counselor, or clergy. Having professional help or just another perspective can help you check on your own feelings.

Learn about Your Child Together

Often one person in the couple ends up doing most of the reading, searching, and leg-work needed to find out more about their child's visual impairment. This may be because one spouse has more time, or because it seems to be the expected role for one person. If only one of you is actively involved in looking at this new situation, however, you may be isolating your best ally. You both need to keep current on information about your child's visual impairment as well as on what doctors, teachers, and therapists are saying. Otherwise, one of you may end up making more of the decisions about your child's ongoing care, treatment, and future. Just because one parent may be going to more of the doctor's appointments or educational meetings does not mean that the other parent has to be excluded from the decision-making process.

We've heard some parents say that they approached gathering information as a treasure hunt and were excited to be able to share new information with each other as they found it. We found that at different times each of us took primary responsibility for researching and compiling necessary information. You may discover that one of you has no patience for information about laws and legal issues while the other is overwhelmed by the medical part. Try to identify what you are good at and specialize in that information while letting your partner specialize in something else.

If you are a single parent, you may find that another family member (maybe your mom or your brother) would appreciate being assigned responsibility for something useful. You will probably need to be the "keeper" of the information, but don't hesitate to accept help from others who care about you and your child.

Become Confident in Your Parenting Abilities

If doctors, teachers, therapists, family members, and even strangers are always giving you suggestions about caring for your child, it is easy to wonder just who is the expert on your child. In fact, *you* are the most important expert on her. Other people may come and go in your child's life, but you, the parents, are the ones who care the most about her well-being, and who have the most at stake in her learning the skills she needs to be independent.

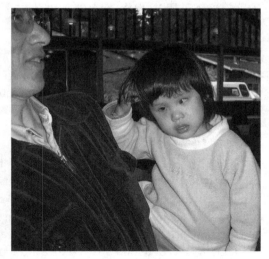

When Ethan was first diagnosed with a visual impairment, we quickly realized that it was in Ethan's best interest for us to be the same take-charge, involved parents that we would have been if he did not have a visual impairment. We had to take responsibility for things that we found a little scary at first, but we quickly became confident in our ability and in our commitment to Ethan. We were lucky because Leslie had danced all of her life and had taught dance for many years, so she felt confident teaching Ethan movement and how his body related to other objects in space. Still, we listened to all of the ideas and suggestions the specialists tossed out. We also felt comfortable asking questions and challenging certain orientation and mobility philosophies and techniques. For instance, as mentioned above, we advocated for Ethan to begin using a white cane long before his O&M specialist thought he was ready.

We also took the lead in Ethan's early literacy education. After his highly regarded TVI had worked with Ethan for six months, we asked her when braille books would be incorporated into his twice-weekly home visits. She said that at 27 months, Ethan was just too young to start with braille. We simply did not agree with that. Ethan was 18 months old when I first noticed him pick up a book, open it, and touch the pages as if reading. He seemed to instinctively know that to read, you must touch the pages to find the words.

Neither my husband nor I were braille literate at that time, so I devised a trick plan. Whenever I read to Ethan during the day, regardless of what I was reading (from a print book), I gave Ethan a braille book. Even though it wasn't necessarily a braille version of the book from which I was reading, Ethan would be reading along with me. Even when I read to him when he was lying down in bed at night, I made sure to have a braille book close at hand because sometimes he would reach over to look at the books I was reading. He seemed to effortlessly grasp the concept of finger reading.

Although we weren't getting the vision services support we wanted at home, we felt confident we were doing all we could as parents of a very young child to ensure that he would become a steadfast reader. Today Ethan reads everything that his classmates read and he enjoys reading and writing stories of his own.

Listen to Your Inner Voice

As a corollary to the point above, get expert advice, but trust your intuition if what the experts tell you does not seem right. No matter how much experience an expert has, he or she does not live with your child 24/7 and may discount subtle cues that seem meaningful to you. For example, as our son's second birthday passed, he became increasingly whiny. He'd always been happy and contented, so we were a little concerned, but not worried. Then in the fall he awoke one morning with a sore throat and slightly swollen left eye. We began a circuit of doctor's appointments that would last six weeks before we were finally told he'd developed glaucoma. When the pressure was alleviated, he was better, but still not quite right. Yet another round of appointments ensued while our son endured another three and a half months of discomfort that the doctors seemed to discount.

Finally, at our insistence, the pediatric ophthalmologist performed an exam under anesthesia and discovered many complications that brought on a great deal of pain, nausea, and dizziness. Approving the surgery recommended (enucleation, or removal of our son's eyes) was a difficult decision to make but watching Ethan experience so much pain and discomfort was equally difficult.

Divide Responsibilities Fairly

Before your child's visual impairment was diagnosed, you and your spouse may each have routinely taken care of specific household chores and responsibilities. It will be important to take some time to rethink these assignments, given the time necessary to take care of the medical and educational issues facing your family now. There may be some chores that no longer seem all that important to do and that could be dropped from the list. For instance, making everybody's beds every morning may no longer seem necessary.

You might want to consider assigning some chores to people outside of the family. For example, you might decide that the outlay in cash is worth the savings in time to have a neighborhood teenager mow your lawn or to have the drycleaners wash and press your dress shirts. Paying close attention to the responsibilities of each spouse will help avoid over-taxing one spouse and causing exhaustion and resentment.

Take Time Out

Even when your child's disability is relatively minor, it's probably still going to be a strain in the beginning. There's such a lot to learn, yet you've got to work just as hard at being a happy person and a happy couple. This is true even in families where no one has a disability. It may be tempting to make your child the center of every activity you do, but this is a mistake. Everyone needs to take some time off from the demands of parenthood every once in a while. This helps recharge your batteries and may give you a fresh perspective on life with your child. It is also important for you and your spouse to have a chance to reconnect as a couple.

Sometimes it is not possible to physically get away from home, but this shouldn't stop you from setting aside some time to spend time together—to watch a movie on TV, eat a special meal, or simply have a conversation about something other than visual impairments. Some couples try to take one hour after the children are put to bed to have a leisurely dinner and quiet conversation.

It may be difficult, at first, for you to feel comfortable leaving your child with a visual impairment in the care of someone else, but it is important that you find a way to do so. In the beginning, most parents feel more comfortable leaving their child with someone they know well. Find someone you trust and arrange a convenient time for him or her to take care of your children. Go to dinner or a movie. Forget the kids for a couple of hours. If you've got someone who's able to watch them for a couple of days—even better! Just get out and be together without the stresses children can put on you.

I remember that at the beginning, I hated leaving Ethan with anyone because I was afraid he would just lie quietly in bed and not be stimulated at all. He was a very easy baby, but I believed that he needed almost constant attention to make sure that he was involved in life. I was afraid that if we left Ethan with anyone else, even someone who loved him, he would not receive the same attention that he would if I was with him. I got a little angry when people tried to convince me that I should change my mind about this. Eventually, I realized that I didn't need to change my mind about the importance of stimulating Ethan, but I did need to loosen up and realize that an afternoon or evening without my attention wouldn't harm him, and, in fact, might give both him and me a nice rest.

Here are some suggestions that may make you feel more comfortable about leaving your child with someone else:

- *Try leaving your child with a relative or a good friend you trust.* You may feel most comfortable dropping your child off at your relative's or friend's house for an hour or so; or you may feel that it is better to have the person come to your house.
- *Start with small amounts of time*—an hour or an hour and a half in the daytime may seem like a much less stressful trial.
- *Compile a small notebook with information that a sitter might need,* including your child's likes and dislikes and any special methods you use to help your child when she becomes upset.
- *Leave clear instructions on all activities to be carried out while you are gone.* Will your child eat, brush her teeth, go to bed? Will there be an opportunity for the sitter to read your child a book or play a game? Make sure that the sitter

is comfortable with all of these activities and you will feel more reassured.

- *Be sure to leave information about how to reach you.* It will help you relax if you know that the sitter has your cell phone number and the name and number of a couple of neighbors and friends just in case they are needed.

Support Each Other's Private Times

Regardless of how close you are as a couple, everyone needs some time alone. If you can, take a little time just for yourself and relax! Go for a walk or to a bookstore or park. Take a class that interests you. The more time you can steal for yourself—even if it's to catch up on much needed sleep—the better everyone will be!

If one of you works outside the home and the other doesn't, it may be especially important for the parent who is gone during the day to give the stay-at-home parent at least a short break from childcare duties in the evening. Sometimes it can feel like a luxury just to be able to cook a meal without your children clamoring for your attention. If both of you spell each other when it comes to childcare duties, your child won't become too dependent on one of you for her care, and you are both less likely to feel burnt out.

Be Kind

This may seem overly simplistic, but it is the best advice we can give you. Be kind to each other and be kind to yourself. Remember that most of the time we all do the best we can with the information we have, and that most people have their hearts in the right place. We have found that if we continue to show and expect kindness from ourselves, each other, and from other people, we find it!

:: Effects on Family Life

It is difficult to anticipate what impact having a child with a visual impairment will have on family life. At first, you will base your beliefs on whatever experience you have had with visual impairments. Unless you have spent quality time on an ongoing basis with a person who is blind or visually impaired, you probably won't have an accurate picture of what people with visual impairments can do.

As mentioned earlier in this chapter, my first thoughts about Ethan's blindness were concentrated on loss. I looked at that fish tank in the doctor's waiting room and could only imagine that Ethan would never see those colorful fish. I still have thoughts like that every once in a while, but now, I am more likely to pay attention to what is added to our family. We are much more keenly aware of the other ways (besides vision) that we can enjoy the world and we work together, with Ethan, in powerful family problem-solving to make sure that we support and have fun with each other.

We have also come to appreciate some of the old maxims we had heard for years. Taking things "one day at a time" can really help, especially at first. While you will want to pay attention to how you can plan for your child's future, worrying too much about challenges that may never come to be can paralyze your efforts to enjoy today.

▪▪ Strategies to Keep Your Family Strong

Listed below are some strategies that we have used to help our family. Of course, some of these may be more appropriate to your situation than others, and the most effective strategies will be the ones you determine for yourselves.

Get Out into the Community

It is very important that families of children with visual impairments participate fully in community life. This includes both day-to-day routines like going to the grocery store or post office, and fun, special activities like going bowling or to a concert. We are fortunate to live in this day and age. A long time ago, people with disabilities were shunned and were often cloistered at home. In the more recent past, people with disabilities were so rarely seen in public that they were often treated as oddities. But today, due in large part to efforts of generations of people with disabilities, their families, and advocates who pushed for landmark legislation, people with disabilities are seen as full and important members of our society. While you may need to learn how to deal patiently with ignorance, you should not have to deal with discrimination.

Still, it is understandable that some families may feel reluctant to participate in community activities with their child who is visually impaired. One reason is that you may encounter people who are curious or even sad about your child's disabilities. Parents often report getting tired of constantly having to address this public attitude when they are out in the community.

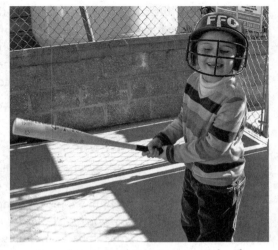

Another reason that parents may have concerns about participating in community activities is a fear that their child may have difficulty or take more time to complete something. For example, if your community sponsors an Easter Egg Hunt, you may want your child to participate but feel that it would be difficult to arrange. We believe that most organizers would be happy to explore ways that your child could enter into the fun, especially if you can help them figure out the best way to make this happen (like giving your child an advanced orientation to the hunting space and including special "beeper" eggs just for her). Your child's early intervention specialist or teacher of students with visual impairments will probably be excited about helping you find ways to include your child in community activities!

A third reason that parents may be concerned about community involvement is if they feel that their child may not be safe, especially relating to orientation and mobility. This is a real concern, but with some advance planning and instruction for your child, there may be a way to help your child participate in activities that will also help develop abilities and confidence.

We used to go to different places when our son was a baby and wonder where the other blind kids were. What would our child be like in one year, or two, or five? The truth is, you most likely won't see other blind kids just out and about with their families. If you're in a larger city, you may be fortunate to have access to a school for the blind that has an infant program, but in the beginning, your child is going to attract more attention than most people's kids. Almost every parent with a child who's blind can recall strangers asking about their "sleepy child." And yes, it does attract even more attention when your child begins using a white cane. (I actually thought this point would be a big emotional hurdle for me. Quite the opposite has happened, though. I am so proud when my son uses his cane properly and struts alongside me down the aisles of local stores!) You may need to spend some time and effort in connecting with other parents and families with children who have visual impairments. You and your child will benefit greatly from these connections

Keep a Sense of Humor

There will always be days when you wish you could just go to the grocery store and not have people stare at you; we all have our difficult days. For the most part, though, people are simply curious. I believe it's in everyone's best interest if you use the stares and awkwardness as an opportunity to change some minds. Sometimes just looking someone in the eye will give them the courage to ask a question (like "Is your baby OK?"). This can then allow you to make a direct, but appropriate response ("Oh yes, she is fine! She has a visual impairment that causes her to look sleepy but she is very aware of who and what is around her.")

Although smiling and being gracious in the face of embarrassment sounds great, it's not always easy. There will be times when you simply lose patience. Even when those times occur, try to forgive *yourself* and laugh about it later with someone who understands. This is one of the most common topics of conversation between parents who have children with visual impairments (and really, any disabilities), so save up your stories to share with others who understand how you feel and can commiserate.

Encourage Friendships

Parents of children with visual impairments often report that they are concerned about their child developing friendships with other children. We have often heard fears from parents that children can be cruel and they worry that their child will be teased, or just as bad, will be excluded from social opportunities. This is a very real fear. These days the news is filled with stories about bullying, but there are far more stories that don't make the news about kindness and true friendship. It is important for all children to have friends outside of family members. Our lives are richer and better because of our friendships.

Children with visual impairments may have unique challenges related to the development of friendships. First, they will not be able to see what a child or a group of children may be doing across the room, so they may not be able to make an independent decision about joining in. Second, children who do not have visual impairments may be initially reluctant to approach your child because of unfamiliarity with visual impairment. Third, some parents of other children and other adults may be fearful about your child's safety or accessibility issues. It may seem silly, but your child may not be invited to a birthday party because the parents of the other child don't know whether they can send a print invitation or may not be able to figure out how your child will enter into party activities. Eventually your child will take on responsibility for developing and maintaining her friendships, but you may have to be more involved while she is young. The next two sections address friendships, your child's friendships and your own.

Your Children's Friendships

Of course, friendships are important for everyone. But for a child with a visual impairment, friendships may take on special importance. First, it is important for your child to know that people outside of her immediate family know and care about her. Second, friends can boost confidence and self-esteem and can be an important shoulder to cry on when things are not going well. Third, good friends can be a social barometer. ("Is this skirt too long?" "Is it cool to play this game?" And eventually, "Do you think that boy likes me?") Fourth, if you have other children, it is important that they don't feel that they have to take total playmate and sibling responsibility. A brother or a sister is different from a friend and uniquely important!

Initially, we worried about whether Ethan would be able to make friends easily, or if peers would say hurtful things to him. Eight years into this, we no longer worry about it. He's a great kid with a good sense of humor and likes many of the same things his sighted friends like. Now that he's in school, we see that he makes friends pretty easily. He has several friends from school whose houses he goes to and who enjoy visiting him and sleeping over.

Kids are usually pretty easy to work with when it comes to informing them about blindness and the things our son can do. We try to generously share information about walking safely with Ethan and about simple ways to communicate through braille with him. Ethan's teacher of students with visual impairments generally does an introduction lesson early in the school year and some children become fascinated with it all and want to know more. Truthfully, it's more often the adults who have the hardest time!

In the early years, you will want to make sure your child has plenty of opportunities to meet and play with other children. Your neighborhood or community may sponsor "play groups" where children and parents get together for a couple of hours once a week to just play and interact. If you can't find an appropriate play group, consider forming one yourself. You can even do this in your home with just a few other children and their parents. This is a relatively small commitment, since all you need are some toys and maybe some snacks. Some parents arrange an outing for their child and others by sending out email notices for everyone to meet at a park or playground. By arranging the activity, you have some control over it and can make sure it is appropriate for your child and gives her the best and most comfortable opportunity to play with the other children.

Calming a Friend's Parents' Fears

When your child is younger, it may seem difficult to help parents of your child's friends understand things aren't really very different for her. It certainly did for us. Over time we learned it was best to let them know straight away the things they could do that would be helpful for Ethan. We've found that it helps to be the first to invite a friend over. This way, Ethan is in his own home and can be comfortable showing his friend what he can do (for example, find his own toys, walk comfortably and independently around the house, get a snack by himself). By the time Ethan goes to visit his friend as his friend's house, the two of them have a pretty clear understanding of how things work and the friend's family often easily joins into the flow of things.

Parents will probably want some specifics about what your child can and can't do. Start with the "can do" list and then, instead of talking about "can't do" things, frame it by talking about what support she needs to be able to do certain things. For instance, the first time your child spends the night with a new friend, you might say, "You'll find that Jessica can completely take care of herself. She won't need any help eating, dressing, or brushing her teeth. Since Jessica has never been to your house, you'll want to tell her and show her where things are and then watch to see if she needs help until she becomes more familiar with you home." Then allow lots of time for questions and information exchange. Many times, parents will tell us later how amazed they are about how well our son gets along in new environments. Basically, if you're easy about it and don't act as if your child will break if things aren't just right, then others will, too.

From our experience and from talking with other parents, we realize that every situation is different. Some people are incredibly flexible, while others need step-by-step instructions on the most routine tasks. Your best bet is to try to respond to the parents of your child's friends with honesty, openness, trust, and the understanding that this may be a long-term relationship that will develop over time.

As your child gets more involved with friends at school, the friends will become such pros at how to play with a child who is blind or visually impaired that their parents will learn from *them*. We've had parents tell us they would try to walk with our son when they were all out together and their own child would tell them, "No, Mom. That's not how you do sighted guide."

We usually try to put parents at ease by injecting humor into our answers. It's just our way of handling their fears. They will sometimes ask if there's something special they should know, and we'll tell them to just be sure and let Ethan know if there's a pool or any other large holes he might want to be aware of.

Your Own Friendships

Parents need friends outside of the family, too. Just like your child, you need to have meaningful relationships with people who can provide you with things that your family cannot—whether that be a shared appreciation of rock music or modern literature, assistance in improving your golf game or your quilting skills, or just providing a sounding board. Just like your child, you need to have the satisfaction of knowing that other people find your company enjoyable and a feeling of connectedness with the world. As the parent of a child with visual impairments, you may also need the support, listening ear, or helping hand that most friends freely give each other.

Friendships *can* sometimes suffer when a child is diagnosed with a visual impairment. You may perceive your friends as backing away emotionally. If that appears to be happening, it may be because they don't know what to say, or they want to fix things and feel they can't in this particular situation. It may also be that your feelings of abandonment and isolation are leaving you feeling a bit defensive.

It will be difficult, but try not to shut out friends' feelings as you manage your own. They will probably come around to understanding the situation if you give them a little help. While you might not want to overwhelm them with every detail you find out, they will probably want to know much of what you are thinking and exploring. They may also need specific tasks to do in order to feel helpful. Perhaps some of your friends say, "Please let me know what to do," making you feel like you have the responsibility to find something for them to do. That something to do could be as simple as setting up a periodic, scheduled time to check in with each other. That way you can support each other and not feel that your friendship is one-sided.

You may also find that you develop new friendships with people (other parents or professionals with whom you work) you meet along your journey. Some of these friends can be long-distance friends that you meet and connect with through email or conferences. Both old friends and new friends have a role to play in enriching your life.

Help All Your Children Feel Special

Everyone has heard comedians joke about siblings arguing about who was Mom's favorite or who received the most affection in a family. We laugh at this, but it really is a big concern for all families. We believe that it is important that everyone in the family feel special and loved. This helps with family harmony by minimizing sibling rivalry.

Some parents have trouble balancing their attention so that all children feel their worth. In extreme cases we have heard that parents actually keep track of the amount of money and time that they spend with each of their children and try to equalize it. We believe that this kind of accounting actually draws attention to possible disparities in attention, and would rather create a natural environment in which every family member's unique talents are appreciated. Adult siblings of people with disabilities often comment that they did indeed get less of their parents' time and attention. At the same time, however, many show greater compassion and understanding than people who did not have this experience.

Be careful when you praise one of your children not to make it a comparative praise. Be sure to say, "You are so athletic" rather than "You are the athletic one in the family" (which implies that others are not as athletic) or, "I love how creative you are" rather than "You are more creative than your brother."

It could be easy to let everything your family does revolve around the needs of your child who is visually impaired, and there may be certain times when this is necessary. However, making a concerted effort to avoid this will help your other children feel valued and will give your child with visual impairments opportunities to be thoughtful and involved in your other children's activities and interests. We have found that our instincts are good if we just make sure to pay attention to this issue along the way and periodically check-in with both of the boys to make sure that they are feeling as special as we think they are.

Make Sure Everyone Pulls Their Weight

One of the most important things we learned when Ethan was young was how important it is to make sure that everyone pulls his or her own weight in family chores and responsibilities. We talked to a teacher of students with visual impairments at a conference who told us that she worked with an elementary age student who couldn't tie his own shoes and didn't know how to make his bed. Even worse than this, she said that this child didn't believe that he should have to do these things because he had never been given that responsibility at home. Well, we were determined that this would not be true for Ethan. Soon, through talks with other teachers and parents, we learned that children who are visually impaired can and do learn to complete household chores like any other children. We believe that this is important for life-long independence.

All parents have to struggle with the question of whether to allow their young child to do something for herself or to just do it for her. Of course, there are times, when you are in a hurry to leave the house, when you have to just put your child's coat on her. But it is important to make sure that most of the time your child has the encouragement and the time to complete tasks as independently as possible, given her age and development. Just like you will examine the family "to-do" list to determine which chores are most appropriate for your older and younger child, you will want to examine the list for appropriate tasks for your children with and without visual impairments. Even if your child who is visually impaired is your only child, make sure that she is assigned responsibilities that benefit the family.

A good way to approach chore assignments is to go through the day and think of all of the responsibilities that someone must take on. While parents are usually responsible for meal preparation, for example, children can be taught to set the table, put ice in glasses, clear the table, and wash dishes. You may separate the assignments by meal (one child sets the breakfast table, the other sets the table for dinner) or by day of the week. There are plenty of household tasks to go around—think creatively and realize that all children have to be taught and supervised to do any task at first.

Have Fun Together As a Family

As you are learning about your child's visual impairment, you may wonder whether your family activities and outings will be limited, but you will quickly learn that this does not have to be the case. Your child will be able to enjoy and benefit from almost any family activity you can think of. If you are a sports enthusiast, there are countless ways to adapt games so your child can participate. While it is true that a fast-paced ball game like baseball might be difficult, even those games can be adapted so that your child can participate. Young children often use a tee to bat from and a sighted guide can run the bases with your child. Of course, if you enjoy watching baseball and football games, an easy adaptation is to have the picture on the television while the sound is turned down and a radio is used instead. Since radio doesn't rely on a picture, the announcers will explain things more thoroughly. As your child grows older, she will enjoy being included in these family activities.

Maybe your family likes outdoor activities such as hiking, swimming, and picnicking. All of those activities are completely available and enjoyable to children with visual impairments. Horseback riding, gardening, singing in a choir, skiing, playing board games—the list of activities available to you and your child is almost endless. An important thing to know, also, is that not only are these things enjoyable for your child; participation in recreation and leisure is very important for your child's development of independent living skills and self-confidence.

Our first teacher of the visually impaired/orientation and mobility (TVI/O&M) instructor was terrific. She was always easy to be around and fun-loving. We felt pretty helpless in the beginning, since Ethan was our first baby. Her twice-weekly visits were like a big social get-together, with café au lait and fresh-baked muffins for everyone! She quickly taught us to have fun with Ethan and to let him be himself. We hung on every word she had to say about what things to do to encourage his movement, teach him to rely on his hearing, and prepare him to be an explorer, confident about his surroundings. From the time he was eight months old, we would play the soundtrack from the musical *Gypsy* and dance him around the room until we all collapsed giggling!

Brothers and Sisters

It would be disingenu-
ous to pretend that having a
brother or sister with a visual
impairment is no different
from having a sighted sibling.
Your other children's lives
will be different because of
your child's visual impairment. But different doesn't
automatically mean difficult
or unenjoyable. In fact, I know
from personal experience that
siblings with and without
visual impairments can have

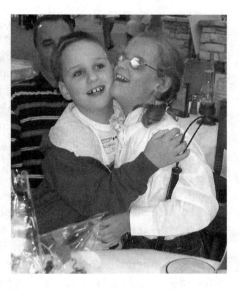

strong, close relationships and enjoy each other's company immensely.
Our younger, sighted son is only fifteen months younger than Ethan is.
They're so close in age they think they're twins! They play well together
for hours at a time.

There is no magic formula that will guarantee that your children
will get along—but then again, there is no single strategy that will ensure
that anybody's children will. All you have to do is go to any bookstore
and look at all the books that have been written about siblings to know
that there are some complex issues involved. We can, however, offer you
some words of advice based on our experiences and you can choose the
ones that seem as if they might be beneficial to your family.

Share Information

It is important to talk openly about your child's visual impairment with her siblings and to answer your children's questions about
it according to their information needs. Don't overload them with
information, but make it clear that you are happy to talk about anything at any time. By making sure your children know that this is not
embarrassing or wrong to talk about, you are allowing them to ask
any question they want and also modeling appropriate attitudes about
the situation. It will also be important that you have frank and open
discussions about how they can respond to questions from adults and
other children. Thinking ahead about the questions your children

may encounter can help you be proactive about making sure they feel comfortable and supportive of each other.

At our sons' current ages, there are few times I feel our older son's blindness plays a factor in a particular situation, so for the most part, we rarely mention blindness as a difference between them. When blindness does put our older son at a disadvantage (for example, when cleaning the room and picking up only those things that are his) I explain to our younger son how difficult it might be right now for Ethan to distinguish what belongs to whom and that he can use some help while he learns these things. Then I make sure that I work with Ethan and expect him to begin picking up his toys on his own.

I do see our younger son gaining insight into various differences we all have. I tell both boys that most everyone has some "thing" that makes them different. It may be height (or lack, thereof), weight, speech, learning, or interests. We're all different from each other and that is one of the things that makes the world so interesting.

Encourage Sharing and Discussing of Emotions

Just like you, your children may have many strong emotions about their sibling's visual impairment. These emotions will likely change with age and circumstance. Even though a child may seem fine with it for awhile, something may happen to make him feel sad, or angry, or resentful. It is tricky to know how to balance letting your child know that it is OK to express negative feelings with your desire to protect your child who has a visual impairment from feeling guilty or responsible.

It will probably be helpful to make sure that your children have plenty of opportunities to talk to you when the two of you are alone. This will give them chances to express and get feedback on the feelings they have about different situations. Of course, you can always consider getting counseling for your children if they seem particularly distressed or if you are having trouble dealing with their emotions. You may also be able to take advantage of sibling support groups in your community or even possibly online. If you can't find one, you may consider starting a group yourself.

Let Siblings Be Siblings

It is important to examine the relationship between your children to make sure that it is appropriate. It can be tempting to put more re-sponsibility for care-taking on your children who are sighted but this can cause several problems, not the least of which is the message to your child who is visually impaired that she needs to be taken care of. If your child who is sighted is oldest, it may be appropriate to assign him or her some "babysitting" tasks when you are briefly gone from the house. But it is not a good idea to have a younger sibling "babysitting" for an older child who is visually impaired.

Try to strike a balance that allows your children to help each other (which we expect from all children) without assigning responsibilities to your sighted children that are usually the responsibility of parents. Encourage and appreciate that your children need to do sibling-like activities together, such as playing and giggling about a joke, and even, maybe, arguing a little bit!

Don't Insist You Do Everything As a Family

Although it is important to have fun as a family, it's also important to let siblings have alone time and time with other friends. Don't automatically reject an activity because your child with visual impairments could not participate in it. Sometimes let the brother or sister do things like this with friends or one parent.

Likewise, don't insist that your child with visual impairments go to all of her sibling's activities, if one or both would be happier doing something else. By creating an environment that values all of the different relationships (parent-child, child-child) in your family, you will give everyone a variety of options for support.

Responsibilities and Privileges

Some parents report that they have difficulty deciding how much responsibility to give to children and when to give it. Of course, you won't give the same tasks to a two-year-old that you will give to a five-year-old, but by breaking tasks down into parts, you can guide each child to take some responsibility at almost any age. For example, your child who is visually impaired may not be ready to take the garbage out independently, but perhaps she can scrape her dinner plate into the kitchen garbage. Later, she can carry one bag while a parent or sibling carries another, walking together to the outside garbage can. Eventually, she should be able to complete the entire task independently. The procedure for increasing responsibilities is the same for all children, but you will need to pay attention to your children's individual needs and abilities.

Paralleling the question about responsibilities is the question about the privileges you allow for each of your children. Giving privileges to children is a way to show them that you trust them. Children who have visual impairments have the same need to know that you think they are becoming more responsible and that they are trusted with privileges. Allowing your child to spend the night at a friend's house or have a friend spend the night at your house will give you a chance to show your child that you trust her to be independent.

One issue that seems to complicate both responsibilities and privileges is overprotection. Your child will likely have to deal with overprotection all her life. There will always be people who want to protect individuals who are blind or visually impaired. In a way, that is a nice thing, as this is often done out of concern. But in reality, it can limit your child's freedom and confidence. There are important safety issues that must be considered and addressed, but, if an activity can be made safe (and it almost always can), then your child should be allowed and encouraged to do the same things that a sighted child would do at the same age. For example, if your other child was allowed to walk down the street to a friend's house when she was eight, then your child who is blind should also be allowed to do this at about the same age. This will take some instruction and practice, but your child will benefit from having an age-appropriate level of independence and the social situations that this allows. In turn, this will help her build confidence in her abilities and in your trust of her.

Understand Conflicts Before You Intercede

It's normal for siblings to have arguments and disagreements but this can be disturbing to parents. Resist the temptation to step in and solve conflicts for your children—they need to learn to deal with other people and to work out problems for themselves. There may be some situations that will make it important that you intervene, for example if your child who is sighted is taking advantage of your child who has visual impairments in some way (hiding from her or using her as an unjustified scapegoat). On the other hand, you will also want to be careful that your child who is visually impaired does not take advantage of the situation by acting helpless to get her sibling to give in to her.

■■ Deciding to Have More Children (Or Not)

One of the most important and difficult decisions that any couple makes is how many children to have. Now that you are experiencing parenting with a "twist," you are right to make your decision about having other children in the light of the current demands and your lifestyle as well as your own personal feelings and your finances.

There are three major issues that you will want to consider. First, you will want to gather information about whether or not another child might also be born with a visual impairment. Some conditions have a genetic basis and there would be an increased likelihood that a second child might have the same disability or disabilities as your first child. Your decision to have another child or not should therefore include a careful examination of genetic issues and how you feel about having a second child with disabilities.

Second, you should carefully consider the emotional, social, and financial impact of having a second child. Do you have the personal and financial resources necessary to provide support for your family? For instance, if one of you has stopped working outside the home to care for your child with a visual impairment, can you support another child on your family's income? Especially if your child has other significant disabilities besides a visual impairment, do you feel as if you have the energy and emotional resources to care for another child?

Third, you will likely also think about the implications of having other children in relation to your family dynamics. Do you believe that children should have siblings to provide family support throughout life? If you originally thought that you would like to have just one child (or two or three), does having a child with a visual impairment change your previous reasoning?

Perhaps you can ponder these questions and make a completely logical decision. Then again, you may find that in the end you have to go with your gut feelings. This is how it was for us. Before Ethan was born, we'd thought we would like to have at least two children. After we learned that he would most likely be blind, however, we went through a period of several months when we reconsidered this goal. As we mentioned before, our early thoughts were that Ethan would need a sibling to "take care of him." We had such limited experience with people who were blind that we didn't know that this would not be necessary, but that a sibling relationship with mutual care and support would be more likely and valuable.

When Ethan was about six months old we heard about a baby girl who'd been born with anophthalmia (absence of the eye). The baby's mother was very young, had no partner to help her raise her daughter, and was living at home with an older sister and father who were unsupportive. As it was reported to us, this young mother had said, "Well, I'd have put her up for adoption, but who'd want her?" We were all horrified by her attitude and thought long and hard about this baby. We discussed the situation and decided that if the young mother's current attitude prevailed, we would definitely consider adopting the baby. Although we never heard about the little girl again and hoped the mother had changed her outlook, we experienced an important realization. That is, we realized that even if we had another child with a visual impairment (or some other disability, for that matter), we would be all right. This added to our conviction that we should go ahead and have another child of our own.

▪▪ Communication and Support

As you can see from reading this chapter, there are endless issues that parents and families encounter every day. This is true for all families who are guiding their children to full, productive lives. Parents of children who are blind or visually impaired face the same challenges as all families with some added twists and turns. Keeping a sense of humor and an understanding of your priorities can be difficult. Here are some general suggestions for getting through the celebrations and the challenges:

- *Rely on yourself.* Regardless of your situation and whether or not you have other people to support you and your child, you have personal resources that will allow you as an individual to do the best you can for your child.
- *Rely on friends and family.* If you are fortunate enough to have supportive friends and family members, be sure to use them as a sounding board and a shoulder when you need it. They can be your best critics and strongest allies.
- *Rely on others who have had similar experiences.* Make sure to connect with other parents of children who are blind or visually impaired to share experiences, advice, and resources. Also get to know some adults with visual impair-

ments; they can provide excellent mentoring opportunities and give you great advice as you help your child develop.

■ *Rely on professionals.* There are many people who will be there to help you and your child get the resources and support necessary to fully participate in educational and community experiences. Connecting with a teacher of students with visual impairments early can save you a lot of time and effort. In addition, make sure to seek out other professionals (for example, social workers, therapists, or genetic counselors) when you need them. They are there to help.

:: Conclusion

Throughout this chapter we have tried to provide some information about creating a positive family environment based on our own experience and the experience of others with whom we have had contact. As our children grow, we are constantly revisiting what our family needs and how we can best support each other. It takes some trial-and-error experimenting to find out what works, but in the end we've always found that we can accomplish what we set out to do, and both the journey and the destination have been rewarding.

You will probably make decisions about what is best for your own family based on your family heritage, religious beliefs, and cultural history. The issues related to how you create a family are highly individual, and each family will be different, maybe in subtle but powerful ways. The important thing to remember is that you and your child or children share a connection that is different from any other relationship in life, and by concentrating on these family connections, you can create a positive foundation for your child's future.

:: Parent Statements

The other day we went to a community picnic. After we ate, the whole group started a game of pick-up softball. We really wanted to play but were a little reluctant at first. Then one of the fathers saw us just sitting on our blanket and he stopped the game and asked if we wanted to play. There are four of us—me, my wife, my daughter Leti, and my son Louis. This neighbor asked Louis if he wanted to bat the ball and then he and I showed Louis how it was all done. Louis swung the bat and actually hit the ball. I ran the bases with him. I can't believe how exciting it was. Louis was a real part of the game and everyone had so much fun. I think it was even more fun for everyone because Louis was included. In a way, I'm sorry I didn't think of it myself, but really, our neighbor is so proud of himself and I think he and Louis have become fast friends as a result.

❧

We like the challenge of finding activities for the entire family. It can be difficult because my children are years apart in age and have very different interests. Add to that Maria's visual impairment and our choices become more limited. Still, we are committed to spending time together and the children now help us find special activities we all enjoy.

❧

My children don't always get along. It is so much easier when they are not arguing, but I guess this is just a part of being siblings.

❧

We used to get a babysitter and go out with friends every once in a while but ever since T.J. was born I have been reluctant to give that responsibility to anyone. I just don't think I could enjoy myself—I'd be too worried about him.

❧

The first time my husband and I went out alone together was when Colleen was about a year old. A friend came over and basically made us go out to dinner. I was scared at first, but I really enjoyed it. Now we have a regular date night every couple of weeks.

❧

My husband and I don't have much of a life outside of work and our home. I don't think we've been out to see a movie in two years. Usually, we're too tired to even rent a video. I'm hoping this will change as the kids get older.

❧

Sometimes I think my other children get short-changed. Damian needs so much of our time and attention.

❧

We started a braille class for parents. We would meet once a week and the purpose of the class was to learn braille but it turned into so much more. I couldn't believe how much support we all gave each other. At Christmas we brailled the gift tags for the presents under the tree. It was great for our children to figure out which presents were theirs!

❧

I've never been much of a "joiner," so it's hard for me to go to parent group meetings. There are a couple of parents I email with, though.

❧

I try to make sure other parents are comfortable with my child. I don't want him to be left out of birthday parties or sleepovers.

❧

I always want to do everything by myself. It's so hard for me to ask for help.

❧

I didn't feel up to going to a parent group until my daughter was seven or eight months old. It took me that long to feel like I was ready to talk about things with strangers.

❧

I couldn't do it without my mother. She has been great. She always loved Jimmy, from the moment he was born. His blindness just doesn't matter to her.

7

NURTURING YOUR CHILD'S SELF-ESTEEM

Dean W. Tuttle, Ph.D., &
Naomi R. Tuttle, B.S.N.

One of the most important jobs of parenthood is nurturing your child's understanding of himself. This includes a healthy appreciation for his strengths as well as a recognition and acceptance of his weaknesses. It may be difficult, but as adults, most of us are able to describe ourselves pretty accurately ("I'm a kind and loyal friend, but I'm disorganized and a little sloppy," or, "I am good in a crisis but tend to procrastinate too much"). As a parent, you have a great deal of influence over how your child comes to view himself. This is important, because how your child views himself is intimately connected with his self-esteem, or feelings of self-worth. Healthy self-esteem is an essential ingredient for your child's sense of well-being.

People with high self-esteem feel competent to meet the day-to-day demands on their lives. Therefore, they feel as if they have control over themselves and their lives. Rather than waiting helplessly or passively to see how events will turn out, they take active steps to influence the events. They feel good enough about themselves to set high goals, and they have the persistence to keep trying even if there are disappointing setbacks. They are able to make decisions for themselves and to live with the consequences of those decisions.

Children with visual impairments are just as capable of developing high self-esteem as other children. Because of their vision loss, however, they may encounter more than the usual number of obstacles on the road to increased self-esteem. Many, if not most of these obstacles, are thrown in their way by other people. For example, your child may not be included in the neighborhood game of hide-and-seek. The other children may not mean to be insensitive, may not know how to include your child, and may not understand that he would enjoy participating in their fun. Also, some parents tend to want to do things for their child with a visual impairment because it often seems easier, quicker, and more efficient. But this prevents their child from learning to do things independently and from experiencing success for himself. Parents may overprotect their child to shield him from making mistakes, from experiencing failures, or from encountering danger. But once again, this inhibits the child's ability to learn and grow from the types of experiences that other children have. Further blows to developing self-esteem can come from unthinking or ignorant remarks made in the child's presence. These remarks could be made by anyone—someone passing in the street, a store clerk, or a classmate. Some of these comments can be shrugged off, but others, especially from someone who matters to the child, can be hurtful.

Obviously, parents cannot (and should not) intercept every passing comment that might bruise their child's self-esteem. But they can nurture feelings of self-worth in their child in many ways. These feelings will help him feel comfortable and secure with himself and his abilities regardless of others' opinions. This chapter describes suggestions that might help you provide support for developing your child's high self-esteem.

❚❚ Nurturing Your Child's Self-Esteem

Developing good self-esteem is a life-long task, and can be plagued by many setbacks. Experiences or events that cause your child to question his self-worth can occur at any time, forcing him to work through his feelings about himself once again. The groundwork for healthy self-esteem, however, is laid during the early years. Young children depend almost exclusively on feedback from others, especially parents, teachers, and friends, in forming conclusions about their own self-worth.

Your child's self-esteem will tend to rise and fall with what people say and do and how these words and actions are interpreted. As he grows and matures, however, he will increasingly rely on his own judgments of success and worth for his sense of self-esteem.

As a parent, you are in the ideal position to shape your child's self-perceptions in a positive way. You can help him begin to find meaning and purpose to his life, establish a strong set of personal standards and values, and begin setting goals for himself. In so doing, you can pave the way for him to become a mature adult, capable of objectively judging his own strengths and weaknesses.

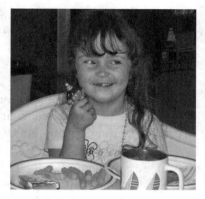

The Life-Long Adjusting Process

Because of the ever-changing demands in your child's life, he will continue to strive toward self-acceptance and self-esteem throughout his life. Although some days will be better than others, you can help your child by understanding that he will continue to deal from time to time with a variety of issues related to his visual impairment. He may, for example, need to think through and respond to unexpected difficulties or to demeaning stereotypes about individuals with visual impairments.

Your child may not experience all of the emotions described below when he encounters a problem or crisis stemming from impaired vision. However, when he becomes uncharacteristically angry, moody, or withdrawn, you may want to consider the possibility that he is wrestling with another personal predicament.

Trauma. From time to time, your child may experience the sting of being different. This may be caused by other people's reaction to his need to use adaptive techniques that are not used by his classmates: low vision devices, slate and stylus, or a talking calculator. For the teenager, the trauma may occur when his friends obtain their learner permits to drive.

Another type of trauma results from encounters with the social stigma of blindness within the community. Many insensitive remarks are rooted in the false notions that people with visual impairments are helpless, unthinking, and unfeeling. One horrified mother tells of an encounter at a party with an elderly gentleman who patted her five-year-old on the head and said, "Bless his poor heart. I just want to cry when I see children like him."

Shock and Denial. After your child has experienced a trauma similar to the one described above, he may be stunned or numb. Or he may simply deny that it ever happened. He may be unable and unwilling to talk about it. Feelings of unreality, detachment, and disbelief are common during this phase. Within reason, both shock and denial are normal and healthy parts of the adjusting process. Shock and denial allow your child to buy time to sort things out before dealing with the consequences of the trauma. Your role as a parent during this phase is to provide continuing emotional support and let some time pass.

Mourning and Withdrawal. As the numbness fades, your child may express feelings of sadness. You will want to allow (and even encourage) him to vent his frustrations concerning the painful encounter. This is usually a time of self-pity, when your child may withdraw from family and friends—a lonely time. Along with the feelings of sadness, there may be expressions of anger and hostility. Try not to become defensive if you just happen to be around when your child lashes out at the closest person around. Your child is reacting to a difficult situation, not directing his anger at you personally. You need to be a good listener, to try to understand your child's point of view, and above all, to give him an extra dose of tender loving care.

Succumbing and Depression. Your child may then begin to verbalize, one by one, the activities or relationships he feels he has lost or cannot achieve. Frequently, your child's perceptions of inabilities or losses are not grounded in fact. It is a good idea to help him sort fact from fiction. For example, he may conclude, after being teased on the playground, "I will never have another friend in my whole life." Or, as a teenager, he may say, "If I can't drive, I can't date." This is the "I can't" phase. Before your child gets too depressed, try to help him by establishing some short-term goals that are easily attainable. For instance, if he is worried about making friends, invite one child over to play a game with him, or to accompany your family to McDonald's.

If it seems that your child cannot get past his depression or if you don't feel comfortable supporting him through this, you should seriously consider getting support from a qualified therapist or counselor. Your child's teacher of students with visual impairments may be able to give you information about some local counseling resources.

Reassessment and Reaffirmation. If your child is feeling sorry for himself, sooner or later he will get tired of this feeling and want to get on with his life. This is often a time to reexamine the meaning of life and prioritize the things considered most important. "It's more important that I get my work done with pride than it is to be embarrassed about using my slate and stylus in public." "It's more important to develop friendships than it is to drive." Since your child will be searching for affirmation as a person of value and worth, you will want to provide approving and confirming feedback.

Coping and Mobilization. Once your child's desire to live life to the fullest reawakens, he will be ready to learn additional techniques and strategies for coping with life's demands. Your child will be more willing to identify himself as "different" with respect to his vision, freeing himself to learn and use the adaptive skills and devices essential for a productive, satisfying life.

Also during this phase, your child will begin to use the available resources in the country, in the community, and within himself. Help him develop a system for obtaining and organizing information about service agencies, specialized programs, companies that sell adapted materials and equipment, and consumer groups, and teach him how to access these resources. Early and continuous exposure to a variety of technological devices, such as a CD player, a talking calculator, computer games, or blindness-related sites on the Internet, help your child with his knowledge and competence and his sense of being in control. Your child's teacher of students with visual impairments can help with this task.

Self-Acceptance and Self-Esteem. With the confidence that competence brings, your child will begin to develop or regain self-esteem as a person of dignity and worth. Rather than seeing himself as a visually impaired person, he will see himself as a person with many characteristics and traits, only one of which is related to his impaired vision. As much as possible, you should structure situations that will encourage and reinforce these positive perceptions. Your goal is to help him to become comfortable with himself—to like himself. It will be worth all of the effort when your child has acquired or regained self-acceptance and self-esteem.

Acceptance of others is based on self-acceptance. Your child will find it very difficult to appreciate and accept others until he has first learned to appreciate and accept himself.

Your child's journey toward healthy self-esteem will be facilitated by a warm and caring home, by genuine acceptance, and by a freedom to express thoughts and feelings. His self-esteem may fluctuate from day to day, depending on his experiences of the moment. Do not be surprised or alarmed when your child periodically cycles back through some or all of the emotions described above.

:: Guidelines for Fostering Self-Esteem

The suggestions below should help you foster healthy self-esteem in your child. Admittedly, it is impossible to stick to all of the guidelines all of the time. But if you can follow most of these recommendations most of the time, you will be doing you and your child a favor.

1. Don't neglect your own self-acceptance and self-esteem. Studies have shown that children are more likely to grow up with high self-esteem if their parents have high self-esteem. The reason is easy to understand. Unless you have some self-acceptance and self-esteem yourself, you will find it very difficult to accept and support your child. If you doubt your own abilities to make good decisions, you are less likely to trust your child to make decisions for himself.

Unfortunately, having a child with a visual impairment can be a threat to many parents' self-esteem, at least at first. In the beginning, some parents may lack the knowledge and coping skills essential for handling the new situation. They may feel overwhelmed by the emotional, physical, and financial stresses of raising a child with a disability, and may doubt their ability to manage. In addition, if they feel as if they have to rearrange their lives around their child's needs, they may feel as if their opportunities for personal growth have been stifled.

Chapters 3 and 6 describe some of the feelings and attitudes that can color your outlook on life when you have a child with a visual impairment. The suggestions in these chapters may help you begin to regain what self-esteem you may have lost so that you can better support your child.

2. Treat your child as a child first; focus on the child, not the visual impairment or other disabilities. Your child needs to know that you see him primarily as a child—your child—with the same basic needs of love, acceptance, and feelings of worth as everyone

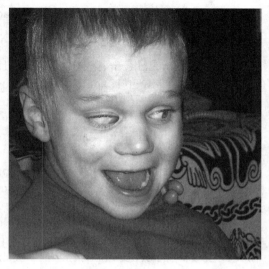

else. If you don't, you risk making your child feel separated from the family emotionally or physically, and he may become increasingly isolated and lonely. As you interact with your child, talk about experiences, friends, and emotions that he has in common with other children. He feels the cold snow on his nose, devours pizza, and likes to be hugged. Don't deny the fact that he has a visual impairment, but emphasize that this is only one of his many attributes. He is also five feet tall, has brown hair, and is a good trombone player.

3. Accept and respect your child's way of perceiving the world. Just because your child cannot see the things you can see does not make his interpretation of experiences any less real or valid than yours. The sound of a cardinal singing or his teacher's encouraging tone of voice can be just as thrilling for your child as the flash of red feathers or gleam of a smile is for a sighted child.

Don't point out what he cannot do. For example, don't tell him it's a shame he can't see the colored fall leaves. Instead, emphasize the different shapes of the leaves and the crunching sound they make as he walks through them. Encourage him to use the senses he can—for instance, by identifying what's cooking for supper by the smells and sounds in the kitchen.

4. Emphasize what your child can do while recognizing possible limitations. For the most part, you should have high expectations for your child. You should expect him to meet the same standards as other children his age. Your child's disability (or disabilities) may have an impact on *how* he accomplishes tasks, but not on whether he is capable of accomplishing them. Some people argue that expectations should be "realistic." But, really, it is almost impossible for us to know what is realistic for anyone. Our accomplishments depend on our skills, abilities, and talents along with the support we receive from other people.

We must somehow find a middle ground between setting expectations that are too low and expectations that are too high. To reduce discouragement and frustration, you will want to help him establish goals that are not too high. On the other hand, you do not want to set your sights too low, or your child will not be challenged to grow and you will foster helplessness. For example, if you don't really expect him to learn to use a knife and fork, you may let him give up after only a few attempts, rather than searching for another way to teach him. The end results of both overly low and overly high expectations are the same: your child's self-esteem suffers and his feelings of worthlessness increase.

Goals that can be achieved with effort and ingenuity will give your child a sense of accomplishment, a desire to keep on trying new activities, and a boost to his self-esteem. It is important for you as his parent to help him find his strengths and capitalize on them.

5. Speak clearly, without relying on facial expressions and body language to convey meaning. If necessary, and with your child's permission, you may need to manipulate his body to show him what you want him to do. Children who do not have visual impairments pick up cues indicating approval and encouragement from smiles, winks, and other body language of others. Children with visual impairments need to rely more on the spoken word and tone of voice to feel included in interactions with family members and peers.

Keep conversations with your child as natural as possible. There is no need to avoid visually oriented words such as "look" and "see," as they are also part of your child's vocabulary.

6. Encourage your child to do things independently. As his parent, you might be tempted to protect your child from all danger, physical or emotional. Your motive may be a genuine desire to shield him from failure. However, it is impossible to shield him throughout life and it is important to allow him to experience difficulty while you are around to support and encourage him. He also learns that failure to accomplish something does not mean he is a failure. He can learn the joy of finally completing a task by himself after repeated attempts, trying harder, and perhaps adapting his method of attack.

Do not rush to help your child at the first sign of difficulty. If he seems to be struggling, especially with a new task, ask him if he needs help, rather than assuming that you need to step in and help. Although it may be quicker to dress him each day, this conveys a subtle message that he is not as capable as his peers who can put on their own clothes. Until he can perform a task successfully, it is better to break up the task into smaller, achievable steps and to allow more time to finish. Praise his accomplishments and compare his achievements today with what he could do a month ago, not with what his sighted peers can do.

7. Praise your child for genuine accomplishments and tasks well done. Praise encourages your child to keep on trying a task that is initially difficult for him. Praise him when he completes a task even if it is not done perfectly, but done to the best of his ability. A child is never too young to understand that he is a source of joy to Mom and Dad.

Try to avoid false praise for achievements that are ordinary or routine. Phony, excessive flattery can have two possible consequences: the child's self-esteem might be unrealistically inflated, or a more mature child might perceive it as a demeaning and devaluating attitude toward blindness.

8. Do not accept blindness as an excuse for unacceptable behavior. Your child needs to understand and keep to the same behavioral standards as any other child. Avoiding discipline because your child has a disability is likely to damage his self-esteem. When a child knows he has done wrong, he expects his parents to respond appropriately. In addition, siblings and peers are quick to pick up on subtle differences in behavior standards and may resent your child if he is allowed to get away with behavior they are not.

9. Be honest with your child about his appearance and behavior. When his appearance or behavior is not socially acceptable, let him know in a tactful, caring way. In some situations, you will need to serve as his mirror, letting him know and teaching him what clothes match and don't match, when his hair looks uncombed, or his fly is unzipped. Help your child to keep current with clothing fads and hair styles so that it is easier for him to be a part of his peer group. Be sure also to teach socially acceptable behavior: how to shake hands when greeting an adult or how to face someone when in conversation. When your child is comfortable and confident with his appearance and social behaviors, he will be comfortable and confident when interacting with others.

10. Give frank and accurate answers to your child's questions about how his visual impairment will affect his life. As he grows up, your child, like every child, will wonder about careers, sex, relationships, and so forth. And like every child, he has a right to know what possibilities lie ahead of him so he can plan realistically for the future. All children are naturally curious, and if your child is unable to get satisfactory answers from his parents, he will seek answers from his peers. This can lead to faulty, distorted, or prejudicial information that would undermine his self-esteem even more.

If you don't know the answer to a question, admit it. Then make an honest attempt to find someone who does know the answer. There

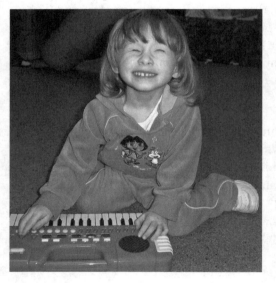

are a number of resources that can help. On the local level, your child's teacher of students with visual impairments or the rehabilitation teacher who works out of the state department or rehabilitation services would be more than happy to answer your questions. On the national level, such organizations as the American Foundation for the Blind, the National Association for Parents of the Visually Impaired, the American Council of the Blind, and the National Federation of the Blind all have knowledgeable people available to assist you.

11. Encourage your child to be involved in community activities. Active participation in school activities, club programs, sports, and other group activities will help him become a real member of the community. This leads to two important outcomes. In the first place, your child will gain a sense of belonging to a group. Fulfilling the need to belong is fundamental to healthy self-esteem. Second, peer interactions within these groups provide your child with many more opportunities to practice and reinforce his emerging social skills. Such opportunities to socialize outside the home may be just as important for your child as school work. For this reason, every effort should be made to involve your child into youth programs in the community outside of school hours.

12. Be aware of your feelings and attitudes toward blindness and be careful not to inadvertently communicate negative attitudes. As parents learn to cope with the demands of raising a child with a visual impairment, it is normal for them to feel a wide range of emotions. Some of these emotions will be positive—pride in their child's accomplishments; admiration at the way he handles challenges; appreciation for the warmth of a hug from their child's loving arms; pleasure in his spark and spontaneity; gratitude for support services.

Other emotions will inevitably be negative. At times, for example, you may resent your child for taking up so much of your attention and energy. You may find yourself blaming him because you have less time to socialize with friends or pursue your interests and hobbies. Some parents may even blame their child's disability for all the problems in the family, from money woes to sibling rivalry.

Whether or not negative feelings about your child's disability are justified, it is important not to communicate them to your child. If your child senses negative or hostile messages from you, he may conclude that he is bad because he is blind or he is unwanted because he is a burden. Respond to your child as a person, not to his visual impairment, and your child can avoid associating negative values with his visual impairment.

13. Help your child develop a healthy sense of humor. The ability to laugh at yourself, at your mistakes or blunders, or at the absurdities of life helps to relieve stress and boost self-esteem. Like any child, your child will learn to laugh from the example of others around him. He may, however, need some explanations. When Dad breaks into laughter as he is heading out the door for a meeting and discovers he has on one brown and one black shoe, the situation will need to be described for your child. The absurdity of a little cat keeping a large dog at bay with one swipe of his paw is funny, but not to your child until someone interprets the absurdity for him. Although these explanations take time, they will help your child develop a healthy perspective of himself and life.

One note of caution: when modeling a sense of humor for your child, steer clear of humor that depends on sarcastic or caustic remarks. For example, if your child knocks over a glass of milk at the dinner table, don't say something like "For a blind person, you're doing just fine." Remarks that are intended to be funny but are really put-downs are damaging to the self-esteem of the one who is the brunt of the joke.

14. Don't make your child the focal point of the family. Although your child may sometimes need more attention and help than other members of the family do, he needs to understand that family life cannot always revolve around him. Like every child, he must learn that other people have needs and desires, too, and that these needs and desires will sometimes take precedence over his. If he does not learn these lessons, he will be in for a huge blow to his self-esteem when he enters the real world of school and work. In the real world, everyone competes as an equal. Everyone is expected to take turns, wait in lines, share, and pull their own weight; so your child may as well learn to do these things within the family.

■■ Conclusion

Most parents share similar dreams for their children. They want their children to be happy. They want them to have rewarding, fulfilling lives. And they want them to grow up to be capable, independent adults. How much you can do to help these dreams come true for *your* child depends on many factors. Some of these factors—such as the extent and nature of his disabilities and how they affect his ability to learn—are out of your control. But other factors are very much under your influence. One of the most important factors you can influence is whether your child has the self-esteem to enable him to keep striving for success even when he is occasionally confronted with overwhelming odds.

Building self-esteem in your child is not a difficult job, but it is an ongoing job. As this chapter explains, almost any interaction you have with your child can be an opportunity to encourage the development of healthy self-esteem. The key is to become aware of how your actions and attitudes can affect your child's perceptions of himself. With the right kinds of support from you, your child can develop healthy self-esteem and look forward to a rich, rewarding, and satisfying life.

∷ Parent Statements

I want to protect my child from all those people who say hurtful things. But at the same time, I know that it will help his self-confidence and self-esteem to learn how to deal with comments himself.

❦

My child's grandparents love him unconditionally. Sometimes I think that they spoil him, but their honest affection for him is really wonderful.

❦

I think the way I react to blindness will make a difference in how my child feels about himself.

❦

I feel sure we will be able to take care of Joey's physical needs but I worry about his self-esteem. I have less control over that.

❦

The more independent Patty is, the better she will feel about herself.

❦

This past summer I went to a camp for visually impaired preschool children and their parents. There were several adults who were blind at the camp. We ate together, played together, walked on the beach, and sang camp songs. I loved meeting these adults who were very honest and generous with us. I know that Megan will have some challenges, but these adults have made it and so can we.

❦

My son, my daughter (who is blind), and I were shopping at a local mall recently. I had just taken them to get haircuts at a shop in the mall and we were walking back to the car my son said "Daddy, why are all those people staring at us?" Well, I took a deep breath and was about to explain that maybe they had never see anyone who was blind when my daughter put her hand up to her head and said "They probably like my new hairdo!" What a great self-concept!

❦

It's hard to think about working on self-esteem when we have so many other problems to address.

❧❀❧

My child is certainly his own person. He has a strong sense of what he likes and doesn't like. Some people think that Wayd is stubborn, but I think he is confident! I look forward to watching him grow!

EARLY INTERVENTION

AND

SPECIAL EDUCATION

Bob Brasher, M.S., &
M. Cay Holbrook, Ph.D.

Like all children, children with visual impairments have diverse learning abilities. Some are talented in many academic areas, some excel in a few areas, some are pretty much "average" students, and some find learning most things a struggle. Regardless of abilities, however, most children with visual impairments will need some extra help to succeed in school due to the challenges that visual impairments (and sometimes additional disabilities) pose to learning.

Many children with visual impairments begin receiving educational support in infancy to help them learn to cope with our visually oriented world and to prepare them for formal education programs. Others may be enrolled in a formal educational program during the preschool years or later.

More and more we have realized that the experience of all children during the preschool years lays the foundation for later learning. This is particularly true for children with visual impairments. Some parents receive early assistance and become aware of their child's educational needs and how to meet those needs right from the start. Other parents may be at a loss as to what to do before they are able to hook up with professionals who can help.

This chapter will provide general information on educational services. Some of the information in this chapter will be applicable now, some will be helpful to you as your child grows, and some of this information will not apply to your child at all.

◼◼ What Kinds of Help Are Available?

As Chapter 9 explains, a very important federal law guarantees children with visual impairments the right to special educational help, if necessary. The Individuals with Disabilities Education Improvement Act (IDEIA or IDEA 2004), P.L. 108-446, mandates educational help for children with disabilities aged three and over, while Part C of IDEA provides educational assistance for children birth to two years of age.

If your child is three years of age or over and qualifies for assistance under IDEA 2004, she will receive what is known as "special education." If she is under three years of age, she will receive "early intervention." As the sections below point out, early intervention and special education services are basically the same, no matter what they are called. However, there may be some differences in how often and where the services are provided. From an administrative standpoint, there may be a difference in the source of funding, but finding financial support for appropriate programs is the responsibility of agencies, centers, schools, and/or departments administering the law. While you may be curious or interested in how funding is allocated, it is not your job to solve the problems of funding and you should never be made to feel uncomfortable or guilty about the cost of specialized services.

What Is Special Education?

There are many reasons that special education can be considered "special." The main reason, however, is that special education programs are tailor-made to fit the unique learning strengths and needs of the individual child. Teaching rates and styles, instructional materials, and educational goals are all designed to fit the child's specific learning abilities. This is in contrast to "regular" or "general" education programs, where teachers teach many children the same subjects using the same methods and materials.

A major goal of special education is to teach children the skills and knowledge that they need to become as independent as possible. For this reason, special education programs are not limited to traditional "academic" subjects such as reading and math. They also include special therapeutic and other services intended to help children overcome difficulties in all areas of development. For example, special education can help a child improve mobility or communication skills. For children with visual impairments, the set of skills that are needed in addition to the general education curriculum is called the "Expanded Core Curriculum." The box on page 204 describes and lists areas of the Expanded Core Curriculum. Additional information about the Core Curriculum and Expanded Core Curriculum can be found in Chapter 13.

By law, a child's special education program must include all the special services, or "related services," she needs to benefit from her educational program. These services are provided by one or more professionals trained in working with children with special needs. For children with visual impairments, special education services may include instruction from a teacher of students with visual impairments, an orientation and mobility instructor, a speech-language pathologist, an occupational therapist, a physical therapist, and/or a psychological services professional.

As discussed later in this chapter, special education and related services may be provided in a variety of educational settings. For example, a child might receive special education services within a regular classroom or within a classroom of only children with visual impairments, or in many other classroom settings. Where a child receives services depends on how and where she learns best.

What Is Early Intervention?

Early intervention can typically be thought of as special education for children birth to three years of age. It consists of special instruction or therapy designed to help infants and toddlers with special needs improve their developmental skills. This intervention is intended to optimize a child's abilities and build a foundation for further learning. Just as in special education programs, the therapeutic and educational services a child receives are tailored to meet her unique learning needs. Educational services for infants with visual impairments often include instruction and support from an early intervention specialist and/or a teacher of students with visual impairments who has training in early

██ The Expanded Core Curriculum

Most people are familiar with the general education core curriculum. It includes areas like language arts, mathematics, social studies, and science. In the past ten years, professionals, parents, and people who are blind have outlined nine unique areas of learning that are important for children who are blind or visually impaired to learn in order to be independent and productive adults. The expanded core curriculum for children with visual impairments includes:

- Compensatory or functional academic skills, including communication modes (e.g., braille, use of tactile diagrams, listening skills)
- Orientation and mobility (understanding where you are and how to move safely from one place to another)
- Social interaction skills (e.g., making friends, interpreting social conventions that are largely based on visual input)
- Independent living skills (e.g., dressing, money identification and management, organization skills)
- Recreation and leisure skills
- Career education
- Use of assistive technology (e.g., use of braille notetakers or video magnifying devices)
- Visual efficiency skills (e.g., learning to use near and distance magnifiers, electronic magnification systems, educational video games, the use of light sources such as light boxes and variable intensity lamps)
- Self-determination (e.g., self-advocacy, development of self-esteem)

Paying attention to the expanded core curriculum from the very beginning can be very helpful. You can help your child develop a strong foundation for each of the areas of the expanded core curriculum by discussing them with other members of your child's educational team.

childhood; physical, occupational, or speech-language therapy; or counseling services for your family.

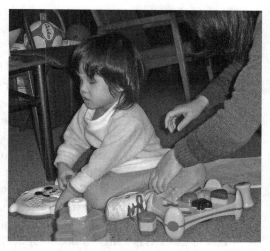

It has been estimated that 80-90 percent of learning occurs through vision. A sighted child learns about the world through observation of the people, places, and things around her. She watches her mother salt her food, so she picks up the salt shaker and imitates the motion. She sees Daddy come into the living room and wipe his dirty shoes on the mat, so she tries to do the same thing. Sighted children use their vision to begin learning about the world from the day they are born.

Children with visual impairments also begin learning about their world from the day they are born. A visual impairment has an impact on learning, however, by limiting opportunities to benefit from the experiences that are farther away than the child can reach, or that do not make noise. Children can and do learn effectively by using their senses of touch, hearing, smell, and taste. The sound an egg makes as it is fried is very different from the sound a boiling egg makes. Even so, this type of learning is different. It requires parents and teachers to become more efficient at using experiences that emphasize hearing and touch, smell and taste.

Early intervention is important for children with visual impairments because through instruction and modeling, children (and their parents) can learn how to best interact with the world using all of their senses—thus minimizing the possibility of delays in learning.

Effective early intervention programs not only help the child, but also the family. Parents learn about their child's eye condition and about the services available in the community. Teachers and therapists show them ways to help their child develop. In addition, counseling support may be available to help parents and other family members as they learn to deal with the challenges and rewards of raising a child with a visual impairment.

■■ Getting Started

Eligibility for early intervention and special education differs with each state's interpretation of the federal law. In general, however, your child is probably eligible for services if she needs special materials (such as braille or large print textbooks), or help learning special skills needed to compensate for her loss of vision (such as developing concepts, orientation and mobility skills, or listening skills).

As you get to know other parents, you will find that there are many different ways to enter into "the system" of early intervention or special education services. Children with more noticeable disabilities may be identified at birth or shortly after. In such cases, parents may be referred for services by a physician or healthcare professional. For other parents, the process is a little more complicated and they may need to take the initiative in finding helpful services for their child.

A good starting place in your quest to obtain early intervention or special education services is to call your state department of education, your state department of health, your state school for the blind, your state division of services for the blind, and/or a local disability organization such as Easter Seals. Addresses and phone numbers for the schools for the blind for each state can be found in the Resource Guide at the back of this book. If you live in a state that does not have a school for the blind, do not hesitate to call a school in a neighboring state, since they may have a regional program. This first phone call may lead to many others before you find the specific local resources that can help your family. Some parents have reported that this is a difficult time. Try not to get discouraged. The information that you uncover during this fact-finding time can help you become familiar with the range of services available to individuals with visual impairments.

Once you are connected with professionals in early intervention or special education, your child will go through assessment procedures to determine her eligibility for services. At the very least, you will be asked to provide documentation from an eye care specialist (ophthalmologist or optometrist) or other doctor(s) about your child's visual impairment. Your child may also be given a variety of tests by teachers, therapists, and other professionals. The purpose of any assessment is to determine your child's strengths and weaknesses so that an education program can be developed to help meet her needs while capitalizing on her abilities.

▪▪ Your Child's Education Program

After your child is found to be eligible for special education or early intervention services, the next step is to plan an individualized educational program. That is, this is the next step if you consent to have your child placed in early intervention or special education. As a parent, you cast the deciding vote as to whether—or when—your child should receive specialized services.

Assuming that you agree to your child's placement in early intervention or special education, a document will be drawn up describing educational goals for your child, as well as what will be done to help her reach her goals. If your child is receiving early intervention services, this document will be called an Individualized Family Service Plan (IFSP). If she is receiving special education, it will be called an Individualized Education Program (IEP).

If it is felt that your child primarily needs adaptations to the environment, a school district might instead develop a Section 504 plan for your child. Section 504 plans are for children whose disabilities have less of an educational impact than those who qualify for IEPs, and are developed to remove barriers that keep children from accessing educational services and curriculum. A 504 plan might specify, for instance, that your child is to receive adaptive textbooks and other equipment to make regular curricular materials accessible.

If your child is in a special education or early intervention program, you will become very familiar with IFSPs or IEPs. Basically, both the IFSP and IEP serve as written documentation of the yearly plan for your child. Both contain long-term goals for your child's education, as well as a statement of your child's current level of functioning. They also include decisions about the setting where your child is to receive services (in a regular classroom, at home, at the school for the blind). Chapter 9 provides a more comprehensive discussion about the elements of an IEP/IFSP.

The actual writing of your child's IEP/IFSP will generally occur at an annual meeting. Under IDEA 2004, some states may offer families the option of writing a new IEP only once every three years. Writing an IEP/IFSP is sometimes stressful and time consuming, but it allows you and the rest of the members of your child's educational team to review your child's progress and plan the best instructional program possible to meet her needs. Even though the option of writing an IEP every three years may be available, you will want to carefully consider the implications of allowing such a long time between formally writing a new IEP. There may also be legitimate and important reasons to request a meeting of the team between mutually agreed upon meeting times and that is your right.

You are a very important part of this process, so the special education or early intervention personnel should make sure that the meeting is scheduled at a convenient time for you to fully participate. You may wish to ask a family member, friend, or other professional to attend with you for advice and moral support. It is your right to bring such supporters to these meetings, and you will probably be encouraged to do so.

To help you take an informed role in planning your child's education, the next sections discuss the three most important elements covered in an IEP or IFSP: 1) educational goals; 2) services that can help a child reach her goals; and 3) educational settings where services can be provided.

What Will Your Child Learn?

What your child is taught in her early intervention or special education program depends on the goals determined in her IFSP or IEP based on her individual needs. As explained above, it is best if

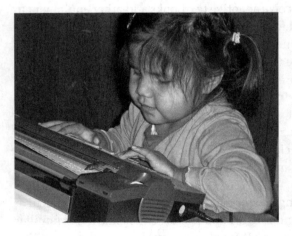

these goals are set *jointly* by educators and parents. Teachers and therapists will have one picture of your child's unique strengths and needs. This picture will be based on their assessment of your child and on any experience they have had working with her. You will also have a picture of her strengths and needs, based on your parenting experiences. If you and the educators can pool your ideas about what your child can and should learn next, she is more likely to end up with appropriate, sustainable goals.

Types of Goals

The specific goals for each child with a visual impairment vary greatly depending on readiness levels and whether there are additional disabilities. In general, however, three types of goals may be set for children with visual impairments:

1. academic,
2. functional, and
3. adaptive.

Academic goals are set for skills related to educational areas such as emergent literacy, reading, writing, and mathematics. Your child may have specific needs in any academic area where mastery of concepts is dependent upon vision. For example, without good vision, it may be difficult to tell the difference between a cow and a horse; grasp the difference in height between a tree and a skyscraper; or even understand what a bumper on a car is. Most children with sight learn these concepts by using their vision instead of exploring the objects by touch.

Functional goals address skills that your child needs to live as independently as possible. These might include eating skills, dressing skills, and toilet training. As your child grows, her goals for functional skills may become more and more complex, reflecting her increased abilities and her increased need for independence. For example, in the area of dressing, a very young child might work on putting on a coat or pulling up socks, while later goals may focus on tying shoes or buttoning a shirt. Still later goals may be to use make-up and learn hair care skills.

Adaptive goals cover specialized skills needed by your child because of her visual impairment. These include orientation and mobility skills, as well as tactual and auditory readiness skills. These goals include plans for addressing areas of the Expanded Core Curriculum. Instruction in these areas will help your child make maximum use of all her senses to gain independence and confidence.

Selecting Appropriate Goals

In planning your child's educational program, her educational team will consider goals that are considered "long-term" as a way of planning for your child. In addition, there will likely be a discussion about how these long-term goals will be accomplished. Historically, educational plans have included both long-term goals and short-term objectives related to each goal. The legal requirements of listing both long-term goals and short-term objectives are changing. However, you and your child's educational team will want to continue to discuss how your child's goals will be accomplished.

Your child's individualized education program (IEP) is a written statement that is developed and reviewed by her educational team. The IEP will include the following:

- a statement of your child's current level of educational performance (including how her disability or disabilities will have an impact on her involvement in the general education curriculum and assessments);
- a list of measurable annual goals (both academic and functional);
- a description of how your child's progress will be evaluated and when periodic reviews will be made;
- a section documenting the decision regarding your child's use of braille (new regulations require that braille be taught to children who are visually impaired unless the education team decides that braille is not the most appropriate media; see Chapter 10 for more information about literacy);
- a list of the special services that will be provided to your child to help her meet her annual goals and participate in the general education curriculum;
- an explanation of the educational team's decision regarding including your child in the general education classroom;
- a description of the accommodations that your child needs to participate in state- and district-wide assessments;
- a statement of dates for the beginning of services, and the frequency and duration of special education services; and
- when your child is 16, a plan for transition to postsecondary goals.

Children with multiple disabilities may participate in alternate achievement standards (meaning that they will not be participating in a general education classroom curriculum because of the impact of their disabilities). For those children, the IEP team will be required to include benchmarks (similar to behavioral goals) and short-term objectives that are reviewed annually to determine how the child is progressing in her educational plan.

Typically, goals are broad statements about areas that will be focused on. Goals might be phrased like this:

- Tony will explore his environment with all his senses.
- Jennifer will become more independent in dressing herself.
- Justin will feed himself independently.
- Stacy will play with other children.
- Kyle will demonstrate an understanding of "large" and "small" related to objects in his environment.

In contrast to broadly stated goals, objectives are more short-term and specific than goals. They are measurable (your child's accomplishment of the objective can be measured) and observable (you can watch your child's activity and know whether she has accomplished the objective). Usually, several objectives are associated with each goal. For instance, these objectives might be set for Jennifer to help her reach the goal in the example above:

- Jennifer will be able to zip the zipper on her jacket up and down ten times in a row.
- Jennifer will be able to tie her tennis shoes without assistance five days in a row.
- Jennifer will put on and take off her mittens independently ten times in a row.

Goals and objectives are written in a prescribed way. Your child's teacher or early intervention specialist can help you understand and become accustomed to the way that goals and objectives will be written for your child. Understanding this is important so that you can fully participate in planning your child's program.

Of course, the objectives for each child will be different because they will depend on each child's individual needs and abilities. You will not be able to look at any other child's IEP/IFSP and predict what your child will be working on. Objectives should be written in such a way that everyone understands not just what the child should be able to accomplish, but also *how* everyone will know if she has met the objectives.

For every objective or goal set for your child, a timeline for reaching that objective or goal should also be set. For example, the IFSP might specify that your child is expected to learn to zip her jacket in one month, or to learn to put on her mittens in three months. Or the IEP for an older child might list goals for improving reading or math skills to a certain grade level by the end of the school year.

As mentioned earlier, goals must be reevaluated every year at an IEP meeting, unless you live in one of the states that is trying out three-year goals. Even in those states, goals must be reevaluated annually, or more often, if you request such a meeting. If your child has met old goals, then new ones will be set. If your child has not met goals or objectives set for her, they may be restated, modified, or just carried over to the new year to give her more time to work on the skill. You must be invited to attend this meeting and will be encouraged to actively participate. You may also call a meeting to discuss the program and your child's progress at any time during the year.

▪▪ Who Will Work with Your Child?

Depending on their needs, children with visual impairments may receive special instruction or therapy from a variety of professionals. Some of these professionals are trained to work exclusively on issues related to visual impairments, while others have a broader background in working with children with disabilities in general. Both types of professionals will tailor their teaching methods and materials to best meet your child's needs and goals.

Described below are professionals who might work with your child at some point. Titles may vary somewhat from state to state, but areas of expertise should be the same.

Teacher of Students with Visual Impairments (TVI)

A teacher of students with visual impairments (also called vision teacher, VI teacher, teacher of the visually impaired, TVI) is a certified teacher who has received specialized training in meeting the educational needs of children with visual impairments. He or she may work directly with your child in such areas as:

- Encouraging movement by introducing toys that are visually or tactually interesting;
- Stimulating the use of all your child's senses;
- Teaching pre-reading skills such as tracking and finger positioning;
- Teaching braille reading and writing;
- Helping her with daily living skills development in areas such as eating and dressing;
- Assessing academic and social learning;

- Assessing functional vision and learning media (braille, print, or a combination of braille and print).

The TVI will have a major role in planning and implementing an educational program for your child. In some cases, the TVI might be your child's primary teacher. More often, the TVI might directly provide your child with targeted instruction (i.e., operating a piece of adaptive technology or working on braille reading and writing) or indirectly, by advising others about ways of enhancing your child's learning. He or she might consult with the regular classroom teacher about ways to adapt activities and materials to your child's ability. For example, the TVI might suggest to the regular classroom teacher that when the weather for the day is discussed during circle time, the children dress up in appropriate clothes instead of using a paper "weather doll" and pretend clothes.

A TVI can play a significant role on the team that creates your child's IFSP/IEP. This person may advocate for additional services and the purchase of appropriate technology and other needed materials.

TVIs are also great resources for parents because they can share their knowledge and understanding of how a visual impairment may affect many areas of learning and daily life. Generally, TVIs have experience working with many children with visual impairments and can therefore share how other families cope with the challenges of a visual impairment. A TVI might help you by suggesting ways to organize your child's toys or books so that she can locate them independently. Or he or she might recommend appropriate chores for your child to do around the house. By working together, parents and a TVI can create an environment that encourages independence.

Vision Consultant

Your child may also encounter a vision consultant. A vision consultant is trained in visual impairments and travels from preschool to preschool and/or school to school, providing technical assistance and support to educators. This consultant may help the preschool or classroom teacher choose appropriate toys and educational materials, may brainstorm with teachers and parents about effective adaptations, and may bring the newest instructional innovations to teachers for use with their students. Usually a vision consultant doesn't work directly with children with visual impairments, but provides suggestions to preschool staff, regular classroom teachers, program administrators, and families.

Orientation and Mobility (O&M) Specialist

The O&M Specialist (also called COMS or Certified Orientation and Mobility Specialist, O&M teacher, travel instructor, mobility specialist, peripatologist) is a certified instructor who has received special-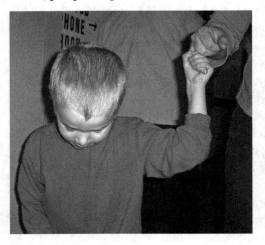ized training in teaching people with visual impairments to travel safely and efficiently. Usually the O&M specialist works with children individually. At first, instruction time is spent learning basic concepts relating to space and direction (over and under, left and right). Later, the O&M specialist begins work on independent travel skills (within a room, from room to room, to the cafeteria and bathrooms, to the playground, and, with your permission, into the community). The O&M specialist will teach your child when it is appropriate to use a sighted guide, when to use a cane, and, when your child is much older, when and if a guide dog might be useful.

Eventually, your child will master the skills that allow her to travel safely through her environment. With the assistance of an O&M specialist, it's possible and likely that a child who is totally blind will learn to cross busy streets, catch a bus, and locate a new travel destination independently.

See Chapter 11 for more information on orientation and mobility.

Clinical Low Vision Specialist

A clinical low vision specialist may be an optometrist, an ophthalmologist, or a university-trained professional. He or she specializes in helping children with limited visual ability optimize their remaining vision. The clinical low vision specialist will work with your child to find the best way to enhance her vision—whether through handheld magnifiers, monoculars (telescopes), special high-powered glasses for reading, or electronic magnifiers that enlarge print onto a screen.

Children typically see this specialist when someone (a parent, vision specialist, classroom teacher, the orientation and mobility specialist) determines that a low vision device might be helpful. If your child's vision or her educational needs or performance have changed, then she may be referred for a visit (or follow-up visit) to the clinical low vision specialist.

The clinical low vision specialist is not usually the child's primary eye care specialist. He or she will generally work with the TVI and orientation and mobility specialist to determine which low vision devices are effective for a child. The TVI and orientation and mobility specialist will then help the child learn to use low vision devices. Low vision devices may assist your child with near tasks or with locating objects at a distance.

It may be difficult to find a low vision clinic in your area. Some residential schools for the blind, state departments of health, rehabilitation facilities, and local hospitals or clinics operate low vision clinics. Some states also have readily available "for profit" clinics operated by trained low vision eye care specialists. The cost of such services varies widely. While some clinics offer low vision evaluations free of charge or at a nominal rate, others are very expensive. In addition to the above resources, you may wish to contact the American Foundation for the Blind for a listing of low vision clinics in your state.

Early Intervention Service Coordinator

A service coordinator is the professional with the major responsibility for guiding your child's early intervention or preschool education program. He or she also usually coordinates all the services your child needs. The service coordinator can assist with a variety of issues, from scheduling your child's therapists to arranging for an appointment with an eye care specialist. Federal law mandates that all children who qualify for early intervention programs be assigned a service coordinator who has expertise in the area of primary disability.

Other Specialists

If your child has additional disabilities, other therapists or specialists may work with her. These special therapists could include:
- an occupational therapist (for help with fine motor skills such as holding a pencil or fork or fastening buttons);
- a physical therapist (for help with gross motor skills such as holding up her head, sitting, and walking);

- a speech-language pathologist (for help with comprehending and expressing communication);
- a special education teacher or infant education specialist (for help with pre-academic and academic skills such as shape recognition, reading, and math).

If a visual impairment is your child's only disability, it is unlikely that these professionals will work directly with her. Her TVI or O&M specialist, however, may consult with them if your child is having difficulty in a particular area.

Paraprofessionals

There has been a recent trend in special education to assign an individual paraprofessional to children identified as having special needs. Paraprofessionals are also called teaching assistants, aides, educational assistants, and other terms. There are many appropriate roles for paraprofessionals to play such as production of braille or accessible materials and assistance to the teacher to free him or her for instructional time. It is not appropriate for paraprofessionals to provide your child with her educational program. Most paraprofessionals are not trained teachers and should not be providing instruction. Please note that knowledge of braille for personal use or production does not qualify a paraprofessional to teach braille to your child.

Parents are often relieved that their child will be getting extra attention from an adult at school without considering the possible negative consequences of this one-on-one assistance. Ultimately, you want your child to learn to complete tasks on her own. Yet if she receives too much assistance from a paraprofessional, unexpected negative results can include increased dependence, lack of self-confidence, and barriers to naturally occurring social interactions with classmates. Before you allow a paraprofessional to be assigned to your child, ask the following questions:

- Does my child have the appropriate and necessary level of direct instruction from a qualified teacher of students with visual impairments?
- Is assignment of a paraprofessional a "band aid" because services from a qualified teacher are not available, or are considered too expensive?

- What are the specific responsibilities of the paraprofessional related to my child? Are these responsibilities appropriate for the qualifications of the person who will serve in this role (e.g., if the paraprofessional will produce braille material, does he or she have qualifications as a braille transcriber)?
- How will reliance on the paraprofessional be phased out? What is the plan to teach my child to be independent by learning to accomplish these tasks independently (e.g., moving safely throughout the building, accessing classroom information)?

∷ Where Will Your Child Receive Services and Go to School?

The professionals described above work with children in both early intervention and special education programs. Where your child sees these professionals, however, may depend on her age. Infants and very young children often receive educational services in different kinds of settings than school-aged children do. The sections below discuss some of the many options that may be available in your community.

Early Intervention and Preschool Settings

Early intervention and preschool programs are usually held in one of two locations: either in your home, or in a "center"—a school, clinic, hospital, daycare center, or other building with classroom space. Some children receive a combination of home- and center-based intervention. Other children may go to an early intervention program several days a week, and to a regular daycare center or nursery school the rest of the week. This will depend on the programs available in your community and the educational setting specified in your child's IFSP or IEP.

Home Intervention

Home intervention services are generally provided when a child is very young or when medical conditions prevent her from participating in a program outside the home. In this type of program, parents receive scheduled visits in their home by a qualified early intervention or preschool specialist. A qualified preschool specialist may be a teacher with training in early childhood/special education who receives help from a TVI, or he or she may be a TVI with experience or training in early childhood issues. The specialist assesses your child's developmental needs and then works on activities with her to address them. The specialist also educates parents about the ways visual impairment may affect their child's development and their family life, and refers them to other appropriate services.

As mentioned earlier, if your child has other disabilities in addition to a visual impairment, she may need services from a variety of therapists and educators. Your case manager or service coordinator may help coordinate these visits, or the specialists may call you directly and make appointments to visit you and your child.

The scheduling of visits will depend on the type of services your child needs, as well as on her unique goals. You may see one therapist once a week, while another may visit less often.

Having therapists/specialists visit you at home can have many benefits. Your child is in a comfortable, familiar environment, surrounded by many of her own toys. Her teachers can demonstrate activities to you in your own home. They can offer specific suggestions about how to make your child safer and more comfortable, perhaps by suggesting changes in lighting or the way furniture is arranged.

There are also disadvantages to home intervention, aside from the obvious inconvenience of having strangers in your home. Probably the biggest disadvantage is the isolation. Your child needs to learn how to socialize with other children, to play, and to share. You, as a parent, can also benefit from time around parents of other children. It is often comforting to know that other parents (of children with and without visual impairments) have the same questions, concerns, and dreams for their children that you have for your child.

Center-Based Programs

No two center-based programs are exactly alike, so it is difficult to generalize about their characteristics. Some center-based programs serve children with visual impairments exclusively; others also serve children with other disabilities or no disabilities. Some programs are run independently by churches or private companies, some by federal agencies such as Head Start, some by state or county agencies, and some by the school district or state residential school for the blind. And, as mentioned above, programs can be housed in many different places, ranging from schools, to churches, to daycare centers, to hospitals.

Center-based programs are usually offered in a centralized place where therapists can come to provide therapy and instruction. Because center-based programs have a concentrated number of students, they can sometimes hire or train specialized personnel and obtain specialized equipment. The center may also use the services of consultants in the area of visual impairments or other special needs. If your child's IFSP specifies that she is to receive consultation or direct services from a TVI, the specialist will usually travel to the center to provide instruction there.

Your child may go to the center all or a portion of every day, every other day, or just once a week. How much time your child spends at the center will depend on the plans developed by you and your child's team. How much you are involved will likewise depend on the program developed for your child. At times, the center's staff may be very interested in your input and assistance, and at other times your child will need to show her independence by having a little distance from you. Participating in a center-based program will help your child learn to interact with other children and adults. This does not necessarily mean your child won't also need some home intervention activities, but her home activities may be supplemented by center-based activities.

Settings for School-Aged Children

By the time your child graduates from preschool, she may already have been in special education for several years. Still, beginning kindergarten or first grade will mean many changes for her, and taking steps to ease the transition will be crucial. She will probably have new teachers and therapists, meet many new friends, and have new goals added to her IEP. One of the biggest changes, though, may be in where she goes to school. In many communities, there are more placement options for school-aged children than for preschoolers, so deciding what is best for your child may be more complicated. Below are some educational settings frequently available for school-aged children.

Homebound or Hospital Instruction

This type of program is usually a temporary program designed to provide services for students who cannot attend regular classes, most commonly due to medical problems.

Homebound Instruction. Children in this kind of program receive instruction in all academic subjects in the home. A qualified teacher and therapists travel to the home on a scheduled basis to help the child work on her individual educational goals. The scheduling of visits by the teacher(s) depends, of course, on your needs as well as her health concerns. Often, parents need to take on some teaching responsibilities when the teacher(s) are not in their home.

Hospital Program. If your child has problems that require hospitalization, a qualified teacher and therapists can provide instruction in the hospital. This is usually a temporary measure until your child is discharged from the hospital.

Home Schooling

Home schooling continues to grow in popularity. Reasons pro and con run the gamut. For more information on this option, and on meeting the standards of your state, contact your department of education. If you decide to use the home schooling option for your child with visual impairments, you will want to make sure that her special needs related to her visual impairment are carefully addressed. Some districts provide TVIs and other services to students who are home schooled.

Residential Schools

A residential school may be a state-supported or private school for children with specific disabilities (vision or hearing impairment, for example). Students attend classes at the school and may live there during school terms. Children often attend such schools to gain important adaptive skills such as orientation and mobility, braille reading and writing, daily living skills, and use of adaptive technology (speech synthesis for a word processor, braille notetaker, etc.). Sometimes these skills are easier to learn in a residential program because intense specialized instruction is more likely to be available there than in a public school. Students at residential schools may also have more opportunities to practice the special skills they are learning under the watchful eyes of trained professionals.

Another advantage of a residential school is the opportunity it provides for socializing with other children with visual impairments. Many offer a wide range of extracurricular activities, including Scouts, sports, and special interest clubs. Especially for children who live in rural areas, a residential school may provide the only opportunity for such social interactions.

After they have picked up the needed skills, many students return to their home school or enjoy a split schedule between public school, for higher academic coursework, and the residential school for compensatory skills development. Sometimes students return to a residential school for short stays as their needs require throughout their school careers. Many schools offer short courses during the year, as well as summer courses of study.

Often, residential schools act as resource centers to the state's local schools, providing valuable consultation, information, and educational materials.

Special Day Service Facility

This is a community-based public or private school that serves children with disabilities exclusively. Some of these facilities serve children with a mixture of disabilities, while others serve children with only one type of disability. Usually specially trained teachers and therapists provide intense, individualized services throughout the school day.

This option is not widely available except in some large cities where there are enough students with similar needs to support such a facility. Typically, children may be placed in these schools on the basis of specialized services required. Often, they may attend the school for a short time to meet specific requirements.

Self-Contained Classroom

A self-contained classroom is a room in a "regular" or neighborhood school. The primary purpose of these classes is to provide specialized instruction to students with disabilities. These classes usually have a smaller student-teacher ratio than classes for students without disabilities in the same school. Teachers in self-contained classrooms are usually qualified in both general and special education.

Students enrolled in a self-contained classroom usually complete at least half of their classroom work there. Students may leave the self-contained classroom throughout the day to receive special instruction (such as orientation and mobility or speech therapy) or to participate in activities in the regular classroom. Some students participate in regular classroom activities to benefit from social opportunities with children who do not have disabilities. Others participate in regular classrooms to work on academic skills.

Self-contained classrooms solely for children with visual impairments are rare, except in large cities where there are enough students with similar needs to fill a class. Children who have other disabilities besides visual impairments may be placed in self-contained class-rooms for students with multiple disabilities, where they can receive additional support.

Resource Room

A resource room is a classroom where special skills are learned and reinforced. For example, a child might receive specialized instruction here in academic areas that are difficult for her. Or she might receive instruction in special skill areas, including braille reading, use of technology such as computers and braille printers, or concept development. No more than 50 percent of classroom work should take place in the resource room. The majority of the day should be spent in the regular classroom, receiving instruction from the regular classroom teacher.

Resource rooms may serve students with several different disabilities (non-categorical classrooms) or serve only students with a specific disability (categorical classrooms). Any resource teacher who provides services to children with visual impairments should have special training and certification in visual impairment.

Regular Classroom with Additional Direct Instruction

In this setting, a student receives most of her instruction in the general education classroom alongside students without disabilities and, perhaps, with other disabilities. On a daily or weekly basis, she receives supplemental instruction within the classroom or in a special classroom from a teacher of students with visual impairments, orientation and mobility specialist, or other specialist, as needed. Besides providing instruction to the child, the teacher of students with visual impairments provides technical assistance to school staff. For instance, he or she may hold workshops to help teachers learn to work with children with visual impairments or consult on specific questions from regular classroom teachers.

Regular Classroom

Some students with visual impairments are able to succeed in the regular classroom with no outside consultative assistance. They may use adaptive equipment such as a word processor with speech output, but do not need assistance to maintain grade-level performance.

Although independence is a goal that is very important for children with visual impairments, the need for special assistance inside or outside of a regular classroom should, in no way, be considered a failure. In fact, some children who are successfully educated in the regular classroom for years may only need assistance from a teacher of students with visual impairments or O&M specialist during transition times—when moving from preschool to kindergarten, from elementary to junior high school or middle school, or from high school into college, vocational training, or the world of work.

Choosing the Right Educational Setting

Depending on the options available in your community, there could be anywhere from a few to a bewildering number of settings in which your child *could* be educated. The chal-

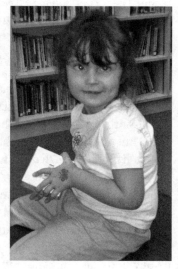

lenge is to pick the setting where your child is likely to make the best progress. Fortunately, federal education laws have set some guidelines that make choosing an appropriate setting a little easier. The most important of these guidelines is the requirement that children with disabilities be educated in the "least restrictive environment" (LRE).

The least restrictive environment is the setting which allows each child the most contact with typically developing peers combined with the most opportunity for educational progress. There are many issues related to LRE. You and your child's educator must consider the following questions when making decisions about placement:

- What settings will give your child the best chance of experiencing educational success and of accomplishing the goals and objectives of her IEP?
- What settings will best prepare your child to meet future educational, vocational, and social demands?
- What settings will best prepare your child to be fully integrated in society?

Those questions are not easily answered. The LRE for one student is not necessarily the LRE for another student. In determining the most appropriate educational setting, each child's specific needs and abilities should be taken into account. It is also important to remember that needs and abilities may change throughout a student's educational career. Therefore, the least restrictive environment for a particular student may change through the years.

Any given placement option is sometimes the least restrictive environment, sometimes the most restrictive environment, and sometimes somewhere in between. It all depends on the student. The resource room may be a more restrictive environment for one student; a less restrictive environment for another. For this reason, professionals often refer to the ideal setting as the "most appropriate placement," rather than the "least restrictive environment." You may also hear the term "most inclusive environment," which means placement with children who do not have disabilities.

The variety of placement options is often referred to as the "continuum of services." Teachers and parents must consider this continuum, beginning with the least restrictive options, as they consider the best possible match of educational services and individual needs. For example, the resource room might be the best place for your child to learn braille skills. But that doesn't mean that the academic subjects must or should be taught in that setting. In other words, sometimes there isn't just one "right" setting for a child; rather, there is a combination of "right" settings.

As your child progresses, her settings will be constantly monitored and changed. Federal laws require that your child's settings be reviewed at least once a year during the IEP meeting to make sure that she is not spending time in the wrong settings. (The exception is if your state has implemented three-year IEPs and you have consented to your child having such an IEP.) Again, you may request reviews of your child's placement at any time. See Chapter 9 for information on changing placement.

Making Decisions about Inclusion

Today, more and more efforts are being made to ensure that all children with disabilities have the chance to interact at school with children who don't have disabilities. The practice of including children with disabilities in classrooms with children without disabilities has come to be called "inclusion." Sometimes children are said to be "fully included," meaning that they spend all, or almost all of their time in a regular classroom with typically developing children.

Where individual children are concerned, there is no one answer to the question of whether inclusion is the best option. For children who have a visual impairment, the answer probably lies in a balancing act. You and your child's teachers must balance her needs for social interactions with her educational needs and requirements for special education.

Below are some unique issues that must be considered when thinking about the general education classroom for children with visual impairments.

Social Considerations

Placing children with visual impairments in a regular classroom provides an opportunity for them to interact with children who are sighted. This is certainly important. We live in a sighted world and children who are blind or visually impaired must be able to feel successful in social interactions with sighted people.

An integrated classroom setting provides common experiences that could initiate understanding and bonds of friendship. Children with visual impairments deserve the chance to form rich and rewarding friendships with other children their age who share similar interests, regardless of whether those children have "normal" vision or not. They can also benefit from feedback from sighted peers as to what is and is not "cool" behavior. In addition, if we want other people to learn to accept people with visual impairments and to feel comfortable with them, it is extremely helpful for them to meet and interact with peers with visual impairments as children.

On the other hand, children with visual impairments—especially those who live in rural areas—may have limited contact with other people with visual impairments. We all like to know that we "are not alone," and that some of our concerns are shared by others. Children benefit from interaction with other children (and adults) who have had similar experiences and concerns. It may be possible that a parent organization, a larger school district, your state or regional division of services for the blind, or your state residential school will provide opportunities for children with visual impairments to interact with one another, through topical meetings, camping or other recreational events, summer programs, athletic competitions, or pen pal programs. If a child with visual impairments is an active member of her community, regularly participating in recreational, church, volunteer, or other community activities with sighted peers, school inclusion may not always be as crucial for her for social inclusion. Below are other factors to consider when examining the issue of inclusion.

Academic Considerations

The number one purpose of schools is to teach "academics" to students. For children with visual impairments to succeed and compete with their classmates, two things must occur. First, they must have access to adapted materials. If your child reads braille, for example, she must be given braille textbooks and classroom materials. Ideally, she will have creative teachers who will find ways to modify other types of class materials, including workbooks, handouts, tests, maps, and bulletin boards. Your child must be included in all classroom activities in order to benefit from them.

Second, children with visual impairments need to know how to skillfully use adapted equipment and skills. Using a talking calculator or an abacus might help your child complete her mathematics assignment more efficiently; using a computer with speech output might help her express her ideas in writing more independently. Merely having adapted equipment is not enough, however. Your child must know which equipment will be helpful and feel comfortable using it.

When considering a placement for your child, ask yourself whether she is prepared to succeed academically. Does she need special equipment to handle the academics? Does she need intense special instruction to learn to use the equipment? If she reads more slowly than other students her age, what adaptations will be made so she will be able to keep up with written assignments? Some students do better if they are placed for a short time in a program designed to teach how to use special equipment before they enter a classroom where they need to use the equipment.

Particularly if your child has another disability in addition to a visual impairment, ask yourself whether the instruction in the classroom will be specialized to match her abilities. If she has a hearing loss, how will instruction be adapted so that she can learn information that the teacher presents verbally? If she has developmental delays, what professional will adapt materials for her and provide academic support if her academic goals differ significantly from the other students'?

Special Skills

Children with visual impairments typically receive instruction in special skills that sighted classmates do not. These skills, which are collectively called the Expanded Core Curriculum, may include orientation and mobility, braille reading and writing, daily living skills, listening skills, and adaptive physical education and recreation skills. These skills may be taught outside the general education classroom, or when appropriate, the teacher of students with visual impairments may work on them in the general education classroom (e.g., at snack time or during classroom recreation activities).

When deciding which placement is best for your child, it is important to consider her strengths and weaknesses in these special skills, and determine which placement will best help her build her skills. Although some instruction, such as O&M, must take place outside the regular classroom, for some children it is preferable to minimize time outside of the classroom. Some children do not mind being "pulled out" of a regular education classroom to work on special skills and are able to make up work they miss in the classroom when they are pulled out, but other children have a harder time making transitions in and out of the regular classroom, or may have trouble feeling as if they belong in a class if they are frequently pulled out.

Questions to Consider

You should have a great deal to say about whether—and to what extent—your child is placed in a general education classroom. For many parents, finding the most inclusive setting for their child is *the* most important factor in choosing a placement. But there are also other factors that you may want to consider in determining the most appropriate setting for your child. Factors to consider for school-aged children are summarized in Figure 1 (page 228); for preschool children, in Figure 2 (page 229). Some factors that you may want to give extra weight to include:

- *Are there sufficient numbers of staff per child?* Do children in the class receive the assistance they need to accomplish their educational goals?
- *Is the staff trained to work with children with visual impairments?* If not, is there a TVI or other expert that staff members are willing and able to consult? Are staff members willing to seek out in-service training opportunities to learn more about visual impairment?
- *Does the staff seem comfortable with your child, and vice versa?* Sometimes teachers ask children to attempt tasks that might be a little frightening at first (walking up and

down steps, reaching for something). Your child may be more likely to try unfamiliar activities, movements, etc. if she likes and trusts the teacher and therapist.

- *Do you agree with staff about the educational goals that are important for your child?* Minor differences of opinion such as about classroom routines can usually be worked out at the meeting to plan your child's IEP. But if you have major disagreements such as about the introduction of braille reading and writing, you might want to seek a program where you are more likely to see eye to eye with the staff.

❚❚ FIG. 1–QUESTIONS TO CONSIDER IN SELECTING A SCHOOL PROGRAM

- What is the student-teacher ratio? Are there sufficient trained personnel (for example, paraprofessionals, parent volunteers, certified specialists, etc.) to support the teacher in providing individualized attention when necessary?
- What are the qualifications of the teaching staff and administration? Have they had experience with including students with disabilities in their school?
- What opportunities are available to teachers for in-service training or workshops on new teaching techniques (including techniques useful for the education of students with visual impairments)?
- Do the teachers and administrators seem to accept and respect differences in students? Are they open to the opportunity of working with a student who is visually impaired?
- Are there opportunities for students with disabilities to participate fully in extracurricular activities in school?
- Is a trained TVI, as well as other certified personnel, available to provide appropriate instruction to your child and consultation to your child's classroom teacher? (O&M, OTs, etc.)
- Are there opportunities for alternative, short-term placements (such as to work intensively on O&M skills)? Are teachers and administrators flexible in providing placement options?
- Are adaptive equipment and materials (including large print and/or braille textbooks) readily available?
- Are physical facilities safe, clean, and accessible?

∷ FIG. 2–QUESTIONS TO CONSIDER IN SELECTING A PRESCHOOL PROGRAM

- Are there sufficient numbers of staff per child?
- Is the facility licensed by the state with a good reputation?
- Are there workers trained to work with children with visual impairments, or do they have a resource to assist them? Do they seem willing to seek out in-service training opportunities to learn more about visual impairments?
- Does the staff seem to accept children with visual impairments?
- Are other parents satisfied with this program?
- Does the program allow open, unscheduled visits by parents?
- Are motivating toys and materials (high contrast, interesting texture, bright colors) used with the children?
- Are written materials available that describe safety and emergency procedures?
- Do staff members provide a safe environment while encouraging independence?
- Are physical facilities safe, clean, and accessible?

- *Is there a commitment to provide educational materials in accessible formats in a timely manner* (at the same times as her sighted classmates receive their materials)?

∷ Becoming an Active Member of Your Child's Education Team

So far, this chapter has touched on several ways that parents are typically involved in their child's education program: they help teachers and therapists set appropriate goals; they have a voice in choosing the right educational setting; they may help their child work on educational and therapeutic goals at home. But if you choose, you can play an even more important role in your child's educational team. You can have a say in virtually every decision made about your child's education. By doing so, you become your child's advocate.

The idea of becoming an advocate may sound intimidating to you if you have only heard the word used in a legal context before.

But, to advocate simply means to speak up on someone else's behalf. This is something you have likely been doing for your child, wittingly or unwittingly, since her birth. For example, every time you take your child to the grocery store, the shopping mall, or Sunday School, you are advocating for her right to be fully involved in the community. When you answer questions from other children, parents, or professionals, you are also being an advocate.

To be an educational advocate for your child means, in simple terms, figuring out how she can get the maximum benefit possible from her educational program. And it means doing whatever it takes to ensure that she gets that benefit. Some of the many ways you might advocate may include: talking informally to teachers and therapists about your child's strengths and needs; requesting specific educational services at an IEP meeting; investigating different placement options and then asking for the one you think would be best for your child; joining other parents in requesting that your school system offer more and better services for children with visual impairments.

You don't need any formal training to advocate for your child. But here are some pointers that can help you get started on the right foot:

- *Review assessment results prior to educational meetings.* This way you will be able to ask appropriate questions and make informed recommendations.
- *Gather as much information as possible relating to your child's needs.* Read books and articles such as those recommended by organizations for the blind and in the Reading List of this book. Watch educational films. Visit websites or join email list services for families of children with visual impairments or other special needs. Talk with other parents about their experiences with the school system and services that have helped their child. As you gather information from other parents, it may be helpful to ask open-ended questions: What has been most helpful to you? What books would you recommend?
- *Ask doctors to clearly explain all medical conditions.* Don't hesitate to keep asking questions until you understand every term relating to your child's condition. Keep in mind, however, that medical doctors are rarely educational specialists. Although their suggestions are well intentioned, you should rely primarily upon qualified educators to as-

sist you with educational decisions. Remember, if a doctor expresses a personal opinion about the use of braille, large print, or regular print materials, it is just that: a personal opinion. Be sure to get other opinions, especially from experienced TVIs.

- *Consider compiling a one- or two-page summary of information pertinent to your child's needs which you can distribute to new teachers and other appropriate educational staff.* (See pages 232, 233 for two sample summaries.) Of course, they will continue to gather more information on their own so that they will get to know your child better. Through sharing this information early with your child, she will eventually become her own advocate, easily sharing her needs for appropriate adaptations with others.

- *Keep a resource file to share with educators.* This file might include names and phone numbers of helpful people and organizations, catalogs of adaptive materials, and copies of helpful articles.

- *Cultivate a relationship of mutual respect with your child's teachers and therapists.* Be accessible to teachers if they want to communicate with you about your child. Show your concern by periodically visiting the classroom or by becoming involved in parent activities when possible. If your schedule permits, volunteer to grade papers or assist teachers in other ways. If you and your child's teachers learn to treat one another as equals, negotiations will go more smoothly when disagreements arise.

- *Document formal and informal contacts with school personnel.* If you jot a note to yourself about each meeting and what happened during the meeting, you will not have to rely on your memory when you have questions.

- *Try to remain objective in meetings with your child's teachers and administrators.* Listen carefully to what others have to say and consider their points of view. While you may not change your mind, you will at least come to a better understanding of the views of the other people on your child's educational team.

- *Try to learn the meaning of common educational terminology to facilitate communication with school personnel.*

▪▪ FACT SHEET EXAMPLE 1

Name: Maria Teresa Gonzales   **Birth Date:** October 2, 2002

Mother: Lydia Gonzales   **Office phone number:** 555-7404
Father: Richard Gonzalez   **Office phone number:** 555-0229
Home Phone: 555-2742

Siblings: Catherine, 14 years; José, 8 years

Visual Impairment: Cataracts; Secondary Glaucoma

Maria was born with cataracts (this is sometimes called "congenital cataracts" because it was present at birth). She had surgery to remove the cataracts when she was less than a year old. The surgery was successful, but because they removed the lens of her eye she wears glasses to replace the lens.

Maria has developed glaucoma as a secondary result of her congenital cataracts but she takes special eye drops, so her glaucoma is controlled at this time.

Maria's visual acuity with her glasses on has been measured at 20/200. She does not appear to have difficulty seeing things that are near to her. Maria will probably have difficulty seeing the board or people's expressions from more than a few feet away. She will be able to tell you when she has difficulty seeing something and will feel comfortable moving closer to the board if she is allowed to do so quietly.

Additional Disabilities: Maria has no additional disabilities.

Concerns: Maria must wear her glasses at all times. We are beginning to look into the possibility of contact lenses for her. Maria should be able to participate in all activities along with other children, including physical education lessons, unless there is very rapid movement such as a baseball coming toward her. We would like for her to participate as fully as possible, so please let us help discuss possible alternatives for activities which may be difficult for Maria.

We are most concerned about the secondary condition of glaucoma. As Maria continues to grow, we will have to watch her carefully to make sure that her medication is correct. Please notify us immediately if she begins to complain about headaches, becomes nauseated, or complains of feeling sick to her stomach. If you notice any other behaviors which would indicate that she isn't seeing as well as usual (such as rubbing her eyes, squinting, watery eyes) please let us know as soon as possible.

Strengths: Maria is a curious child. She makes friends easily and enjoys exploring new places and activities. She will let you know if she has difficulties seeing something.

∷ Fact Sheet Example 2

Name: Joseph Allen **Birth Date:** February 6, 1999

Mother: Mary Kay Allen **Office phone number:** 555-1809
Father: Steven Allen **Office phone number:** 555-1997
Home Phone: mother—555-2303; father—555-2223

Siblings: no siblings

Visual Impairment Cortical visual impairment

Additional Disabilities: Developmental Delay; Cerebral Palsy

Joseph was born with severe multiple disabilities. At first, we did not know that he had a visual impairment, in part because we were focusing on his other disabilities. It is still difficult for us to determine exactly what Joseph sees and doesn't see. As with other children with cortical visual impairment, Joseph has variable vision—in other words, sometimes he sees better than other times. He is also light sensitive, so he will not be able to work if he is facing a bright light or a window.

Some teachers have thought that Joseph was lazy or not motivated, but that is not true. He will do better if he has frequent breaks to allow his eyes to rest. He also responds better to work and environments that are not very cluttered.

Concerns: Our major concern is that some people don't have very high expectations for Joseph. We believe that he will be able to accomplish a great deal if he is provided with a rich environment of stimulating activities.

Strengths: Joseph has a great sense of humor and enjoys teasing others. He has quite good receptive language and is progressing in expressing himself through use of assistive technology.

Whenever a teacher or therapist uses unfamiliar jargon, ask for clarification.

- *Know your rights and the rights of your child.* Find out about the laws, regulations, and school policies that affect her. Chapter 9 provides an overview of the most important federal laws you should know about. If you know what you and your child are entitled to, you will feel confident in asserting your rights and in requesting appropriate educational assistance.

- *Find out about advocates and organizations that can assist your efforts in the educational process.* A list of national

organizations can be found in the back of this book. Some
of these organizations publish newsletters or email updates
that keep parents abreast of new and pending federal legislation and other issues relevant to parents. Local organizations may be able to help you more directly. For example,
they may be able to refer you to people (lay advocates,
parents, lawyers) in your area who can give you advice or
help you advocate for something. On a smaller scale, you
may simply want to find an experienced parent who will
help you talk to your child's teacher or go with you to IEP
meetings to lend moral support. Ask your doctor about support groups for parents of children who have visual impairments, or whether he or she knows of other families that
you might contact. You can also call your state residential
school for the blind, state department of education, state
department of human services, state health department, or
state rehabilitation agency for the blind.

Remember, although the school professionals who work with your
child have good intentions, *you* will remain the best advocate for your
child. School personnel will come and go, but you will be the constant
in your child's life; you will be *the* expert on her strengths and needs.
It will be great if others help you advocate, but even so, it will always
be important for you to directly oversee your child's education. Keep in
mind that the more you know, the less frightening the process will be.
Compile and store information in your memory and a kitchen drawer for
the time that you will need it. If you forget or don't know a crucial piece
of information, don't be shy—ask for help…from an advocacy group…a
fellow parent…your spouse…a neighbor…or an interested friend. Don't
try to take the world on alone; there's usually help if you look for it.

:: Conclusion

For most parents and families, early intervention and special
education are uncharted territories. The terminology, assessment and
eligibility procedures, special services, classroom settings, even the
subjects taught all seem very different from what you encountered during your own school years. Over time, however, most parents come to
see that there are very good reasons for these differences. Good early

intervention and special education programs give many children with visual impairments the best shot at mastering the knowledge and skills to become productive members of their community.

As you become more familiar with the worlds of early intervention and special education, you will begin to see how all the parts fit together. You will begin to see the importance of setting appropriate goals for your child's IFSP or IEP. You will also begin to see which professionals can help your child and how. And perhaps most importantly, you will begin to see how you can work with these professionals to ensure that your child makes the optimum progress. It might seem like a tall order at first, but if you take things a step at a time, you can learn to use the special education system to your child's best advantage.

⚏ Parent Statements

It's great when the special education system works!

⚜

I've learned that when someone (a doctor or teacher) uses an acronym that I don't understand, I just ask what it means. I don't even hesitate.

⚜

I don't know what we would have done without Marilyn, our preschool consultant. She was so patient. She really helped us know what we needed to know and prepare for the future.

⚜

The most worrisome thing about the preschool years is that my son will grow out of them! I feel like this time when he is a preschooler is a peaceful time compared to what will happen when he goes to school. Matt has cognitive disabilities in addition to his visual impairment and it just doesn't seem fair that everything will change when he turns five. He's not ready, and I don't think I'm ready either.

⚜

Our first meeting with the early intervention team was a nightmare. I feel like I had to prove that I was a good parent. I don't think it has to be that way.

⚜

It seems as if our son is constantly being tested. I know they have to know where he stands so they will know what to work on, but sometimes it seems as if they do more testing than teaching.

❧

Sometimes I feel outnumbered by all of the special education experts with long titles. It is hard not to be intimidated.

❧

In our school district, the early intervention team comes to your house. I hate having to tidy up all the time so they won't think I'm a bad housekeeper. But I think it's good that they can see our son in his natural environment and make suggestions about adapting our household to his needs. They also show us fresh ways to play with his toys.

❧

We've gotten support from the school for the blind all along. Even though my child is not going to school there, they still take the time to answer questions and even sent some people to help my child's teachers out when everything was new to them.

❧

In some IEP meetings, teachers seem to think my comments are unimportant. I'm trying to get more forceful in communicating my thoughts. It helps to think through in advance what I want to say.

❧

I guess my biggest fear is that when Madison goes to school, other children will make fun of her.

❧

Our school district does not have a vision specialist. The special education supervisor says that Caitlin will go to the resource room, but I know that teacher does not know braille. I'm afraid Caitlin will fall through the cracks.

❧

We feel like we are in control of our daughter's educational plan. We make sure that we are prepared before the meeting and take careful notes dur-

ing the meeting. We find that our strong involvement in DeeDee's educational team is critical to making sure that her needs are met.

❧

I'm glad that Gracie will be in a regular classroom in her neighborhood school. I think that is the best place for her and she already knows some of the children.

❧

Each time we had IFSP meetings, we were asked what our goals were for our son. We would say, "He's our first child. What are other kids doing at this age?" They would tell us and we'd say, "Well, that's what we want our son to do." Even when a child has more than one disability, I believe it is far better to aim for the norm than to expect only what experts and others suggest your child is capable of. Our philosophy is to always try to keep hopes and goals for our child high.

❧

Teachers and therapists at school meetings tend to use a lot of acronyms. We started a notebook of acronyms that are most often used, which helps us feel more in control of those foreign-sounding terms.

❧

You have the right to maintain your privacy. Your need to share sufficient information in order to receive the best possible services for your child should be balanced with your right to privacy. Remember that some kinds of information are just no one else's business. You may need to practice saying "No."

9

AN OVERVIEW OF
LEGAL ISSUES

Tom E. C. Smith, Ed.D., &
Tanni L. Anthony, Ph.D.

It may seem like an understatement to note that there have been many positive changes for people with disabilities, including those with visual impairment, over the past several decades. There was a time when people with disabilities were severely restricted in the types of educational programs they could participate in, the types of jobs they could train for, and their abilities to travel and obtain information. It is only thanks to the ongoing contribution of parents, consumers, advocacy organizations, and dedicated professionals that laws and practices have changed to improve the education, daily life, and work outcomes for persons with disabilities. Parents' voices have been central to national reform efforts and change within individual schools and communities.

It is important for you to have current information and an understanding about the major laws that provide basic rights, protections, and benefits for you and your child. Such information will help you ensure that your child is receiving all of the services and benefits that he needs and is entitled to as a person with a visual impairment. This chapter covers information about these laws and offers guidance in using them. It also provides information on other legal issues such as taxes, governmental assistance programs, and becoming an advocate for your child.

In reading through this chapter, remember that each state has its own guidelines for implementing federal laws. Check with the Department of Education in your state to find out about the guidelines for early intervention and specialized education programs. You may also want to investigate whether there is a parent training center or parent clearinghouse center in your state that provides ongoing information about federal laws, any changes in these laws, and places to find legal support. In the Resource Guide, you will find contact information for agencies and organizations that can help you determine how to locate state-specific information.

:: Education Laws

The Individuals with Disabilities Education Act (IDEA)

In the past, people with disabilities, including visual impairments, were often isolated and not allowed to participate in the mainstream of public education. Prior to the 1970s, many students with disabilities were excluded from their neighborhood schools and the general education curriculum (the curriculum used with students without disabilities), or were not provided an appropriate or effective education. In the early 1970s, parents, advocacy organizations, and civil rights attorneys challenged state and local school officials for denying students with disabilities the right to an education equal to that of their nondisabled peers.

By 1975, Congress enacted a federal law to protect the educational rights of students with disabilities. The original law, Education of All Handicapped Children Act (Public Law 94-142), has been amended several times and now has a revised name more in keeping with what is called "person-first language"—the Individuals with Disabilities Education Improvement Act of 2004 or IDEA (Public Law 108-446). IDEA is perhaps *the* most important law for you to know about, as it guarantees all children with disabilities the right to a free and appropriate public education. Over the years, the law has been modified to promote more efficient early identification of disabilities, more integrated service provision to children with disabilities, improved access through the general education curriculum, and a strengthened role of parents and parent/professional partnerships in educational settings. Key provisions in the law are explained below.

Coverage

IDEA applies to all children who have a disability resulting in the need for special education services. The disability must interfere with the ability to learn or to access information for purposes of learning. For example, blindness or low vision will likely prevent or limit a student from gaining information that is typically presented through print (textbooks, words on chalkboard, handouts), resulting in the need for specialized materials or instruction.

Children with qualifying disabilities are covered by Part C of IDEA from birth through age two and by Part B of the law from age three through twenty-one. Children who qualify for special education receive specially designed instruction, supports, and services to meet their unique needs. The details about what special education includes are in Chapter 8.

To determine whether your child is eligible for special education services, a comprehensive evaluation by a team of professionals, including an eye care specialist (an ophthalmologist or optometrist) and a teacher of students with visual impairments (TVI), will be completed. Depending on your child's needs, other professionals such as a school psychologist, a physical or occupational therapist, a speech-language therapist, and/or a general education teacher may also be involved in these educational assessments.

Your child will be found eligible for special education services if he meets two criteria. First, his physiological abilities to see must fall within your state's guidelines for visual acuity (how clearly a person sees) and/or visual field (how wide a person can see while looking straight ahead). Most school programs for children with visual impairments have an entrance visual acuity of 20/70 in the best corrected eye. Eligibility based on visual field "cut-offs" is based usually on a restricted visual field of only 20 degrees. Some states have eligibility criteria that expand the definition of blind/visually impaired to include any child identified with cortical visual impairment, regardless of his visual acuity or visual field. Eligibility "cut-off" measurements may vary from state to state. Most states will consider a child as eligible for special education services if his visual acuity and/or visual field are expected to get worse over time.

The second part of eligibility involves your child's need for specialized services in order to obtain reasonable educational benefit. If loss of vision adversely affects educational performance to the degree that special education services are needed, then your child will be eligible

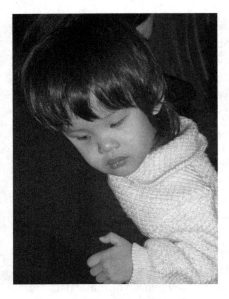

for services that will enable him to compensate for the visual loss (e.g., learn braille, use low vision devices, use a long cane).

Your child should be assessed in all areas related to the suspected disability, including, as appropriate, health, vision, hearing, social and emotional skills, general intelligence or thinking skills, academic performance (if he is school age), communication abilities, and motor skills. Appropriate vision evaluation and hearing screening must precede all developmental or academic evaluations to ensure that care has been taken to protect optimal visual and hearing status of the child. If the child's problems are due to either auditory or vision problems, addressing these needs may eliminate the need for further assessment and interventions.

Tests and materials used to evaluate your child must be appropriate for a child with a visual impairment in order for the results to accurately reflect your child's true learning abilities and educational needs. Further, if your child has limited English proficiency, the assessment materials must be appropriate to measure the extent to which he has a disability that requires special education versus measuring the extent of his English language skills.

If your child has additional disabilities besides a visual impairment, the professionals on the evaluation team will determine to what extent these disabilities affect your child's development. Results related to your child's motor skills, cognitive skills, and communication skills will then be taken into account when planning for your child's special education.

Free and Appropriate Education

By law, all students who qualify for coverage under the IDEA must receive a free and appropriate public education. The "free" part of the phrase means exactly what it sounds like. Your child has the right to receive a reasonable education at public expense, without any cost to you. "Appropriate" means that the education must meet his unique learning needs and allow him to have access to, and progress in, the general curriculum. Students cannot simply receive the same education as other children or even other children with visual impairments of the same age. Students must receive specially designed instruction tailored to their individual learning needs.

Students must also receive all needed *related services*—developmental, corrective, and supportive services necessary to enable the student to benefit from the special educational program. Specialized transportation, physical therapy, occupational therapy, speech language therapy, and orientation and mobility services are examples of related services that might be scheduled for your child based on individual learning needs. All related services must be provided by trained and qualified personnel. For example, orientation and mobility services should only be provided by a certified Orientation and Mobility Specialist (COMS).

It is important to realize that "appropriate" does not necessarily mean "best." Sometimes there may be many different devices, systems, curricula, or programs that could meet your child's educational needs. Your child's school or early intervention program is not required to choose the method that you necessarily think would be best, so long as the one they choose is appropriate.

Least Restrictive Environment

Under IDEA, students must receive their special education services in the least restrictive environment (LRE). The least restrictive environment is the setting that allows the child the most opportunities to access and learn from the general education curriculum, be with nondisabled peers, and to receive needed special education services. As Chapter 8 explains, there are a wide variety of settings that might be considered the least restrictive, depending on your child's needs. For some children with visual impairments, the LRE might be the general education classroom, where none or few of the other students have a disability; for other children it might be a residential school for the blind; and for others it might be something between these two situations.

In considering the LRE for your child, the school is required to start by considering whether the most appropriate setting is the general education classroom. This should be considered first. If it is determined that your child cannot learn and receive needed services in the general education classroom, then other educational settings should be considered. The primary factor that determines placement should always be the needs of your child. In many instances, the ideal placement is a child's neighborhood school. If this is not the case, the child should receive services in another setting that may be considered less inclusive but may be more appropriate for a short or long term. The philosophy of inclusion should never be a more important factor in the placement decision than the needs of the child.

Individualized Education Program/Individualized Family Service Plan

For your child's education program to be appropriate, it must be individualized based on his strengths and educational needs. To ensure that your child's program is individualized, the IDEA requires that a written plan be developed that outlines how his unique needs will be met. For example, if your child's primary literacy media will be braille, the plan should reflect how braille will be taught and how it will be embedded in literacy activities. For children under the age of three, the plan is called an Individualized Family Service Plan or IFSP. For children three and older, the plan is called an Individualized Education Program or an IEP.

There are six areas that the IEP is required to address:

1. *A description of your child's present level of performance or what your child is currently able to do.* This will include a description of skills in all developmental areas.

2. *The measurable annual goals, including academic and functional goals.* For some children, short-term objectives will also be set. See Chapter 8 for examples of goals.

3. *The specific special education services that will be provided to your child.* These might include direct instruction from a teacher of students with visual impairments and/or a certified Orientation and Mobility Specialist.

4. *The date these special education services are expected to begin and a projected date when they will conclude.*

5. *The method(s) that will be used to determine whether goals are being achieved.* For example, progress might be moni-

tored using standardized and teacher-made tests and classroom observations.

6. *The ways in which your child will participate in general education programs and activities, as well as state and district assessments.* This will include any accommodations your child will need—for example, braille or enlarged print.

The IEP also may address parent counseling and training needs, as a related service, if those needs will help the child make greater gains toward meeting IEP goals and objectives *and* this need is agreed upon by the IEP team. For example, if your child is learning braille, it would be very beneficial if you also learn braille. The IEP may therefore state how the school will assist you in learning braille by giving you information about a free correspondence course or a local class, or independent work with a district braillist or teacher certified in the area of visual impairments.

The required elements for an IFSP are basically the same. One major difference, however, is that the IFSP does not focus just on the child's needs, but the entire family's needs. It therefore must also list services that will be provided to help parents and siblings. For example, the IFSP might specify that brothers or sisters will be involved in a support group for siblings of children with disabilities. In addition, the IFSP must indicate who your child's service coordinator (case manager) will be.

IEP/IFSP Meetings. Your child's IEP or IFSP should be developed in joint meetings between you, the teachers, related service providers (e.g., orientation and mobility specialist, physical therapist), and other school or program representatives. At the meetings, you will work together to identify your child's needs and to determine what goals and services are appropriate. The IEP must be written and agreed upon before special education services begin, and must be reviewed at least annually to make sure that it continues to meet your child's needs. The IFSP must be reviewed every six months due to the frequency of developmental changes in children under the age of three years. You, as a parent, have the right to request a meeting to review or reconsider your child's IFSP or IEP at any time.

It is extremely important for you to take part in the IFSP or IEP process. You will recognize needs of your child that the professionals may not see. For example, when your child is young, you may have a much better idea of difficulties related to language developing or dressing, eating by himself, and other self-help skills than educators who are not able to view your child at home. Because of your knowledge you may have important suggestions for activities that are reinforcing to your child. Your role is to make sure these unique needs are identified and included in the IFSP or IEP.

When you first begin attending planning meetings, you may feel nervous about speaking up about your child's needs and how you would like to see them met. Please remember that you are a very important member of the team, and professionals will learn and benefit from your observations and suggestions. It will be important for you to do your homework before you come to a meeting and show that you have put some thought into your child's educational program.

To help prepare for an IFSP or IEP meeting, first gather information about the educational programs available in your community. This will help you go into meetings with knowledge and opinions of what might be best for your child. If your child is under the age of three, ask your Service Coordinator or Case Manager for information services available in your community and throughout the state. If your child is school-age, you may want to observe classes in a variety of programs, such as public schools, state schools, and residential schools. Talk with administrators and officials in your school system and other community agencies about programs and support services available. Parent groups and other organizations can help by putting you in touch with other parents who may already know a great deal about the pros and cons of different programs. It may be helpful to call your state's Department of Education and speak with personnel familiar with service options for school-age children in your state. The Resource guide lists organization that may be able to help.

Second, organize a file that includes all evaluations and any educational and medical reports and records that pertain to your child. This should include copies of letters that you write, as well as receive, teachers' notes, and records of important phone calls. Keep this file updated with any new information, such as the current IFSP or IEP. The file will help you remember the events, issues, and solutions that occur throughout your child's educational program. It will also provide you with a record of who said what—which can be helpful if you ever become involved in a due process hearing or other litigation.

Third, before the meeting consider what goals and services you feel are necessary for your child and in what setting you think they should be provided. If you are unsure about appropriate goals, feel free to consult with other parents or professionals who are familiar with your child's strengths and needs. Remember that it is possible that a child may behave differently in his home and school environment, so there may be different perspectives on your child's strengths and needs.

Write down questions and concerns that you would like to have addressed during the team discussion. During the meeting, be sure to take notes, including the answers to your specific questions. Do not hesitate to ask for clarification of any unfamiliar terms or puzzling comments that come up during the meeting. You have a right to understand what is being discussed.

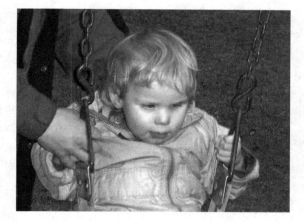

Fourth, consider asking someone you trust to attend the IFSP or IEP meeting with you. You might ask a friend to come along for moral support, to take notes, and to help you remember everything you want to say. You might ask a doctor or private therapist to give their professional advice about your child's need for a particular service. However, it is important to understand that motor therapy services (occupational therapy and physical therapy services) within an educational setting are geared toward the educational and not the medical therapy needs of the child. You may also want to ask an advocate or an attorney to attend the meeting, if you think you will have trouble persuading the school or program staff to see things your way.

Finally, it is quite likely that you will want your child to attend meetings in the later grades. As children get older, it is important for them to take more responsibility for their education by getting involved in the development of the IEP and the placement decision. This helps them develop self-advocacy skills, which are very necessary for adults with visual disabilities. This is actually acknowledged in IDEA by the requirement that all students served in special education must become involved in the development of their IEP by the time they are fourteen.

You can think of your child's IFSP or IEP as a roadmap or a guide to make sure your child receives necessary services. There is no guarantee, however, that all the goals on the IFSP or IEP will be accomplished. It will take hard work and energy from you, from your child, and from the educators who work with him to ensure that he is making steady educational progress. High expectations by you and the other educational team members will continue to be important for appropriate goal planning.

Procedural Safeguards

The requirement that every child in special education have a written IEP is one of the ways that IDEA protects the rights of children with disabilities to a free, appropriate education. IDEA also includes a number of other *procedural safeguards* or rules that are aimed at upholding the rights of you and your child. Under IDEA, every state must abide by these safeguards, if they want the federal government to provide them money to finance special education programs and services (and every state does!). Table 1 on pages 250-251 summarizes nine of the procedural safeguards.

Resolving Disputes

Despite the safeguards outlined above, disputes sometimes arise between parents and early intervention programs or schools. Here are some examples of possible disputes:

- Parents feel that their child needs weekly instruction in orientation and mobility skills, but the school thinks one O&M lesson a month is sufficient.
- The school system believes a child would be best served in a program solely for children with visual impairments, while his parents believe he would make better progress if he received most of his instruction in a general education classroom.
- Parents and the school system disagree about the amount of support the child needs from a paraprofessional.
- Parents want their child to use large print, while the school wants to teach the child braille.

If possible, it is best to work through any disagreements informally during the IFSP or IEP process. Although IDEA includes formal dispute resolution procedures, it is usually easier, quicker, less expensive, and more likely to establish supportive working relationships when disagreements can be settled through informal discussions.

A good first step in resolving a dispute is simply to try to be persuasive and tactful in explaining why you disagree. Take time to understand why the school believes in a certain method, placement, or service delivery. If this tactic does not work, you might talk with school administrators about your concerns. For instance, if you have a disagreement with your child's teacher certified in visual impairment, talk next to the teacher's supervisor, then consult with the person next in the line of authority (e.g., building principal, district Special Education Director). Ask other parents who have worked successfully with the school for advice.

You can also ask the school for mediation services—discussions before one or more neutral individuals aimed at resolving the dispute without going to a due process hearing. School districts are required to offer mediation before a due process hearing can occur. Parents may also file a complaint with their State Department of Education. Contact them for more information about the process of mediation or filing a complaint. Parents should remember, studies have shown that mediation is successful more often than not. Therefore, it is probably a good idea to try to resolve disputes through mediation before going to a more adversarial stage.

If you cannot resolve the disagreement informally, IDEA gives you the right to request a due process hearing. A due process hearing may be requested by a parent, surrogate parent, or a child, if he has turned the age of majority under state law. Early intervention or school personnel may also request a due process hearing, in some circumstances.

You may ask for a due process hearing because of a disagreement about any aspect of your child's educational program. Possible reasons for requesting a hearing may include:

- You disagree with the results of the evaluation of your child.
- You disagree with a proposed IEP.
- You disagree that your child should stop receiving special education services.
- You disagree with the proposed placement for your child or believe it is not in the least restrictive environment.
- You object to a proposed change of placement.
- You refuse to consent to a requested evaluation of your child.
- You refuse to give initial consent for initial placement.

To request a due process hearing, you will need to follow the procedures outlined by your State Department of Education. Most states will ask that you write a letter explaining the nature of the dispute, as well as how you would like to see it resolved.

∷ TABLE 1—MAJOR PROCEDURAL SAFEGUARDS UNDER IDEA

1. **NOTICE**—You must be given written notice when the school district begins, changes, or stops the special education and related services for your child, including the schedule or the location of services.

2. **CONSENT**—You must give written permission or consent for the school district to: 1) initially evaluate your child to determine if he is eligible for special services; 2) initially place your child in a special education program; and 3) release any confidential or personally identifiable information to anyone not authorized by law to be able to review it.

3. **CONFIDENTIALITY OF RECORDS**—You can review any records the school district keeps on your child. Specific school personnel who are working with your child can review these records. Your written consent is necessary to release the information to others who are not authorized by law.

4. **PROTECTION IN EVALUATION PROCEDURES**—Your child must be given a variety of tests or a multidisciplinary evaluation by qualified personnel, both during the initial eligibility evaluation and during later evaluations, to gather information needed to develop an IEP/IFSP. This is to ensure that the educational programming decisions for your child are made based on the most current, accurate, and complete information available. The tests used must not discriminate in terms of race or culture. Testing must also be arranged so that the results are not affected by your child's disability.

5. **INDEPENDENT EDUCATIONAL EVALUATION**—You have the right to have an evaluation of your child done by persons of your choice. If you disagree with the results of the school district's evaluation, you may ask the school district to conduct another evaluation using professionals not employed by the school system. You might want to seek an independent evaluation, for example, if the school district refuses to provide special education services because they did not find that your child's visual impairment has an adverse effect on his educational performance. Or you might seek another evaluation if the school is willing to provide services for problems related to your child's mental retardation, but not for problems related to his visual

impairment. Sometimes the school district may be obligated to pay for this evaluation, but only if you request it from the school district itself. If you go out on your own and personally put together an evaluation team, then you will have to pay for it.

6. **INDIVIDUALIZED EDUCATION PROGRAM (IEP)**—Your child has a right to an Individualized Education Program. This is a written plan that describes the special education and related services that will be given to your child. This plan is based on the needs of your child identified in his evaluation and the goals and objectives that are designed to meet those needs.

7. **EDUCATIONAL SURROGATE PARENT**—If a child is a ward of the state or the parents cannot be located or identified, the school district must appoint an educational surrogate parent to protect the child's rights. Educational surrogate parents must receive training so they can make appropriate educational decisions for the child.

8. **MAINTENANCE OF PLACEMENT**—During any dispute between you and the school district regarding evaluation, programming, placement, or services, your child has the right to remain in the setting or program he was in when the dispute arose. This is called "stay put." Your child has the right to remain in this setting until the dispute is resolved. One exception: If a child has been removed from the school following a behavior manifestation determination, or after the child is removed due to bringing a weapon to the school, possessing, using, or selling illegal drugs, or inflicting serious bodily harm upon another person, then the student remains in the interim alternative placement during any parental appeals.

9. **ATTORNEY FEES**—If you "substantially prevail" (win your case) in any hearing or lawsuit regarding a special education issue for your child and you are represented by an attorney, you may be able to recover your attorney fees from the school district. Note, however, that in situations where the hearing officer or court finds that the child's parents or attorney has filed a frivolous, unreasonable complaint or the complaint was filed for an improper reason, such as to harass or cause unnecessary delay, then the court may award attorney fees to the school from the child's parents or child's attorney.

You should then be granted a due process hearing conducted by an "impartial hearing officer." This hearing officer will be knowledgeable about special education and special education laws, and have training in how to conduct a due process hearing. At the hearing, you will have an opportunity to explain your disagreement or complaint. You should come prepared to present facts, testimony, expert evaluations, and other information to show why the school's decision is wrong and will not provide a free and appropriate public education to your child in the least restrictive environment. You may be represented by an attorney or an advocate, if you wish. While not mandatory, most parents do secure representation to assist in presenting their case.

The hearing officer will consider all the evidence presented by you and the school and make an impartial decision. The decision from the hearing officer must be implemented unless it is appealed. If either you or the school does not agree with the decision, such an appeal may be made to state or federal court. At this appeal, you should present expert evidence to support your position and hire an attorney to represent you. The court will then determine whether the decision made at the district level was proper for your child.

During the due process hearing and any appeals, the IDEA requires that your child stay in his present educational placement. (Again, the exception is if the appeal is due to an alternative placement following a behavior manifestation or the child is removed because of drugs, weapons, or due to inflicting serious bodily harm.) This is known as the "stay put" provision. This is something to keep in mind if the very reason for requesting a due process hearing is to change your child's placement. On the other hand, if you like your child's current placement and are fighting the school district's decision to change it, the provision can work in your favor. In any case, if you decide on your own to transfer your child to another school or program without the school district's approval, you will have to pay any costs involved unless you ultimately win the dispute.

After all the hearings are over, you may be able to be reimbursed for attorney's fees. Under an amendment to the IDEA, parents can sometimes recover these fees if they were found in the hearing or lawsuit to have "substantially prevailed"—that is, that the school district or agency had to alter its behavior as a result of the parent taking legal action. The court, though, can limit or refuse the awarding of attorney's fees, if parents reject a settlement offer from the early intervention agency or school district and then do not get a better outcome. The court can also require that parents pay the school's attorney fees if the child's parents or attorney have filed a frivolous, unreasonable complaint or the complaint was filed for an improper reason, such as to harass or cause unnecessary delay.

As mentioned earlier, a due process hearing can be time-consuming and emotionally draining, as well as expensive. Consequently, experts usually recommend that you request a due process hearing only as a last resort. Experts also recommend that you be represented at such a hearing by an attorney knowledgeable in special education law, since the school district will be represented by such an attorney. If other means of resolving a conflict fail, don't hesitate to assert your rights. Your child's educational welfare could be at stake.

Family Educational Rights and Privacy Act (FERPA)

The Family Educational Rights and Privacy Act (FERPA) is a law that applies to all families with children in school. However, it has special significance for families who have a child with a disability. FERPA was passed to guarantee the confidentiality of "personally identifiable information" in educational records. Personally identifiable information means attaching something that would reveal who the child is, such as the child's name or parents' names, to information such as the public record of state assessment scores that would be available to people who do not have a need for this information. This means that someone who is looking at data from a school district or an educational agency should not be able to identify your child.

FERPA also guarantees that parents have access to their child's records. It is especially important for you to know about this law because of the many evaluations, reports, IFSP/IEP documents, and so forth that will be gathered and maintained through your child's school career.

Under FERPA, you have several rights regarding your child's educational records. They are:

- *The right to know your rights*—You have the right to be told your rights under FERPA.
- *The right to examine records*—You have the right to see the educational records the school or early intervention program keeps on your child. You have the right to see a list of others who have seen your child's educational records. Often there is a sign-in sheet attached to your child's

school record folders. The early intervention coordinator or school administrator should be able to tell you how this information is maintained.

- *The right to consent to release information*—You must give written consent before the school can release personally identifiable information to individuals who are not usually entitled to see it. For instance, you must give consent before a medical doctor, vocational rehabilitation counselor, or school consultant you have hired can see your child's records.
- *The right to challenge incorrect information*—You have the right to request that information that you believe is incorrect or violates your child's privacy rights be corrected or removed from the records. If your request is denied, you have the right to ask for a hearing where you can present your concerns.

■■ Anti-Discrimination Laws

In addition to IDEA, which is primarily a funding law, there are two civil rights laws that significantly affect the lives of children with visual impairments. These two laws, Section 504 of the Rehabilitation Act of 1973, and the Americans with Disabilities Act (ADA), both focus on equal opportunities and equal protections for individuals with a wide array of disabilities, including visual impairments.

The Rehabilitation Act of 1973, Section 504

The Rehabilitation Act of 1973 was the first federal law that focused on discrimination based on disability. This act prohibits discrimination against people with disabilities by programs and activities that receive federal funds.

Specifically, Section 504 states that "no otherwise qualified individual shall, solely by reason of his handicap, be excluded from the participation in, be denied benefits of, or be subjected to discrimination under any program or activity receiving federal financial assistance." Section 504 also requires that reasonable accommodations be made so that individuals with disabilities can participate in programs that receive funding.

Almost all early intervention or school programs receive some funding from the federal government, so this is one place where you should definitely notice the effects of Section 504.

To enable your child to fully participate in educational activities, there might be accommodations such as braille, screen enlargement software, magnification devices, large print, beeper balls for gym activities, desk lamps, or adapted board games with tactile markings or textures. Your child may be given more time to take tests. The classroom environment should be adapted according to the orientation and mobility needs of your child. For example, the classroom may be designed to have clear travel paths. Or, the school building may install environmental tactile warnings (one school district purchased planters to highlight the presence of drinking fountains that could not be detected by a cane).

Another area where your child may see benefits from Section 504 is in parks and recreational facilities that receive federal funding. For example, children with visual impairments (with or without additional disabilities) cannot be excluded from participating in classes or sporting events sponsored by a federally funded recreation program. Parks and the buildings on them must be physically accessible to people with disabilities.

Section 504 will probably be most important to your child if his visual impairment is not considered to be severe enough to qualify for special education services under IDEA. This is because the definition of a "handicapped individual" is broader under Section 504 than it is under IDEA. According to Section 504, a person with a disability is anyone who has a physical or mental impairment that substantially limits one or more of that person's "major life activities such as caring for oneself, performing manual tasks, walking, seeing, hearing, speaking, breathing, learning, and working." Children whose vision impairment is above the "cut-off" measurement your state uses to determine who qualifies for IDEA assistance may still qualify for assistance under 504. Section 504 does not require visual acuity standards for eligibility, only a determination that a substantial limitation in a major life activity, such as seeing, results from the physical or mental impairment.

Children who qualify for educational assistance under Section 504 are entitled to receive a free appropriate education in the least restrictive environment. Schools are required to provide equal access to services, programs, and activities, and to materials, the classroom environment, or instructional methods that will enable eligible students to receive an education "comparable" to the education that nondisabled students receive. Under Section 504, schools are not required to have a written plan describing accommodations that will be provided (similar to an IEP), but they can if they choose to do so. In fact, the Office of Civil Rights (OCR) encourages the use of a written Section 504 Plan.

If your child does not qualify for special education services under IDEA and you believe he might qualify for educational assistance under Section 504, you should ask to speak to the 504 Coordinator in your school system. For more information about Section 504 of the Rehabilitation Act of 1973, call the Office for Civil Rights, listed in the Resource Guide.

The Americans with Disabilities Act of 1990 (ADA)

The Americans with Disabilities Act of 1990 (ADA) is a sweeping piece of legislation that has opened doors and provided opportunities for people with disabilities, including those with visual impairments, to participate more equally in society. The ADA, similar to Section 504, is considered civil rights legislation. While Section 504 only applies to entities receiving federal funds, the ADA applies to virtually everything except churches and private clubs. Some of its provisions will benefit your child from birth on; others will not become important until he reaches adulthood. Becoming familiar with the law now can help ensure that your child is an active participant in his community at all ages.

The ADA prohibits discrimination against people with disabilities in three major areas: public accommodations, public services, and employment. Here is how the provision might help your child now and in the future:

Public Accommodations

The ADA requires that any place open to the public be accessible to people with disabilities unless this is not physically or financially feasible. Restaurants, motels, office buildings, parks, stores, libraries, movie theatres, day care centers, schools, airports, and other public buildings are all affected by this part of the ADA. Any program or facility that is accessible to people without disabilities must also be made accessible to people with disabilities.

For individuals with visual impairments, this provision means that there should be braille and speech output materials available, making it possible for them to participate in community activities. Restaurants must have braille menus or be prepared to have staff read menus aloud to patrons; state and local government services such as courthouses, post offices, and licensing offices should be able to make available personal readers, cassette recordings, and braille materials. Amusement parks, too, must have braille markings, and museums and historical sites must have braille descriptions of exhibits, or perhaps tape recorded tours.

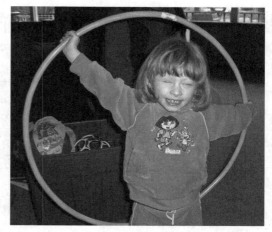

Under the ADA, it is also against the law for individuals with disabilities to only be offered opportunities to participate that are different and separate from the opportunities for individuals without disabilities. That is, your child cannot be relegated to a program, facility, or activity that is only for children with disabilities if he would rather participate in a regular program. For example, a county recreation program cannot stipulate that children with visual impairments could enroll in some activities, but not others. Or the community skating rink could not require that children with visual impairments only skate at a certain time. In rare cases, your child could still be excluded from participation if he was found to "pose a direct threat to the health and safety of others."

Public Services

The section of the ADA that addresses public services requires that architectural barriers found in local or state government buildings or facilities be removed to the "maximum extent feasible." New buildings and facilities must be constructed without barriers. This section also requires that buses, trains, and other transportation services be accessible to individuals with disabilities. In fact, it is a violation of the ADA for state and local governments to purchase vehicles or transportation equipment that is not accessible. Although the majority of these requirements are aimed at increased accessibility for people with physical disabilities, your child will also benefit. Transportation schedules should be available in braille, and public elevators, room numbers, and restrooms should have braille markings.

Employment

All parents think and dream about what their child will be when he "grows up." In the past, parents of children with disabilities have had special concerns about their child's future because of the possibility that employers would discriminate against their child, regardless of his abilities. The ADA prohibits discrimination against a qualified worker on the basis of disability. Specifically, the law prohibits an employer from refusing to hire, train, or promote an employee just because he has a disability. In fact, an employer cannot even ask a prospective employee about his disability. The employer may, however, describe specific core elements of the job and ask if the person can accomplish the requirements of the job with or without appropriate accommodation.

Employers must make adaptations within the workplace that will enable an otherwise qualified worker to perform the job—provided these adaptations can be made without "undue cost." Examples of adaptations an employer might be expected to make for a worker with visual impairments include providing magnifying mechanisms for a worker to use various types of machinery, providing a part-time driver if the job required limited travel, providing special lighting, or modifying the layout of furniture or equipment in an office. This section of the ADA applies to employers with fifteen or more employees.

This section of the law also protects family members of individuals with a disability from discrimination based on "relationship or association." Specifically, people are protected from "actions based on unfounded assumptions that their relationship to a person with a disability would affect their job performance, and from actions caused by bias or misinformation concerning certain disabilities." For example, an employer cannot refuse to hire the parent of a child with visual impairments because the employer fears that the parent will take excessive time off to care for his child.

Making a Complaint

What should you do if you think your child is being discriminated against and you believe that the ADA prohibits such discrimination? The first step is to try to resolve your complaint informally. Talk to the person in charge about what you think the problem is and how you would like to see it resolved. Perhaps they do not even know that they are violating the ADA and will be happy to work with you to change any practices that may be discriminatory.

If negotiating informally does not work, your next step depends on the nature of your complaint. If you believe the school system is discriminating against your child, you should contact the ADA coordinator for the school. Under the ADA, all schools must develop procedures for families to file complaints about discrimination under the ADA. If you have a complaint against a state or local government agency or a private company or organization, you should contact the U.S. Department of Justice. If you have a complaint against an employer, you should contact the Equal Employment Opportunity Commission. For more information about the ADA, you can contact the Disability Rights Section of the Civil Rights Division of the U.S. Department of Justice. Contact information for all of these agencies can be found in the Resource Guide.

▪▪ Government Benefits

A number of federal programs offer financial assistance for people with disabilities and their families. Children with visual impairments may qualify for some or all of these programs, providing they meet eligibility requirements. Since the rules governing these benefits change from time to time, care must be taken to seek out the most current information about the following programs:

Supplemental Security Income (SSI)

Supplemental Security Income (SSI) is a program administered by the Social Security Administration. Its purpose is to provide cash benefits to the parents of children with disabilities and adults with disabilities. As of 2006, the maximum monthly SSI payment was $603 for an individual and $904 for an eligible married couple.

To qualify for SSI, an individual must satisfy three requirements. First, he must be a citizen of the United States or have proper (legal) immigrant status. Second, the disability must be so severe that the person cannot engage in "substantial gainful activity." Because children do not generally work for a living, the Social Security Administration does not apply work standards to them. The medical examiner does not compare a child's conditions with that of an adult. Instead, the disability evaluations specialist tries to determine whether the disabling condition "significantly disadvantages" the child. The law states that a child will be considered disabled if he or she has a physical or mental condition (or combination of conditions) that results in marked and severe functional limitations. The condition must last or be expected to last at least twelve months or be expected to result in the child's death. Also, the child must not be working and earning over Substantial Gainful Activity (SGA).

Substantial Gainful Activity refers to the maximum amount an individual can consistently earn from a job per month. As of 2005, the SGA amount was $830 for a individual with a disability who was not blind and $1,380 for a person classified as blind. This does not mean that individuals should not work; it just means that there is a line that is reviewed before deciding if a claim can be made. The official definition of Substantial Gainful Activity is the performance of significant physical and/or mental activities in work for pay or profit, or in work of a type generally performed for pay or profit. "Significant activities are useful in the accomplishment of a job or the operation of a business, and have economic value."

The third requirement is that the individual's income and assets must fall below a certain level. Income is money you have coming in—parental income, child support for a child with a disability, unemployment, worker's compensation, wages, etc. Resources are things an individual owns, such as vehicles, stocks, and bonds. The resource limit is $2,000 for an individual and $3,000 for a couple. So, a child, under the age of 18, with two parents in the household would have a resource limit of $5,000 ($2,000 for himself and $3,000 for his parents). Income is on a totally different scale. Income is like a dimmer light switch; the more you turn it (the higher or lower the income) the more the light goes up or down (the more eligible or ineligible to receive SSI). When the applicant is a child under 18 who lives at home, his family's income and assets are counted toward this limit. The maximum amount a family can earn and have their child still qualify for some SSI is very complex and different for each family. Parents should call the Social Security Administration at 800-772-1213 to find out if their child and family qualify for this assistance.

Medicaid

Medicaid is a government-sponsored health insurance program. It can be used to pay for medically related services such as physical therapy, speech therapy, occupational therapy, orientation and mobility, and some medical examinations and treatment.

Eligibility is based on income. Income guidelines vary from state to state, but children who are eligible for SSI are also often eligible for

Medicaid. To apply for Medicaid, contact your state's Department of Human Services.

Tax Equity and Fiscal Responsibility Act of 1982 (TEFRA)

There is an alternative to Medicaid for families whose income is too high to qualify for Medicaid. Under a program called the Tax Equity and Fiscal Responsibility Act of 1982 (TEFRA), families in some states can qualify for medical assistance (MA) based on the severity of their child's disability. The family's income is *not* counted when determining eligibility for this assistance.

To be eligible for TEFRA assistance, a child must be under 19 and require a certain level of home health care comparable to care that would be provided in a hospital, nursing home, or an intermediate care facility for persons with developmental delay (mental retardation). It is up to the State Medical Review Team to determine whether a child needs that level of care, based on information they receive about the child from doctors, hospitals, and schools.

Under the TEFRA option, all services medically necessary to care for your child at home are covered, up to your state's payment limits. These include therapy, prescription drugs, medical supplies and equipment, and private duty nursing.

TEFRA is an optional program for states; currently fewer than half the states participate. Contact your Department of Human Services or local social service department for more information on this program.

▪▪ Free Matter for the Blind

If your child is legally blind, he is entitled to send and receive certain materials through the mail postage free. Materials such as textbooks, educational materials, braille letters, and talking books (books on tape from the Library for the Blind or other services) may be mailed without postage. These materials must have the words "free matter for the blind" stamped or handwritten on them. It is important to remember that these materials must be for the use of someone who is legally blind, not simply related to visual impairments in some way. This service is not available, for example, for parent groups to mail newsletters to their members, but can be used for a grandmother to mail a braille letter to her grandchild who reads braille.

◼◼ Conclusion

In the United States, many important legal provisions protect your child's right to an education, access to public environments, and assurance of equal opportunities in the communities. The laws that are currently in place were created due, in part, to the hard work of parents, consumers, and professionals. If we lived in a perfect world, you would not have to learn about disability law on top of all the other new information related to your child's special needs, and people with disabilities would automatically receive the supports and services they need to live full and productive lives. Unfortunately, we do not live in a perfect world. Although laws guarantee your child some very valuable rights and benefits, he will not necessarily receive them unless you make sure that he does. This does not mean that you need to become a lawyer or even on expert on disability-related laws. But you do need to be informed about your child's basic rights and keep abreast of any changes or challenges to them. You, your child, and your family will all benefit from this knowledge.

◼◼ Parent Statements

The laws that we have now have made such a wonderful difference in Bennie's education. I can't imagine going through this fifty years ago.

❧❀❧

We went to a presentation on advocacy at a parent meeting recently. I'm glad that the laws exist now to protect individuals with disabilities, but it seems a little overwhelming to me. Listening to the presenter, I started thinking that I was going to have to fight for everything that Christopher needs. But then I talked to some other parents who told me that I just need to know about these things, I probably won't need to fight. That's reassuring to me.

❧❀❧

Sometimes it seems as if things aren't the way they should be, but I don't know whether I should call a lawyer or not.

❧❀❧

Who gets to make the final decision about where Mike should be educated, us or the school? That's what I'd like to know.

❧⊱

Sometimes I go to meetings and I don't know whether to sign something or not. But everyone is sitting around waiting for me and I feel so much pressure.

❧⊱

"Appropriate" is such a tricky word. The school can interpret it one way, and parents can interpret it another. Getting on the same page isn't easy sometimes.

❧⊱

I live in a small town and I've known the superintendent of schools since I was little. He lives right down the street from me. When I try to question anything the school is doing or not doing, I feel like I am destroying my relationship with the people who work at the school. Even more important, I am afraid of the repercussions that would have for my son.

❧⊱

I really feel that my views are important and that our family values are considered. It is important for me to be able to speak my mind and to feel respected.

❧⊱

My husband and I both went to Jessie's IEP meeting. It wasn't easy because we both had to take off from work and we had to arrange for a babysitter for the kids, but it was worth it because we both heard the school's recommendations, and we were both able to have input.

❧⊱

At every IEP meeting we go to, the school gives us a copy of our legal rights. I know I should probably read them over from cover to cover, but I haven't quite found the time for that yet.

❧⊱

Once when I was a freshman in college, I helped a blind student find her way through the cafeteria line. We ate supper together and had a really lively, interesting conversation. I hate to admit it, but I didn't go on to make friends with her, and never even talked to her again. I guess this was mainly because I felt a little uncomfortable around her—didn't know where to look when I was talking to her, and so on. With today's laws encouraging community inclusion, kids without disabilities will hopefully grow up to have a much more enlightened attitude about kids with disabilities than I had.

❧❀❧

I find myself spending a lot of time thinking about what kinds of jobs my child might be able to do when he grows up. I know the ADA prevents job discrimination, but I still can't help worrying that he may have a tough time finding a decent job.

❧❀❧

I want my child to be in the "real world." I hope the laws that are passed in this country will help us achieve that goal.

10

GROWING INTO LITERACY

Alan Koenig, Ed.D.

Literacy is highly valued in our society, so parents may be concerned about how their child with a visual impairment will learn to read and write. While the way in which children with visual impairments learn reading and writing will be much the same as for children with typical vision, there are differences that will need attention. You can provide a wealth of simple, valuable early literacy experiences in the home that will build the foundation for reading and writing for your child. With guidance and assistance from a teacher of students with visual impairments, the early home experiences you provide will help prepare your child to achieve literacy to the greatest extent of her ability.

Literacy is the ability to use written language—reading and writing—to accomplish a variety of important tasks in our daily lives. Early literacy, sometimes called "emergent" literacy, refers to children's early experiences with, and attempts at, reading and writing. During this stage, children develop an awareness that letters and words have meaning, and that we use them to communicate our ideas. The early literacy period lasts until a child enters a formal reading and writing program, generally in late kindergarten or first grade.

The foundation for literacy actually begins at birth. When an infant begins to understand that crying will get Mom or Dad to come into the room or that "go bye-bye" means a ride in the car, she is developing language skills that will be essential in learning to read and write. As a preschooler begins to master basic skills in understanding and producing oral language, she acquires the foundation needed for developing literacy.

Children demonstrate early literacy skills when they scribble a message and then "read" it back to someone or when they look at a book and tell the story from the pictures. Children also show early literacy skills when they recognize that the "golden arches" mean "a place to eat hamburgers" or that an outline picture of a man or woman on a door means a restroom. Children pick up these early literacy skills because they see print being used around them, and they learn to associate certain literacy events with meaningful things in their lives.

Children with visual impairments also learn through association, but they will rely less or not at all on visually observing events in their environment. For example, a child with a visual impairment may associate the sound of the garage door opening with Mother coming home from work. Or she may pick up a book with a fuzzy patch on the front and associate it with her favorite story, *Pat the Bunny*. Because a child with a visual impairment cannot rely on her vision to imitate others, it is important to take more direct steps to assure that early literacy develops. This chapter will suggest some ways you can help your child gain important early reading and writing experiences. But first, to give you an idea of where your child is heading, the chapter discusses options for reading and writing for people with visual impairments.

▪▪ Options for Reading and Writing

A visual impairment does not prevent literacy from developing, nor does it necessarily make it more difficult to learn to read and write. With appropriate intervention, children with visual impairments can arrive in a formal school program well prepared to learn to read and write. But a child with a visual impairment may need to learn alternatives to reading and writing standard print, depending on her learning characteristics, abilities, and needs.

There are a variety of options for reading and writing, and one or more of them will be appropriate for your child. This section describes the various options; a later section explains how the choice among options will be made.

Print

Many children with visual impairments read and write in print. But because a visual impairment may affect the resolution (or clarity) of printed words, the image must be enlarged so the child can read efficiently. There are a variety of ways to enlarge the visual image that the eye receives. One way is to actually make the print larger. When a book is enlarged, however, the pictures may not be reproduced in color and so become less interesting to children. Fortunately, books for young children are already in large print, so it is usually unnecessary to enlarge them even more.

If a child cannot read ordinary print in children's books, there are various ways of making the print larger. One way is simply getting closer to the book! For example, a child can essentially double the size of print by bringing a book from ten inches away to five inches. Despite common fears that reading at a close distance will harm a child's eyes, this is not true. Increasing the contrast, or sharpness of the words, may also help. Adjusting lighting or using colored acetate filters may help to increase the contrast. A TVI (a teacher who is specially trained to teach students with visual impairments) and your child's eye care specialist or a clinical low vision specialist can advise you about the types of modifications that will be most helpful for your child.

Yet another option for reading print is to use a magnifying glass. A magnifying glass increases the size of letters and allows a child to read more easily. Generally, low vision devices such as magnifying glasses are not prescribed for very young children because they can use other simple modifications to explore books. Also, some children—such as children with restrictions in their peripheral vision (tunnel vision)—may not benefit from a magnifying device. This decision, however, must be made individually for each child. If your child needs a low vision device, an eye care specialist who has special training in low vision will help to choose the most useful one.

There are a variety of ways to write print. Some children with visual impairments are able to use a regular pencil, but others use a black felt-tip pen to provide additional contrast. For many children just learning to write, a soft-lead artist's pencil may be a good option, since it produces a very dark line, but can also be erased. Most children with visual impairments learn typing or keyboarding, usually earlier than children with typical vision.

Braille

Reading in Braille. Children who use their touch and hearing, rather than their vision, as their primary senses generally will learn to read braille. Braille is a system of reading and writing in which letters and words are formed by patterns of raised dots that are felt with the fin-

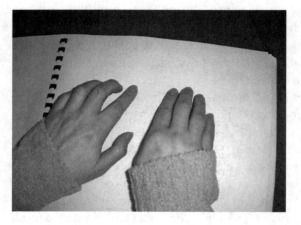

gers. Children usually learn to read braille with the index fingers of both hands, although some people use all fingers except their thumbs.

Braille was invented by Louis Braille in the early 1800s when he was a student at a Paris school for children who were blind. Louis was intrigued by a system used in the military to read by touch at night. This earlier system had twelve dots that were arranged in a grid that was two dots across and six dots down. Louis felt that twelve dots were too many, so he developed a six-dot "cell" with two across and three down. (See Figure 1.) He assigned different shapes to each of the letters. Louis's system of reading was used by the students at the school in Paris, but was not formally adopted or even called "braille" until after his death.

The braille code used in the United States today is based on the tactile alphabet invented by Louis Braille. The braille alphabet is the same as the print alphabet except that a "w" had to be added, however, since the French alphabet did not have this letter during Braille's lifetime. Figure 2 presents the braille alphabet, numbers, and some punctuation marks, as well as a short poem.

In addition to having shapes for each letter of the alphabet, the braille system used in the U.S. and Canada also has a series of contractions. There are a number of ways contractions are made in braille. For example, one or more letters from a word can be used to stand for the whole word, when used in a sentence. Thus, in the braille version of "Twinkle, Twinkle, Little Star" in Figure 2, the letter "s" written by itself stands for the word "so," while the letters "ll" stand for "little" and "abv" stands for "above." Sometimes a special configuration stands for a word or part of a word. For example, Figure 1 shows the configuration that stands for the word "the" and can also be used as part of a word such as "then." Notice that there is a single lower dot in front of each word at the beginning of the lines and the word "I." This is called the "capital dot" and means that the next letter is capitalized. In braille there are no unique shapes for capital letters, as there are in print, so capitals are indicated with the capital sign.

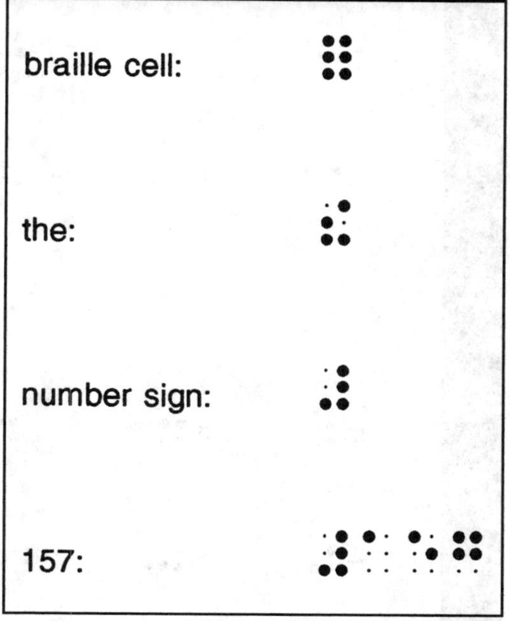

▪▪ FIGURE 1

braille cell:

the:

number sign:

157:

As with capital letters, there are no unique shapes for numbers. Numbers are indicated with a "number sign," as shown in Figure 1. When the letters a through j have a number sign before them, they are the numbers 1, 2, 3, 4, 5, 6, 7, 8, 9, 0, as shown in Figure 2 on the next two page. For example, Figure 1 shows how 157 is written.

Altogether, there are 189 contractions in the braille code. When something is written using all possible contractions, it is called "contracted" braille. If something is in "uncontracted" braille, it means that no contractions are used. In North America, contracted braille is almost always used. Most children begin to use contracted braille in reading and writing instruction from the very beginning. Some teachers are beginning to use uncontracted braille with beginning readers, although this is not yet a common practice. If a child learns uncontracted braille during early reading instruction, then she probably will learn the contractions later on in primary or middle school.

■■ Figure 2

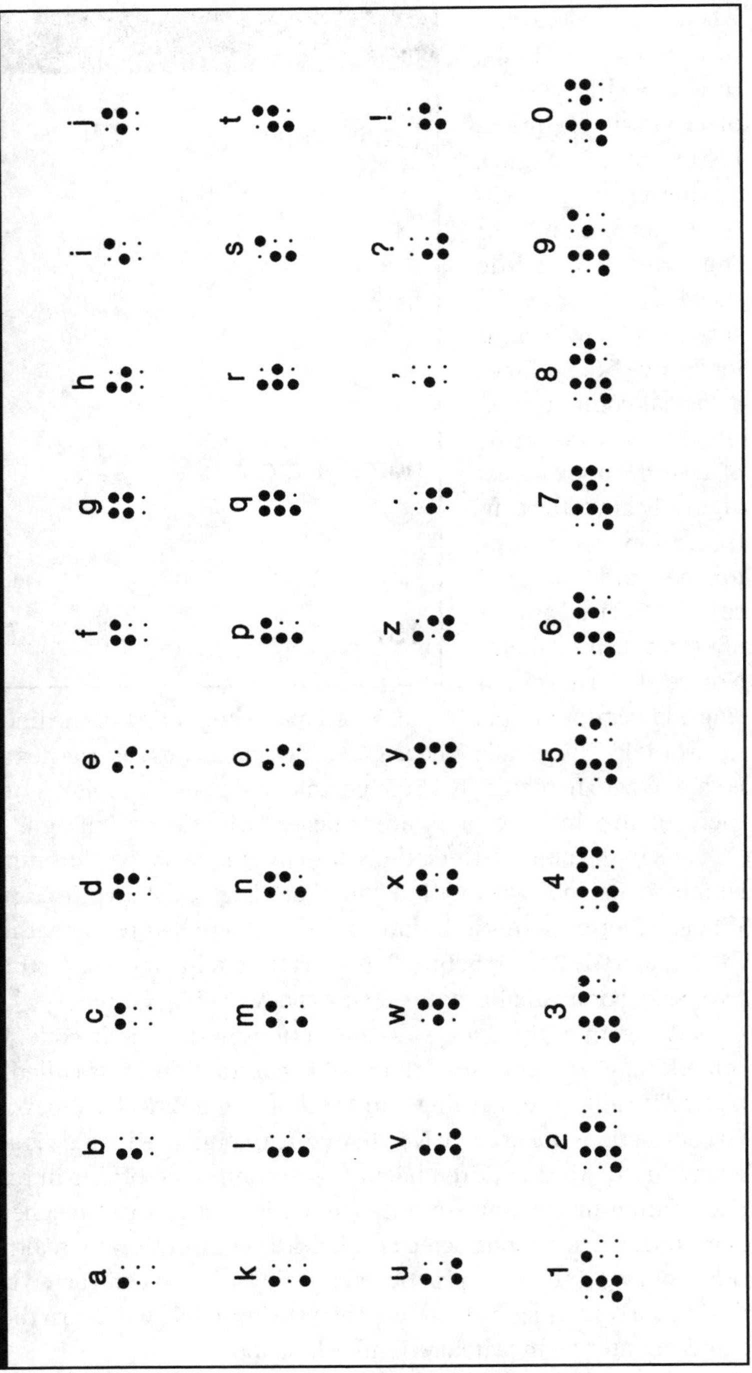

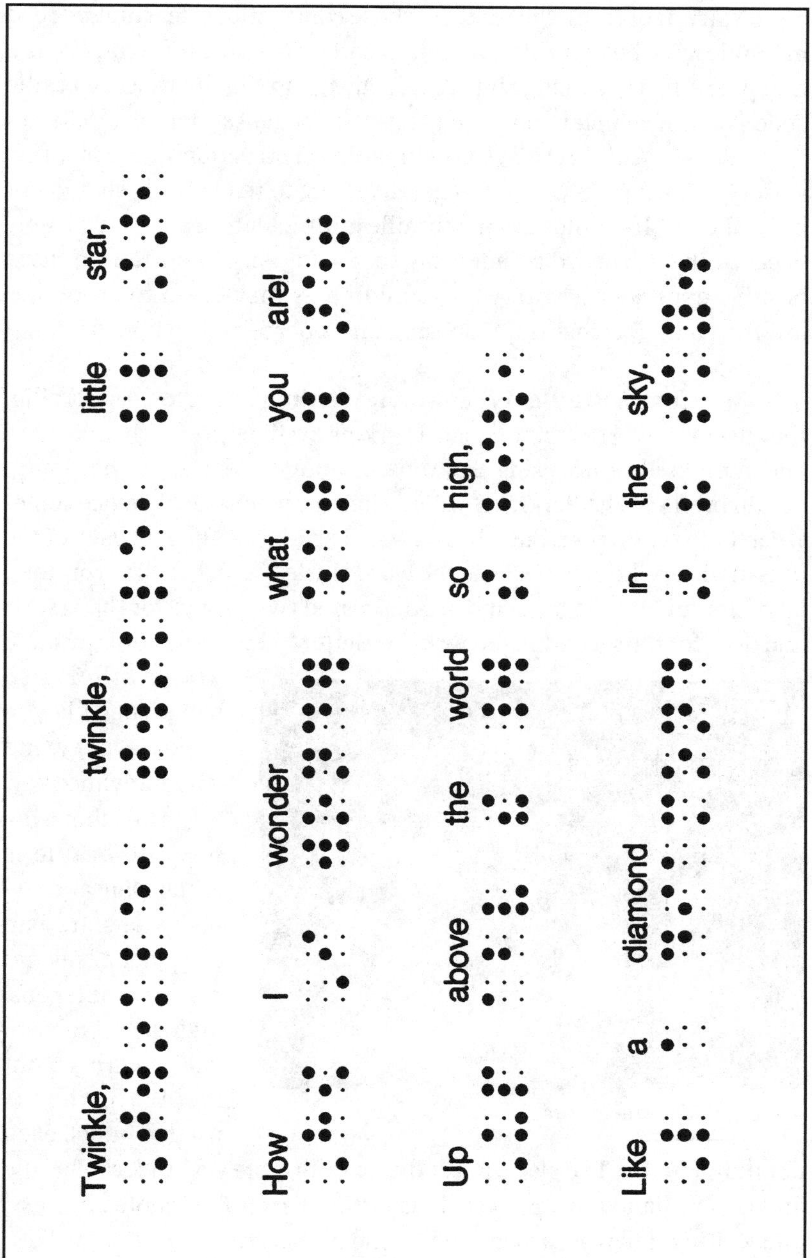
Twinkle, twinkle, little star,
How I wonder what you are!
Up above the world so high,
Like a diamond in the sky.

You might think that with all those contractions, learning to read in braille must be very difficult. But it really is no more difficult, or easy, than learning to read in print. True, some people claim that the braille code is more *complex* than the print code because more symbols are used. But if a child receives good reading instruction and has a rich variety of background experiences, learning to read braille should not be "difficult." If a child says that braille is difficult to read, it is probably because she has heard an adult say so. So it is very important to share positive experiences with young children as they begin to encounter braille reading, rather than focusing on its perceived complexities.

Writing in Braille. When young children begin to write braille, they usually use a machine called a Perkins Braillewriter, although more and more children are using electronic braille devices such as the Mountbatten brailler. The Perkins Braillewriter is a mechanical device somewhat like a typewriter, but it has only six basic keys—one for each of the dots in the braille cell. To write the word "little" (which is "ll" in braille), all of the keys for the left hand are depressed twice, once for the first "l" and once for the second "l." To write the letter "a," just one key is pushed.

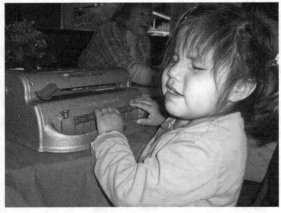

Using a Perkins Braillewriter.

The brailler also has a space key, a back-space key, and a line-advance key.

Another way to write braille is with a slate and stylus. The slate is a template of several rows of braille cells, and the stylus is a device with a blunt metal tip that is used to punch each dot individually. The slate and stylus is a portable way to write braille and is very handy for tasks such as jotting lists, taking notes in class, and writing down addresses and phone numbers.

Usually children master the use of the braillewriter before learning to use a slate and stylus. Learning the slate and stylus usually occurs sometime in the late primary grades or early in middle school, but when your child learns will be a decision made by the team working with your child in school—including you.

Typing or keyboarding is another very important skill for children who read and write in braille. Since it allows them to communicate directly with people who read print, it is very helpful in school and later for employment. Typing is a rather easy skill for a child to learn when good instruction is provided. This skill is generally introduced after a child has learned to write with a brailler, usually around third or fourth grade. With so many computers in schools, however, some children learn "keyboarding" even earlier than third grade. When to introduce keyboarding is another important decision that will be made by the educational team working with your child.

How Can Parents Learn Braille? If your child will be learning to read and write in braille, you probably will want to learn braille yourself. As your child goes through school, this will allow you to assist with homework, as well as write messages and letters to her. Also, as your child comes to realize that you value and respect braille as a way to read and write, she will develop this same value and respect.

Table 1 on the next page outlines some resources that can help you learn braille. *Just Enough to Know Better* is perhaps one of the best, because it was designed especially for parents. This guide introduces the alphabet, punctuation marks, some special symbols such as italics, and all of the contractions. Other programs are valuable as well, although they are generally geared to future teachers or braille transcribers, and therefore go into extensive detail about the rules governing use of various braille contractions. Whichever program you use, your child's teacher should be able to give you valuable help.

Listening

For children with visual impairments, listening is a very important way of gathering information from the environment. Your child will learn to rely more on her listening skills than children who have typical vision. It is a myth, however, that children with visual impairments have "better" hearing. It is more accurate to say that they learn "more efficient use" of hearing.

During the preschool years, your child will learn to associate different sounds with certain activities. For example, she will learn that the refrigerator door opening may mean it is time for a snack! Likewise,

:: TABLE 1—INSTRUCTIONAL MATERIALS ON BRAILLE FOR ADULTS

Title and Source	Description
Just Enough to Know Better The National Braille Press 88 Saint Stephen St. Boston, MA 02115 www.nbp.org	This friendly book was written specifically for parents to introduce contracted braille. It is written in both print and braille and contains a handy guide to all the braille contractions. It even has flashcards to help you practice!
New Programmed Instruction in Braille, Third Edition SCALARS Publishing P.O. Box 158123 Nashville, TN 37215 www.scalarspublishing.com	This book uses programmed learning to introduce small sections of the contracted braille code and allows ample practice before going on. It is written in print and facsimile braille. It covers all letters, contractions, and rules. A supplementary book provides reading practice in real braille.
Instruction for Braille Transcribing American Printing House for the Blind P.O. Box 6085 Louisville, KY 40206-0085 www.aph.org Library of Congress 1291 Taylor St., NW Washington, DC 20542 http://www.loc.gov/nls/	This instructional manual was written for individuals who wish to become braille transcribers. It introduces all letters and contractions in contracted braille and the rules that govern them. It also contains information on basic format techniques for braille materials. The manual can be purchased through APH. Or if you want to become a certified braille transcriber, you can take a free correspondence course from the Library of Congress/National Library Service for the Blind and Physically Handicapped.
Introduction to Braille Braille Reading for Family Members Hadley School for the Blind 700 Elm Street Winnetka, IL 60093 www.hadley-school.org	The Hadley School for the Blind offers two correspondence courses for family members of children who are blind or severely visually impaired. These courses are offered free of charge. The first course presents uncontracted braille, and the second course presents contracted braille.

most of the information she receives while watching television will be through listening to conversation and sound effects.

When your child enters school, listening will become critical to her progress. She will need to listen for and remember things that other children can readily see, such as assignments or other information written on the chalkboard. Later in elementary school or junior high school, your child will learn to "read" books that have been recorded on cassette tapes by listening to them. This will be very important when your child is in high school and college. Some textbooks are not available in braille at the high school level, and very few are available in college. All books, on the other hand, can be received on cassette tapes through a nonprofit organization called Recording for the Blind & Dyslexic (RFB&D). (See the Resource Guide for the address.) As your child enters high school, she will need to learn to order books from RFB&D.

Although listening will be extremely important for your child, it is not a substitute for learning to read and write in print or braille. Listening will be a valuable *supplement* to reading, but will not replace it. Your child will need to learn to use both reading and listening, and then later decide when it would be best to use one or the other for completing certain tasks. For example, if your child is working on a report and needs to read several books in a short amount of time, it may be more efficient to use books on tape rather than to read all the books in print or braille. If, however, she is making a list of friends to invite to her birthday party, she will probably choose to use braille or print to compile her list.

Computers and Other Technology

Computers and other technological devices will also be valuable supplements to your child's primary reading and writing medium. These devices can enable your child to compete equally in the classroom with peers who have typical vision.

There are many different ways for children with visual impairments to use computers. One of the most important ways is through word processing programs. A word processing program allows you to write documents, revise them, and then print out a final product. There are word processors that provide large print on the screen, braille on a special display, or speech sounds through a synthesizer.

Because there are so many useful computerized devices, most children today learn to type on a computer keyboard rather than on a typewriter. However, it is still important to know how to use a typewriter for some tasks. For example, it may be easier to address envelopes with a typewriter than with a computer system. Also, technology may break down sometimes or a computer may not be available, so there may be a need to have an alternative, such as a typewriter, for writing print documents.

Here are some ways technology may be useful to your child:

- A closed-circuit television (CCTV) operates like a small television station. The student moves a regular print book on a moving table under the camera, and the CCTV presents enlarged print on the monitor. Some CCTV models now present images in color.
- Some devices, such as the Kurzweil Reading Machine, convert printed words to spoken words. The speech is "synthesized" by a computer, so it sounds somewhat like a robot.
- There are a number of programs that enlarge print on a computer screen or convert words on a computer screen into synthesized speech.
- There are some devices that can be attached to a computer and allow the user to have a braille display of what is on the computer screen.
- Portable braille note-taking devices allow individuals to braille information into the device and retrieve it later. The devices can be hooked up either to a computer or directly to a printer.
- One type of device allows a child to braille on a Perkins Brailler or an electronic brailler in contracted braille, then produce a print copy for the teacher via an attached inkprint printer.

New devices are being developed so quickly that there is currently a technology explosion. Since any list printed in this book would soon be outdated, the best source of information on available technology will be your child's teacher of students with visual impairments. He or she will discuss the various options with you and help you decide which might be best for your child.

Technology for children with visual impairments ranges in price from a few hundred dollars to many thousand dollars. If the educational team agrees that certain technology is needed and this is placed in the IEP, the school district is responsible for providing the recommended technology, for use at school, at no cost to the parents. Technology used in the home often becomes the financial responsibility of the parents, however. Sometimes state social services can help families with the purchase of technology for home use, although this varies widely among the states. Another source to explore may be local community service clubs, such as the Lions or Kiwanis.

While technology will likely be a valuable tool for your child in school and in adult life, it still will not replace reading and writing in print or braille.

∷ Building the Foundation for Literacy

Now that you have an idea where your child is heading, you can begin to think about ways to help her get there. In other words, what can you do to help foster her literacy development?

We know through research that the essential building blocks for literacy come from early experiences and exposure to reading and writing activities in the home. So parents play an important role in preparing their child for the type of literacy that is taught in school programs. As the parent of a child with a visual impairment, you may have to be more aware of your role in readying your child to read and write. Early home activities that will help prepare your child to read and write include:

1. actively engaging her in first-hand experiences,
2. exposing her to literacy activities in the home and community,
3. reading to her, and
4. encouraging her early explorations in reading and writing.

Providing Experiences

The foundation for literacy—as for all learning—comes from first-hand, common experiences, such as going to a friend's birthday party, helping to clean out the garage, and riding a tricycle. It is through these early experiences that your child will be able to bring meaning to a story or a book. If your child has experienced first-hand the activity or event portrayed in a story, then she will be able to understand the story as it is being read. The meaning of a story doesn't come from the print or braille itself, but from your child's previous experiences.

To understand the importance of early experiences, you might think of words as capsules that are stored in your child's brain. If your child can say a word but does not have any actual experience to back it up, the capsule will be nearly empty. For example, your child may be able to say the word "sheep" because she has heard you talk about sheep on the farm, has heard a story about sheep on *Sesame Street,* or has heard the "baa" sound from a "See and Say" toy. All of these things provide a

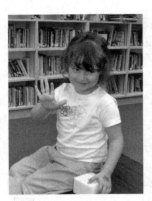

little bit of information, so there is a little bit in your child's "sheep" capsule. However, the capsule is not filled until your child has had an actual, first-hand experience with a sheep, ideally on a real farm. If your child has an opportunity to pet a real sheep, smell a sheep in its natural habitat, hear a live sheep "baa," and so forth, then the "sheep" capsule will be adequately filled.

If your child has low vision, her use of vision will provide some information for the capsule as well. But again, the actual experience is needed to fill the capsule with rich and accurate meaning. In some cases, visual information from pictures in a book or on television will be incomplete or, perhaps, inaccurate. Pairing visual images with information from other senses is accomplished through first-hand experiences. While pictures or TV shows can provide some information, it is nothing like the real thing!

In providing experiences for your child, try to concentrate on common occurrences in the home and the community. To be useful and valuable to your child, an experience does not have to be a major family undertaking, such as a five-day cruise on an ocean liner. While this would be a wonderful experience for any child, it is not necessary for developing an essential base of early experiences. Taking a ride in a paddle boat or row boat would be more valuable as a basic experience!

When your child has an opportunity to actively experience things in the world around her, meaningful language will develop. This can occur when your child associates what she is experiencing with a word that already exists but which she has not experienced before. For example, your child may say "boat" without ever riding in a boat. But after you ride in a boat, she will have a real experience to make the word "boat" meaningful. Or it can occur when you provide a new label as part of a new experience. For example, your child may not know the word "silo." But as part of a trip to the farm, she is able to explore outside of the silo, crawl up the ladder, and play around in the grain inside the silo. As part of this experience, she is told that this thing is a "silo." So your child not only adds a new word to her vocabulary, but also has the background experiences to make it meaningful. Again, the most meaningful way to learn things is through actual, hands-on learning. For example, it is more valuable for your child to learn that most tree trunks are rough and most leaves are smooth during a family outing to a forest than it is to learn to sort rough and smooth blocks.

Here are some types of activities in the home that provide rich experiences:

- helping prepare a snack or bake cookies;
- picking up the morning paper;
- helping stack dishes in the dishwasher;
- helping rake leaves or plant flowers;
- picking up clothes or toys;
- getting the mail from the mail carrier;
- playing with siblings or friends in the backyard;
- calling Grandma and Grandpa on the telephone.

Early in your child's life, these home experiences will likely be the focus for many of your activities. But you should expand your child's experiences outside the home as well. Some common community activities might include experiences such as:

- playing at the city park with siblings and friends;
- splashing in the "baby pool" at the public swimming pool;
- exploring the grocery store and stores at the mall;
- visiting a farm with animals and machinery;
- eating at a fast-food hamburger stand and a "sit-down" restaurant;
- visiting a petting zoo;
- visiting public places such as the post office, fire station, and library.

To assure that your child is gaining the maximum benefit from experiences you provide, keep these important points in mind:

- *Make sure your child is an active participant in the experience.* She should use all her senses, since the more information that is received, the more accurately she will understand and fill her literacy capsules. If your child is a passive participant (for example, by going to a farm but not going into the animals' pens), capsules will not be sufficiently filled with quality information.

- *If your child has vision, visual information should be paired with other types of sensory information during experiences.* Visual information is valuable to store in capsules, but generally should not be the only source of information. Again, the more senses that can be used to learn things, the better.

- *If the experience includes several steps, make sure your child participates in all steps from the beginning to the end of the process.* For example, if you are baking cookies, the first step would be gathering all the ingredients from the cabinets (although you could even make the first step a trip to the grocery store!). And the final step before eating them might be to wash the dishes. Your child needs to experience the whole process, rather than isolated and fragmented bits. For example, if your child only stirred the ingredients when making cookies, then she would think that to get cookies you stir the batter and then eat the cookies. She may not be aware of all the other steps that go into making cookies unless she actually participates in each step.

- *Throughout the experience, be sure to provide your child with the vocabulary associated with it.* For example, a trip to the farm would include names for the various animals as they are being explored, as well as "farm," "barn," "pen," "tractor," and so forth. Then later, when your child hears you read these words, or reads them herself, the previous experience will provide a basis for understanding the story.

- *When you have a chance for some special experiences that might not be so "common" (such as that five-day trip on a cruise liner), take advantage of the opportunity!* It will be a valuable enrichment to your child's life and yours.

Obviously, there are certain first-hand experiences that your child will not likely be able to have. For example, most children will not have an opportunity to visit the Great Wall of China. But if your child has climbed on a fence, opened and closed gates, and compared different types of fences, she can use these experiences—perhaps along with a three-dimensional model—to develop a general understanding of the Great Wall. Without the basic experiences, this would not be possible. So the focus should remain on developing a core of common experiences that will be the foundation for everything your child learns.

Exposure to Literacy in the Home and Community

Children become aware of written language and the way it is used by observing adults and others use it as part of daily life. Children who have typical vision are constantly seeing reading and writing happening around them throughout the day, and, as is often the case, they want to imitate what they see. For example, a child might see Mom looking at the newspaper and hear her say, "Oh, there's a concert tonight at the park—let's go." So the child might pick up a newspaper (maybe even upside-down) and say, "Oh, free pizza tonight—let's go!" Or when the child sees a parent writing something, she might take a crayon and scribble a message (sometimes on the refrigerator). It is through these constant interactions with print that children begin to understand that written language has meaning, and that we use reading and writing to accomplish important tasks in our lives.

Children with visual impairments miss some or all of these incidental exposures to literacy activities, so learning through imitation is greatly restricted. Therefore, you will need to make literacy activities overtly obvious to your child. In your home, you can have your child sit in your lap and help to hold things as you read the morning paper or the mail, "talking your way" through the process. You might say, "Oh! Here's a letter from Grandma. Let's see what she has to say." After opening the letter, you can read it aloud and then encourage your child to react to it in some way. You might say to your child, "Grandma asked if we would like to visit next weekend. Would you like to go to Grandma's? Let's write a letter and tell her!"

In the community, you will need to take time to explore signs and printed materials. If your child has low vision, getting closer to things, coupled with tactual exploration, will be a good strategy. If your child is blind, making direct contact with the materials works best. For example, you might lift up your child so she can explore street signs or signs in stores—many have raised letters. Also, most elevators are now marked in braille, so you can show your child the braille number of the floor you wish to visit and say, "We're going to the third floor, so let's push this button." A growing number of restaurants offer braille menus, so ask your waiter if your child can hold and explore one while you are reading the choices.

Literacy is used almost constantly throughout the day, and your child needs to know this! A child with a visual impairment needs to know the range and variety of reading materials in the home and community, including telephone books, magazines, newspapers, cookbooks, signs, brochures, and church bulletins. At first, you will need to make yourself super-conscious of the literacy tasks you do, because these tasks are generally done so automatically. The key thing to remember is to take active steps to make your child aware of these materials and the ways reading and writing are used.

Reading to Your Child

One of the best ways to build a solid foundation for literacy is to read aloud to your child on a regular basis starting early in life. In many homes, reading to a child during the evening or at bedtime is one of the most cherished activities of the day, and—for developing early literacy skills—one of the most important. As children hear their parents read stories on a regular basis, they begin to understand that ideas can be written down and kept forever in a book.

The first thing you will need is reading material. If your child has low vision, you will find an ample supply of wonderful children's books at the public library or local bookstore. Beginning in infancy and during the preschool years, it will be important to select motivating books that are brightly illustrated but contain relatively simple pictures or drawings. Too much clutter in the pictures may overwhelm your child at first. Be sure also to consider your child's background experiences and the age-appropriateness of the reading materials. For example, if your child has visited a farm, you may choose stories and books about farms and farm animals. Because of the prior experience with a farm, your child will understand and enjoy the story and be motivated to hear more. Also, farms and farm animals are likely to interest young children, while things such as mountain climbing and homecoming dances are not likely to provide the same interest until they grow older. You want your child to be able to understand and enjoy the story and to be motivated to hear more.

If your child is blind, there are a wide variety of reading materials in braille, although the selection is not as abundant as for books in print. Some braille books, called "twin-vision books" or braille-print books, contain both print and braille. These are ideal if you do not know how to read braille yet, since they expose your child to braille *and* provide print for you to read. Twin-vision books are also good if you are not sure whether your child will later read in print or braille. Table 2 on the next page lists sources of twin-vision books, some available for purchase and others for loan. While it is vitally important for your child to have exposure to braille books, do not feel as if you should *only* use braille materials. Other books can be quite motivating to your child, especially if you add some real objects for your child to hold and explore while you are reading. For example, if you are reading "The Three Little Pigs," you could have some straw, sticks, and a brick for your child to explore as you read each section of this delightful story.

After you have found appropriate reading materials, then it is simply a matter of starting! Here are some suggestions for reading aloud to your child*:

- *Start reading to your child as soon as possible.* It is never *too* early.
- *Read from twin-vision books or books with simple, colorful pictures.* Be sure your child is sitting in your lap or right next to you so she can see or feel the book.
- *For infants, use Mother Goose rhymes, repetitive stories, and simple songs.* These stimulate an infant's curiosity and attention. You might include finger plays to actively engage your child in the event. For example, if you are singing "The Itsy Bitsy Spider," you might show her how to use the index and middle finger of one of her hands to "crawl" on her other hand.
- *Set a specific time every day to read a story to your child.* You may find that reading just before bedtime will become part of an enjoyable night-time routine and an important social event for you and your child.
- *Start with simple picture books, then move to longer stories and perhaps even short novels.* Before reading, be sure to describe pictures to your child or help her interpret the pictures. Take time to enjoy the pictures on each page!
- *When you have advanced to longer stories and books that cannot be completed in one reading session, be sure to finish the story the next time or over several successive readings.*

---

* *Suggestions adapted from (and added to): Jim Trelease,* The New Read-Aloud Handbook *(New York: Penguin Books, 2001).*

▪ Table 2—Where to Get Twin-Vision Books

Source	Description
The National Braille Press 88 Saint Stephen St. Boston, MA 02115 www.nbp.org	This company offers a *Braille Book of the Month Club* for children. For the cost of any print book in their collection, you can receive the twin-vision version. These books contain the original print book with braille either on the print pages or inserted in clear plastic sheets. These books are for purchase only.
Seedlings P.O. Box 2395 Livonia, MI 48151-0395 1-800-777-8552 www.seedlings.org	Two types of books are produced. The first has braille labels placed on print books for preschoolers—some with sound buttons! Other twin-vision books are rewritten onto braille paper with print typed above the braille lines (although not necessarily word by word); these books contain no pictures. These books are for purchase only.
American Action Fund for Blind Children and Adults 18440 Oxnard St. Tarzana, CA 91356 www.actionfund.org	This organization offers a variety of twin-vision books for preschoolers through 4th graders on loan at no cost. Write to them for an application. You will provide your child's age and interests, and they will send you books via free matter for the blind. When you finish, you return them the same way, so there is no cost for postage. They also provide free braille calendars!
National Library Service for the Blind and Physically Handicapped Library of Congress 1291 Taylor St., NW Washington, DC 20542 http://www.loc.gov/nls/	The Library of Congress offers twin-vision books on loan through their various regional libraries. If you are unsure of how to contact your regional library, just ask the librarian at your local public library. Your child will need to be registered with the regional library in your area. All books are sent via free matter for the blind. You can also obtain children's books and some magazines in recorded formats and braille through the Library of Congress.
BrailleInk 1704 Holly St. Austin, TX 78702 http://www.brailleink.org	BrailleInk publishes existing high-quality children's books in a format that preserves the originals' print and illustrations in the top portion of the page and adds braille in the bottom portion. In addition, directly above each braille cell is the corresponding print character(s)—for both uncontracted and contracted braille. This arrangement enables print and braille readers to share the same book and makes it easy for anyone to teach or learn the braille alphabet. In each book there is a printed braille glossary that presents the alphabet, numbers, and punctuation. In books with contracted braille, the contractions *that appear in that book are presented* along with very basic rules for their usage.

- *Before you begin a story, read the title and ask your child what the story might be about.* Take some time to recall similar experiences that you and your child have had that relate to the story.
- *Read with plenty of expression, especially the dialog.* Remember not to read too fast, and adjust your rate of reading to match what is happening in the story. During a chase scene, for example, it is OK to read faster to stimulate your child's excitement.
- *Reading aloud is something that takes practice.* You can help yourself by reviewing the book beforehand and maybe even reading it aloud to yourself or to your spouse.
- *Try to add a real object or objects to the story whenever possible.* If you are reading "Jack and the Beanstalk," you may want to have some beans in their pods or some actual beanstalks ready to show your child. It would be ideal to have visited a garden and taken some time to work in it prior to reading the story. Also, scratch and sniff books and pop-up books are interesting and motivating to many young children. Again, it is important that your child have real-life experiences with the activities in the story. For example, if you are reading a scratch and sniff book to your child that has common food smells, you want to make sure that she has had previous experiences with helping in the kitchen.
- *If you find that your child is simply not interested in a book (regardless of whether it interests you), find another book that will bring excitement and enjoyment to your reading sessions.*
- *If your child is becoming acquainted with braille, it would be great to have someone who is blind read to your child.* This modeling of true braille reading is as important to a child who will read braille as modeling of print reading is to a child who will read print.
- *Learn more about reading aloud.* Borrow *The New Read-Aloud Handbook* by Jim Trelease from your public library or buy it from Penguin Books.
- *Most of all, have fun!* This is an important social time for you and your child, and you want it to be a special time.

As you read aloud to your child, you can help her develop a sense of "book behavior." These behaviors are things like holding a book right-side-up, turning one page at a time, reading from top to bottom and left to right, using page numbers, and taking care of books. These are important behaviors your child will use the rest of her life.

Early Reading and Writing Experiences

In addition to reading to your child, there are a variety of early reading and writing experiences that you can use to foster development of literacy. Generally during the preschool years or kindergarten, your child will begin experimenting with reading and writing, so it is important for you to encourage and respond to what she is doing in a nurturing and reinforcing manner. Here are some suggestions for activities you might use with your child:

- *After reading a story with your child, act it out using family members as various characters.* Be sure to use some real objects that were used in the story to make it even more meaningful.
- *Labeling objects that are important to your child is a good early reading experience.* You can label objects according to what they are (toy box, bedroom), or just label them with your child's name. If you are unsure whether your child will read in print or braille, label objects in both. Ask a teacher of students with visual impairments or an adult who is blind to help you make labels in braille using plastic labeling tape. It's a good idea to make a few extra labels for special things that get a lot of use because labels tend to come off after awhile.
- *Make tactile books based on your child's experiences.* Gather objects during the experience and attach the object to pages made of heavy paper or cardboard. Punch holes in the margin of the paper and fasten them together with ring fasteners. Braille or print can be added to provide more information. When finished, "read" the book with your child by having her explore the object on each page and tell about the experience.
- *After your child has an experience, have her tell you a story about what happened so you can write it down in print or braille.* (You may need to ask a teacher or an adult who is

blind to help you with the braille version.) Then make it into a book and put in on the shelf with other books. Re-read this story with your child whenever she would like. Since your child told you the story, she will likely be able to say some of the words that are coming up.

- *After some experiences, you may want to record an account of your adventures onto cassette tape.* These can be kept on the bookshelf and listened to whenever your child chooses.
- *Create book bags or book boxes to accompany stories and books.* Fill the bags or boxes with some of the items from the story. Or if the story was based on an actual experi-ence, fill the bag with items you picked up along the way. For example, if you took a trip to the zoo and later wrote a story about it, the book bag or box might contain a model of a giraffe, a popsicle stick from one of your snacks, and a snake skin you found.
- *Keep plenty of paper, crayons, pencils, and paints around the house for your child to use.* You may want to have a screen on which your child can draw. Just wrap a small piece of window screen around a piece of stiff cardboard or board and secure it. Then when your child draws or writes on a piece of paper taped to the screen, she will receive tactual feedback. If your child is blind, you might want to get a Sewell Raised-Line Drawing Kit from the American Printing House for the Blind. This simple kit has a clipboard with a rubberized surface, sheets of thin plas-tic, and a drawing device like an ink pen, but without ink. When the drawing device moves across a plastic sheet, it creates a bumped-up or raised line.
- *Encourage her to "write" messages using her own spellings or pictures.* If your child is blind, if possible have a braille writer with paper in it so she can practice "scribbling" as well. After your child "writes" something, have her read it back to you. After drawing, have her tell you about the picture. Be sure to post these creations on the refrigerator so she will know you value her work.
- *When you are going to the store, have your child make a list of things she needs.* She can do this with invented spellings or pictures, or you can write the list together. You might

also make a list of "things to do" or write a message to another family member.

- *Your child might want to keep a diary or journal of the important events during the day (or on some special days).* You can write down the events as your child dictates them to you. Your child will notice you writing as she dictates the events, helping her make the connection between what is being said and what is being written.

- *If your child is blind, be sure her fingers are in contact with the braille as you read things together.* Encourage her to "track" along the lines with the pads of the fingers on both hands as you read. It is not necessary for her fingers to be on the same words as you are reading—this will come later with more formal instruction. As your child gets older and more experienced with books, you may want to read only when she is tracking. This way she will begin to understand that to read braille, you must keep your hands moving!

- *If your child has low vision, move your finger under the words as you read.* Let her fill in words she knows or can guess from the context of the story. Also take time to interpret pictures. Your child may need help in picking out the most important things in the pictures and in moving her eyes around the page in a systematic manner.

These are just a few of many early reading and writing experiences you can use with your child. For more ideas, talk to the TVI who is working with your child. Above all, have fun with your child as you begin to explore early experiences with reading and writing. If these experiences become a chore, then neither you nor your child will benefit.

As your child enters kindergarten, she will receive formal instruction in reading and writing. If your child has low vision, the TVI will make sure that she is learning the efficient visual skills needed for reading and writing. Also, the teacher will make sure that appropriate materials and other adaptations, as were mentioned earlier, are made. If your child is blind, it is most likely that the TVI will be the primary teacher of reading and writing. The teacher will provide instruction in tactual discrimination and efficient hand movements so your child can quickly identify braille words and concentrate on the meaning in the story. You will work closely with your child's teachers by helping with reading and writing assignments and activities as they request, as well as by continuing to read aloud to your child and expand her background experiences. The foundation you provide before your child enters formal schooling and your continued cooperation throughout her school career will help assure that she has the literacy skills needed for living and working after graduation.

:: Making Decisions about Print or Braille

During the preschool years, it may or may not be evident whether your child will be a braille reader or a print reader. If it is not clear whether your child should begin formal reading instruction in print or braille, the decision will be made about the time she enters kindergarten. As Chapter 8 explains, this decision will be made by a team of individuals, including you, who are involved in your child's education. The educational team will systematically assess your child to determine which reading medium will be most appropriate.

To make a decision on the best reading medium, the team will gather a lot of information about how your child uses sensory information, and then select an appropriate reading medium to match. If your child is most efficient in using visual information, especially for completing detailed tasks twelve to fourteen inches from her eyes or closer, then she may use print for reading. If she is most efficient in 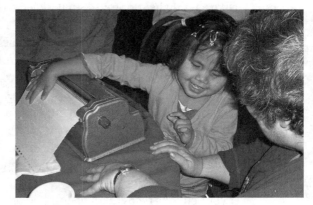 using tactual information to accomplish such tasks, then she may use braille for reading. In the meantime, if there is any question at all, you should present both braille and print to your child and observe how she responds to each.

Because you see your child more often than anyone else does, you will have an important role in helping to gather information on the best medium for your child. Here are some questions to keep in mind:

- When people enter the room, does your child recognize them by listening to them talk, touching them, or seeing them?
- When reaching for a toy, is your child attracted to it visually, or does she use other clues such as bumping into it or hearing a sound from it?
- When exploring toys or other objects, does your child use touch or vision?
- Does your child tell likenesses and differences in toys or other objects by touch or by sight? For example, does she tell her shoes from someone else's shoes by looking at both pairs or by touching them?
- Does your child accurately identify objects at near distances (within twelve to sixteen inches of the eyes) using vision or using other clues such as touch or sound? At intermediate distances (between sixteen and twenty-four inches)? At far distances (beyond twenty-four inches)?
- Does your child accurately identify large objects (like a chair or a bed) by touch or sight? Medium-size objects (like a teddy bear or toy)? Small objects (like a paper clip, coins, or marbles)?
- When your child uses fine motor skills (such as stacking blocks or cutting with scissors), does she use vision or touch?
- When reading from a print book, does your child show interest in the pictures or does she prefer to examine some real object that is associated with the story?
- When reading from a twin-vision book, does your child attend more to the braille or to the print?
- Does your child scribble, write, and draw using her touch or her vision?
- If your child is recognizing her name or other simple words, is she doing this in print or in braille?

For any of these tasks, your child might not show a preference for use of vision or touch, so you should note that she uses both senses. It may be helpful to keep a record of the distances from objects at which your child responds, as well as any observations related to the lighting conditions or the level of contrast that is preferred. Your observations should be shared with the TVI and other members of your child's educational team.

Besides gathering information about how your child uses sensory information, the team will want to consider whether your child's eye condition is stable. If your child has a stable eye condition and makes efficient use of her vision, the educational team may decide that print is the best option for reading and writing. If your child has an unstable eye condition that is likely to get worse, then the team may choose braille as the best option. The educational team will also consider any additional disabilities that may influence development of reading and writing skills. For example, if your child has a motor impairment that affects the way she moves her hands and fingers, then braille reading may not be the best option. Or if your child has a cognitive disability, reading in either print or braille may not be possible, or other important skills may take priority over the development of literacy skills. The team may decide to emphasize important daily living and work skills rather than reading skills. See the next section for more information about how additional disabilities may affect literacy skills.

Based on all this information, a decision will be made about which medium your child will use in beginning reading instruction. Some children might enter a formal reading and writing program in kindergarten or first grade without a clear preference for one medium having been established. Therefore, the team might decide to begin reading instruction in both print and braille and decide which is the most efficient medium later. Some children will continue to read in both print and braille throughout the school years. Remember, any decision on reading medium can be changed as your child's needs change.

∷ Literacy Skills for Children with Additional Disabilities

If your child has additional disabilities, the attention given to developing literacy skills may be different. A cognitive disability in addition to a visual impairment will probably make learning to read and write more difficult. In particular, a severe or profound cognitive disability may make developing literacy skills an unlikely achievement. A motor impairment, if not accompanied by a cognitive disability, may require changes in the mode of reading (such as use of taped materials rather than braille). Other disabilities, such as a hearing impairment or learning disability, may also influence the development of literacy skills. A thorough assessment of your child's abilities and skills will be needed to determine the emphasis that should be placed on developing literacy skills.

In developing an IEP, the educational team will consider all of your child's needs, and then prioritize the skills to address those needs. For children with additional disabilities, social skills, daily living skills, and vocational skills are often considered essential to living as independently as possible. These skills may therefore be considered more important than academic skills, such as reading and writing. Even though reading books and writing papers may not be emphasized, functional uses of literacy may still be taught to increase independence in daily living or vocational tasks. For example, being able to read labels on food products will help in preparing meals, and identifying one's name will help in punching a time card at work.

If the focus of your child's program is functional literacy, then the educational team will need your help to decide which tasks in the home would be easier if your child could use reading or writing. Using literacy in real-life situations is one of the primary keys in developing functional literacy. Also, regardless of the severity of your child's additional disabilities, she will probably still enjoy listening to a story being read aloud. Reading aloud is a form of communication, and communication skills are very important for everyone.

⦂ Conclusion

Fostering growth in early literacy might seem somewhat complicated at first, and you might occasionally wonder whether you are going in the right direction. But really, there are just four things to remember. First, actively involve your child in a rich background of common first-hand experiences. Second, read to your child on a regular basis. Third, give your child opportunities to interact with a wide variety of literacy materials and tasks. Fourth, when your child experiments with early reading and writing, support her enthusiastically. When you have any questions, feel free to ask a vision specialist. Above all, enjoy this time! It will be mutually rewarding for both you and your child.

▪▪ References

Henderson, F.M. "Communication Skills." In *The Visually Handicapped Child in School,* edited by B. Lowenfeld. New York: John Day Company, 1973.

Koenig, A.J. and M.C. Holbrook. "Determining the Reading Medium for Students with Visual Impairments: A Diagnostic Teaching Approach." *Journal of Visual Impairment and Blindness* 83: 296–302.

Lewis, S. and Tolla, J. "Creating and Using Tactile Experience Books for Young Children with Visual Impairments." *Teaching Exceptional Children* 35: 22–28.

Lowenfeld, B. *The Visually Handicapped Child in School.* New York: John Day Company, 1973.

Lyenberger, E. "Reaching for Literacy." In *Realities and Opportunities: Early Intervention with Visually Handicapped Infants and Children,* edited by S.A. Aitken, M. Buultjens & S.J. Spungin. New York: American Foundation for the Blind, 1990.

Miller, D.D. "Reading Comes Naturally: A Mother and Her Blind Child's Experiences." *Journal of Visual Impairment and Blindness* 79: 1–4.

Olson, M.R. and S. Mangold. *Guidelines and Games for Teaching Efficient Braille Reading.* New York: American Foundation for the Blind, 1981.

"Prebraille Readiness." *Future Reflections* 10: 13–16.

Roberts, F.K. "Education for the Visually Handicapped: A Social and Educational History." In *Foundations of Education for Blind and Visually Handicapped Children,* edited by G.T. Scholl. New York: American Foundation for the Blind, 1986.

Stratton, J.M. and S. Wright. "On the Way to Literacy: Early Experiences for Young Visually Impaired Children." *RE:view* 23, 55–63.

Sulzby, E. and W. Teale. "Emergent Literacy." In *Handbook of Reading Research: Volume II,* 727–57. New York: Longman, 1991.

Trelease, J. *The New Read-Aloud Handbook (5th edition).* New York: Penguin Books, 2001.

▪▪ Parent Statements

I'm learning braille now. It's not as difficult as I thought, but it takes time and practice.

❧

I've wondered if I should learn braille myself. I've tried to figure out the numbers on the elevator at work and it seems like it wouldn't be difficult, but I'm not ready to work at it.

❧

I'm not sure whether braille will be important for my daughter but I want her to have the opportunity to learn it.

❧

Janet holds books real close to her eyes to see the pictures or the words.

❧

Katherine loves books! Her sister, Colleen, reads with her sometimes. Katherine loves to be read to and she's beginning to recognize letters and words. I think she'll be a good reader.

❧

My child is two and a half years old. At our local parent group meetings I hear lots of arguments about braille. Frankly, I don't care right now. We have other problems to solve first.

❧

It seems important for Joe to learn braille in case his eyes get worse.

❧

I get sad sometimes when I realize that I can't just walk in any bookstore and buy books for Danny. My sister's kids have hundreds of books but Danny only has a handful.

❧

At first, I didn't see the point of reading to my son. He couldn't see the words or the pictures. But I now know that all children should be read to in order to encourage literacy development.

❧

I wonder how my child will know what's in the newspaper or in magazines or other things that aren't in braille.

❧

I am learning braille through Hadley School for the Blind. My oldest son, Scott (who is not visually impaired), loves it! I can hardly get to the braillewriter for practice because Scott is always doing "his" braille.

❧

We put Janie's braille papers up on the refrigerator just like her sister's schoolwork.

❦

We knew without a doubt that we wanted Justin to be a braille reader. Before we even knew Justin had no vision, we began learning about braille and how to get books in braille for him. We got our first Perkins Braillewriter when Justin was five months old so we could learn braille and so he could begin to play write on it.

❦

I meet many parents from various parts of the country. If talk about braille literacy comes up, I tell them that anyone can learn how to read the braille alphabet in 60 seconds. They usually look surprised or dubious! When I explain the simple code, though, they often see how simple it could be to learn the basic alphabet and numbers.

MOVING THROUGH THE ENVIRONMENT (ORIENTATION AND MOBILITY)

Kevin Stewart, Ed.D.

Most parents of children with visual impairments have questions about their child's ability to move around independently. For all children, the ability to move safely and efficiently from place to place in the home, preschool, and community is unarguably an important life skill to acquire. It is during your child's daily routines and play behaviors in these early years that he begins to move and interact with his environment. Through movement and interactions with people, objects, and events, he begins to learn about his body and position in space, and to refine his movement patterns. These skills provide the necessary foundation for later independent travel in the community.

In typical development, vision helps to motivate a child to explore his physical environment and provide a sense of awareness of body movements in space. When your child has a visual impairment, learning without sight can be fragmented and disorganized. It is therefore important that you and your child's early interventionists begin as soon as possible to facilitate his purposeful movement by creating a meaningful learning environment. Learning to move safely and efficiently is critical to your child's overall development and independence.

The skills that will enable your child to move from place to place are collectively known as orientation and mobility (O&M) skills. The process of orientation involves knowing where you are, where you are going, and how you are going to get there, by interpreting information available in your environment. With young children, orientation involves learning how to use sensory information and problem solving abilities to identify people, objects, and locations. The process of mobility involves the skills of movement and negotiating the environment safely and efficiently. During the early years, mobility is primarily focused on the development of movement patterns and includes specific techniques such as guided travel, trailing techniques, protective techniques, and use of mobility devices. These specific techniques are discussed in more detail later in this chapter.

Although orientation and mobility are complementary, they are not the same. For example, your child may be very mobile but frequently get lost or disoriented. Or, your child may always know where he is, but may not move around safely in the environment. Children need both of the skills of O&M in order to travel as independently as possible as they get older. The foundation of these skills begins to be laid in the infant, toddler, and preschool years and provides the building blocks necessary for independent travel skills during the elementary, high school, and adult years.

This chapter is designed to assist you in encouraging your child to move purposefully and independently. You will be introduced to the O&M skills as they relate to your child's early development, along with specific guidelines to assist you and others who interact with your child, in your home and preschool settings. This is the time for you and your child to learn together and for you to encourage him to develop his natural curiosity about objects, people, and events in his world.

▪▪ Orientation & Mobility Instructors

O&M skills are typically taught jointly by an O&M instructor and parents. O&M instructors are professionals trained to teach travel concepts and techniques to enhance the independent travel skills of people with visual impairments. The ultimate role of the O&M instructor is to support your child as he learns more about his body, positional relationships of objects in the environment, and how to move purposefully and easily from place to place in both familiar and unfamiliar environments. To accomplish these goals, a shared responsibility among the parent, O&M instructor, and other professionals working with your child is critical. Together you can help motivate your child's curiosity and help integrate O&M skills into your child's daily routine in a variety of environments.

Children with visual impairments are often eligible to receive training in O&M skills through their early intervention or special education program. There is no set age at which O&M instruction should begin, but independent travel skills are an integral part of early childhood development, and instruction in these skills should begin as early as possible. Instruction and support in O&M skills may span your child's preschool, elementary, high school, and adult years.

Through O&M training, young infants and toddlers develop environmental and sensory awareness and begin to move with a purpose through daily routines and play activities. During the preschool and elementary years, their purposeful movement patterns and environmental awareness are refined to enable them to travel safely in their classrooms, on the playground, and within their neighborhood. During the late elementary and high school years, children generally learn how to cross streets, ride city buses, plan more complex routes of travel, and travel in unfamiliar areas independently. This independent travel helps build your child's self-esteem and self-confidence by giving him more control over his environments without having to rely on others. If your child learns good O&M skills early, he is more likely to develop into a responsible, confident, and independent traveler as an adult.

Role of the Orientation & Mobility Instructor with Young Children

Many of the O&M skills are heavily dependent on what is naturally happening to your child during these early years, such as the development of movement and language. Consequently, the O&M instructor may work directly with your child or collaboratively with you and your child's early interventionist or preschool teachers. The O&M instructor can help you set up your home so that it supports your child's motivation and curiosity to explore his surroundings in a purposeful manner. In addition, the instructor can help your child develop good smooth movement patterns such as: rolling, crawling, walking, and moving in and out of different postural positions, all necessary for later independent travel skills.

As your child enters preschool classrooms, the O&M instructor may consult with your child's teachers to assist them in setting up a safe learning environment and provide specific strategies to encourage travel independence. This will facilitate movement and help reinforce the specific mobility skills you are working on at home.

:: Components of O&M Skills during the Early Years

Generally, before your child will be able to learn the more formal O&M techniques, he needs to have acquired certain developmental and sensory skills and a basic understanding and awareness of his body and environment. For example, in order for your child to understand position terms (such as behind and under) and use his senses to orient himself to the environment, he must first learn to move and interact with both objects and people. As a parent, you probably work on many of these skills with your child during the course of your daily routine. Thus, O&M skills worked on in the early years must not be taught in isolation, but integrated into your child's daily routine and functional activities as they naturally occur. These skills provide the building blocks that many of the formal techniques rely upon. These building blocks in O&M emphasize a developmental approach—that is, certain skills need to be mastered before other skills. Some principles of the developmental approach include:

- *Sensory before Conceptual Understanding*: Young children need to gain an awareness and begin to identify and inter-pret information obtained through their senses of hearing, smell, touch, taste, and vision (if they have some usable vi-sion), before they understand the properties and functions of objects (such as texture, shape, and color).
- *Body before Space*: Your child needs to gain an under-standing of his body parts, their functions (such as "I use my ears to hear; I use my hands to pick up my cup"), and positions such as: in front, behind, on, and off, before he can comprehend the layout of a room, house, or yard.
- *Familiar before Orientation*: Your child needs to become familiar with his surroundings and movement within

familiar environments, before he can orient himself to new environments.

- *Trial and Error before Problem Solving*: Through natural curiosity, your child will practice and try skills before thinking through sequences to obtain a desired objective. For example, your child will practice pouring (dumping toys out of a box) before he will make the connection and be able to pour cereal from a box to a bowl.

- *Gross Motor before Fine Motor*: Your child will work to refine "big muscle" movements—such as rolling, crawling, standing, and walking—before "small muscle" movements and fine coordination—such as picking up, buttoning, and zipping.

The building blocks so integral to O&M training with young children that are embedded in early child development are:
1. sensory development,
2. concept development,
3. movement and postural development,
4. techniques to facilitate familiarization/orientation, and
5. techniques to facilitate safe movement.

Sensory and concept development are critical to your child's orientation skills. These building blocks assist him in knowing where he is in the environment in relation to all other objects. Movement and postural development and specific guiding and protective techniques pertain to mobility skills. Each of the above developmental areas will be discussed within the context of the child's environment and functional routines.

Sensory Development

Sensory skill development helps young children to better use their senses of vision, hearing, touch, and smell to take in information about the environment. Accessing and interpreting this sensory information helps children understand their world, as well as their location in that world. When helping your child interpret environmental information, it is important to relate one sense to another. Your child will learn to use the information received by one sense to help him interpret the information gathered by another. Take your kitchen, for example: your child may identify the kitchen by the smell of food cooking in the oven in addition to the hum of the refrigerator and the feel of the tile floor. Generally, children with visual impairments must learn to use and develop their remaining senses more than other children do. Thus, it is important to understand what each sense provides.

Vision

Vision allows children to gather a great deal of information in a very short period of time at varying distances. The ability to locate a light source within a room can help a child determine where he is in the room.

Parents and professionals can help children with low vision by providing higher contrasting colors on floor and object surfaces; reducing the visual clutter in the room; and changing the lighting. For example, increasing the color contrast in a room or placing a high contrasting object in the room may help your child function better within this area. Adding extra lighting in a room will also increase existing color contrasts, thereby assisting your child—unless he is sensitive to light. If so, lowering the lighting levels may increase his ability to see specific objects in a room.

Touch

Young children learn about objects through exploration and play. Learning how to touch and gain meaningful information about objects is important to the orientation process. While your child moves and explores within his world, he will be in contact with a variety of objects such as furniture, walls, and floor coverings. By recognizing what he is touching, he will begin to map out his environment. This, in turn, will help him with independent exploration and movement.

Touch augments to some extent what is received from the other senses. Although your child hears the sound of his bedroom door opening and closing, he needs to explore the door through touch paired with sound and activity (going in and out of the door) to help him make sense of the sound. Touch provides your child with a means to identify objects located along travel routes within familiar areas by their texture, size, and shape. Recognizing objects will help your child understand where he is and to determine whether he is moving in the desired direction. Some tactile experiences that assist in the orientation process include distinguishing and identifying carpet, tile, wood, plastic, doors, door jams and casings, walls, and various sizes of furniture.

Hearing

Hearing is a sense that will provide your child with extremely valuable information for orientation purposes. The ability to hear and determine the location and direction of a sound is critical to your child's environmental awareness. The doorbell ringing signals that someone is arriving; the sounds of pots and pans or cans being opened lets him know where the kitchen is; the running of water in the bathtub identifies the location of the bathroom in the hallway. However, before your child can use sound in these ways to help him orient himself, parents and professionals must examine the typical developmental sequence in which sound use in learned.

Using sound to help children with visual impairments while traveling begins very early in life. Infants learn to localize and turn toward the sound of familiar voices, then objects. Eventually they begin to focus on the sound of familiar people and objects and follow them as they move. Toddlers begin to identify and discriminate among familiar sounds, especially those found in your home and community. Preschoolers begin to recognize specific places and activities by sound and question adults about what is happening. During these toddler and preschool years, you can help your child make sense of the sounds he hears. For example, in a grocery store, he may hear the sound of water spraying near the produce section. With your verbal explanations and opportunities to touch, listen, and talk about this situation, the sound of the water spray will take on meaning and be used as a signal, or clue, to the location of the produce.

If your child cannot see visual landmarks, sound also becomes important in helping him maintain his direction of travel and straight line of travel. This ability, too, follows a specific developmental progression. Infants first learn to localize on sound that is presented at ear level, then ear level and downward, followed by ear level and upward. At this point, your child is then able to localize on sound presented in front of his body, and then behind. During the toddler and preschool years, children learn to position sound sources in different positions in relation to the body. They learn to orient by traveling toward, away, or alongside sound sources. These early skills provide the building blocks for your child to maintain his directional orientation through a hallway, along a sidewalk, and, later, across a street at an intersection.

Smell

Smell is not the strongest sense for orientation, since it does not tend to pinpoint the exact location of an object, but it nonetheless provides valuable information. By being exposed to smells and learning to distinguish and identify smells in the environment, your child will learn to relate smells to general areas. This, in turn, helps him know where he is in the environment. The smell of food may indicate the kitchen, whereas the smell of soap and powder indicates the diaper change area in the bedroom or bathroom. Once children are traveling in the community, smell can assist them in knowing the general location of a bakery, hair salon, or a flower shop.

As with the other senses, the information obtained through smell alone will be meaningless unless paired with other sensory information. You, along with others working with your child, need to provide opportunities for him to experience different environments so he can actively explore the sensory information received through all available senses. By interpreting sensory information during daily activities, children begin to learn the necessary body, spatial, and environmental concepts necessary for orientation and independent travel in their environments from infancy through adulthood.

■■ Concept Development

Concept development involves learning about the nature (size, shape, texture, function) and location of objects. Concepts include *body image* such as body parts (hands, fingers), body planes (front, back), and body actions; and *object and environmental relations* such as size (big, little), shape (round, square), position (up, down, behind, under), distance (near, far), time (now, later), amount (more, few), and weight (heavy, light).

Body Imagery

Body imagery, which includes the understanding of body parts, planes, and actions, begins in infancy. As your baby is touched and handled, he begins to sense and become aware of his body parts. It is important to provide him with both light and deep massaging touches and strokes. The best time to do this is while changing, bathing, and cuddling your child. Later, he will learn the names of his own and others' body parts.

As your child begins to move about, he will begin to understand that his body parts have planes (front, back, sides, top, bottom) and specific functions (nose for smelling, ears for hearing, mouth for eating). Initially, children learn to understand planes such as top/bottom and on/off. Later they develop an understanding of more complex terms such as front/back and that their bodies have two sides. Eventually, around the age of five or six, they are able to label their sides as left/right. Similar to learning body parts, planes can also be taught during daily functional activities such as dressing, eating, and bathing. In addition, these concepts can be taught through songs, rhymes, and made-up games that encourage body movements, such as the actions to the song "Head and Shoulders." Understanding these concepts related to body imagery is the first step in understanding where one's body is in space in relation to others and objects.

While your child is beginning to learn about his body, he is also beginning to experiment with movement by kicking, rolling, and moving his arms and hands. Through these actions, young children begin to actively interact with objects and people. Consequently, they begin to relate their bodies to others and objects in their near space (within arm's reach). This leads to learning about spatial relations of objects and people in the environment, so critical to the orientation process.

Object and Environmental Concepts

These concepts involve the understanding of the properties of objects (size, color, shape, texture, and weight), directional terms (such as forward, backward, up and down), and positional relationships (such as in front, behind, left and right). Understanding these concepts is necessary for your child to gain an awareness of where he is in relation to all other objects.

The environment can be thought of in terms of two distinct spatial areas:

1. the area within your child's arm's reach, or near space; and
2. the area beyond your child's reach, or distance space.

As an infant and early toddler your child will interact with objects and environmental events within his near space. During this period, he needs to be encouraged to reach toward, manipulate, and explore objects using all his available senses during play and daily activities. Objects such as spoons, bowls, cups, toys, and bathing and changing items are encountered during daily activities of eating, bathing, changing, and playing. During these activities, your child has the opportunity to explore the similarities and differences among the objects encountered. Consequently, he will learn to distinguish and identify one object from another, and begin to search for desired objects near his body.

By searching for objects, young children learn to relate their bodies to the position of objects around them. You can encourage the understanding of positional relationships by verbally labeling and helping your child locate objects in their near space. For example, during eating activities, you may say, "Your spoon is in front of your hand," while at the same time physically moving your child's hand toward the spoon. During bathing, you can verbally label what you are doing: "I am getting the soap; it is in the water behind you," as you guide your child's hand on yours as you reach. By pairing the label of positional relationships to movement during daily activities, you can help your child gain a better understanding of his body in relation to objects and actions in his near space.

After your child begins to understand his positional relationship to objects and events in his near space, he is ready to understand objects and events in the distance. This typically occurs around the late toddler and preschool years (ages two to four). During this period, your child needs to be exposed to, and encouraged to explore, larger areas, using all his available senses. Rooms of the house, your yard, the neighborhood, preschool, playground, and stores are environments that children at this age typically explore. Children with normal vision learn about their environment and community incidentally as they travel with parents and teachers on errands, field trips, and daily activities. Children with visual impairments, however, benefit most from direct instruction and repeated exposure to the world around them. These experiences not only help children learn important concepts, but also provide the building blocks for purposeful O&M when they are older and can function in the community independently.

Before your child can completely understand where objects are located in the distance space, he must first learn what objects and events are found in each environment and be allowed to actively interact in community experiences. For example, objects in a grocery store include shelves, aisles, carts, checkouts, different food sections, and automatic doors. Later the understanding of these objects (their sounds, smells, textures, and visual characteristics for those with low vision) will assist your child in mapping his environment.

▪▪ Motor and Postural Development

Motor development includes the growth of both gross motor and fine motor skills. Gross motor skills involve large muscle movement and balance, and include such skills as walking and running. Fine motor skills involve using smaller muscles such as those in the hand and wrist for intricate movement and manipulation.

Developing smooth, coordinated motor skills is essential for acquisition of independent mobility skills. For example, the ability to stand and walk allows children the opportunity to explore the environment in an upright position and develop the good balance and fluid walking patterns needed to learn appropriate white cane skills. Similarly, learning to hold and manipulate objects leads to the fine motor skills of holding and manipulating a white cane with the hand and wrist.

The developmental motor skills that are related to mobility during the early childhood years are identified in Table 1 on the next page. Children who are encouraged to purposefully explore their environment and are exposed to a variety of environmental sounds, textures, and other experiences gain a better understanding of their bodies, spatial relations, and the world around them.

:: Techniques to Facilitate Safe Purposeful Movement

Formalized mobility techniques allow children with visual impairments to move about their environment in a safe and independent manner. These techniques include:

1. the use of a human guide,
2. protective techniques, and
3. mobility devices, including the white cane.

Being proficient in one or more of these mobility techniques will greatly increase your child's flexibility and independence.

The introduction of these techniques, regardless of your child's age, should initially take place under the direct guidance and supervision of a certified O&M instructor. Which techniques and how they are introduced are dependent on your child's age, abilities, amount of vision, motivation, and the nature of his current and future travel environments. By working together, you and your child's O&M instructor can choose appropriate techniques to help your child develop safe and purposeful movement within your home and community.

Human Guide Techniques

Using age appropriate guiding techniques, you and your child can learn to travel comfortably in both familiar and unfamiliar areas. When

▪▪ TABLE 1—MOTOR SKILLS ESSENTIAL FOR MOBILITY

Area of Development	Infancy (Birth – 18 months)	Toddler (18 – 30 months)	Preschooler (30 – 48 months)
Gross Motor Skills	• Head control • Protective responses • Rolls over • Sits • Pushes up on hands while on tummy • Crawls • Pulls to stand • Cruises furniture • Stands • Begins to walk with a wide gait with support • Pushes/pulls toys	• Climbs • Negotiates steps • Jumps • Simple motor planning in and out of positions • Throws ball forward • Stands on one foot, demonstrating increase in balance control	• Negotiates steps, one foot on each stair • Jumps off low bench • Hops • Is able to plan and change positions more easily • Imitates more complex movements • Pedals tricycle • Walks forward, backward, and sideways • Climbs on playground equipment • Running refined
Fine Motor Skills	• Responds to touch and textures • Inspects and brings hands together • Reaches and grasps objects • Shakes rattle • Releases grasped object • Hitting/banging/raking objects • Holds objects and transfers objects between hands • Turns head to sound • Picks up small object • Finger feeds • Puts objects in containers • Imitates action with an object • Places one block on top of another	• Wrist rotation develops for manipulating door knobs • Develops pincer grasp (thumb and index finger) • Plays with stacking rings, form boards • Scribbles • Turns pages in a book • Builds a 3-5 cube tower • Begins to unbutton clothing • Plays with simple puzzles	• Copies shapes • Builds an 8-10 cube tower • Unscrews lids • Advanced stacking and sequencing • Size and shape discrimination by touch • Strings beads • Places pegs in pegboards • Opens and closes doors, windows, and drawers.

your child is first learning these techniques, you will act as his guide and verbally describe obstacles and features you are approaching. As your child gains more experience, he will take on a more responsible and active role by learning to pay attention to your body movements (turns, stops, and starts) and environmental information (ground level changes, sounds, and textures). Consequently, the O&M instructor will probably work on this technique with you and your child together, showing you how to monitor and correct the techniques. It is important that all members of your family learn to guide your child in the same manner. Later your child will be able to teach peers, friends, and others how to be good guides.

Basic Guiding Technique

Using this technique, your child grasps the finger, wrist, or arm of another person (the guide) and walks just behind the guide. This gives your child time to react when approaching steps, curbs, and other obstacles. Where on the arm your child grasps the guide will depend upon his size. Small toddlers typically grasp the guide's finger (Figure 1), while early preschoolers grasp the wrist, and older children grasp just above the guide's elbow (Figure 2). At each age, the child holds his upper arm parallel and close to his body, forming a 90-degree angle with his lower arm. This helps him maintain a safe half-step relationship behind his guide. In addition, the child's grip should be secure, but comfort-

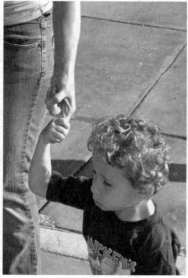

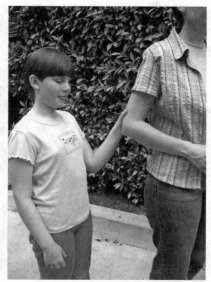

Fig. 1   Fig. 2

able for the guide. This grip and position allow the guide to encounter obstacles and changes in terrain first and to provide maximum safety and reaction time for the child.

If your child is learning the basic guiding technique, that does not mean that you cannot sometimes just hold hands with him. Holding hands provides an emotional connection and is also especially important with young children when an adult control grip is necessary for safety reasons, as in congested public areas. Whenever possible, however, you should encourage your child to use the proper grip while using the guiding procedure. Using the proper grip reinforces and develops fine motor ability and encourages active participation, while holding hands does not.

Narrow Passageway

The narrow passageway technique allows for safe and efficient passage through a restricted space that cannot be negotiated using the basic guiding procedure. (See Figure 3.) Before entering the narrow space, as your child's guide, you move your guiding arm behind and toward the small of your back. This signals your child to then straighten his arm and move directly behind you without stepping on your heels. Initially, young children have difficulties interpreting this signal, so you may need to provide your child with a verbal cue, and exaggerate your arm movement to indicate that he needs to step behind you. In addition, your child may need to hold onto your guiding arm with two hands to assist him in maintaining a safe position (Figure 4). After leaving the narrow space, you return your arm to a normal guiding position and your child resumes the basic guiding position and grip.

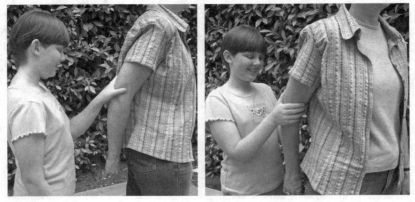

Fig. 3   Fig. 4

For this technique to have meaning, young children need many opportunities to explore what is meant by a "narrow space." By feeling the width of their body, their guide's body, and the space between objects (such as a doorway, aisle, and furniture) young children further their understanding of spatial relationships between their bodies and environmental objects.

Stairways and Curbs

Using this technique, you as the guide squarely approach the edge of steps and curbs, then pause. You next encourage your child to come up beside you and feel the step with his foot. Then, as the guide, you take the first step and your child follows, remaining one step behind. A pause after you complete the stairs or curb indicates to your child that he has one more step to negotiate. This technique is successful when young children are exposed to and explore a variety of stairs and curbs.

Exploring the components of stairs, including the riser, base or step, lip, and railing begins very early in life. Young toddlers with and without visual impairments can begin to experience and negotiate stairways on their bottoms, then later hold onto the railing while sidestepping. Once upright mobility and balance develop, children learn to negotiate steps one step at a time leading with the same foot, with one hand on the railing. With refined balance—typically developed during the preschool years—children begin to alternate their feet while ascending and descending stairs.

Doorways

There are many types of doors your child needs to be exposed to throughout his early years, especially when moving about on his own. They include: manual doors with doorknobs like those found in a house, automatic doors in grocery stores, sliding doors, heavy double doors, and revolving doors. Children need to learn that doors open and close; come in different sizes; can be pushed or pulled; and can be used as entrances to cupboards, buildings, and vehicles. Initially, you will need to verbally and physically explore doors in different areas with your child. You can also help your child learn early concepts about doors by allowing him to play with the doors of cabinets.

Once your child is walking upright with you in different environments, being able to guide him through a variety of different doorways found in the community is critical to his and your safety. As your child's guide, approach doors on your right with your child on the side opposite the door to be opened. Verbally tell your child that you are approaching a door. Open the door and position your guiding arm across your child's chest with your child directly in front of you. This position allows for ease of movement through the door with your child out of the way of other pedestrians and moving doors. Your child is also able to feel your body movements as you traverse through a doorway. Once clear of the doors, you and your child reposition to the basic guiding procedure.

There are other formalized techniques to negotiating doors with a guide, which allow your child to take a more active role. However, these techniques require him to have the necessary upper body strength to hold and manipulate a variety of doors. A Certified O&M instructor can teach you and your child these techniques, when appropriate, and how they are applied in different situations.

Protective Techniques

Using age appropriate protective techniques, your child can learn to detect objects at waist level and above as he travels independently in his environment. At first, your child may need verbal and/or physical reminders to use these techniques where they would be helpful. These techniques are typically used when moving through space to locate a given object and to help protect the body from objects such as open cupboards, chairs, tables, and poles near swing-sets and slides.

Upper Hand and Forearm

The purpose of this skill is to detect objects that may be encountered in the upper region of the body. With young children, this technique may be referred to as the "upper bumper." To form the "upper bumper," the child bends his forearm at the elbow, forming an angle of approximately 120 degrees. He holds his arm in front of his body at shoulder level, parallel to the floor, with the hand aligned in front of the opposite shoulder, palm facing away from the body and fingers relaxed and close together. (See Figure 5.) If your child has difficulties maintaining this position, you can use an interlocking grip to assist him.

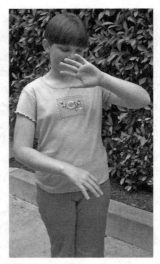

Fig. 5

Lower Hand and Forearm

The purpose of this skill is to locate and provide protection from objects at waist level. With young children, this technique may be referred to as the "lower bumper." To form the "lower bumper," your child extends his hand downward approximately six to eight inches from the midline of his body. His fingers are positioned close together and relaxed. For maximum protection, children sometimes use the upper and lower bumpers in combination.

Mobility Devices

Mobility devices are tools used by individuals with visual impairments to assist them in moving through their environment independently and safely. The white (or long) cane is the most commonly used tool by people with visual impairments. With young children, useful mobility devices are objects and toys used as bumpers and adaptive canes. These devices may be used to assist children with visual impairments in learning to stand, walk, and move purposefully in their environment.

Using Objects and Toys as Bumpers

Often it is possible for children to protect themselves by carrying or pushing toys or objects in front of their bodies. For example, your child might carry a tray out in front of himself while moving or might push a toy grocery cart in front of himself. Using toys and objects this way can make it easier to make the transition to using a cane or one of the alternative mobility devices described below.

Adaptive Cane

Adaptive canes, more commonly called alternative mobility devices (AMDs), are popular for use with preschool children who have outgrown the toddler push toys. These devices are pushable protective devices made of plastic tubing (PVC pipe). An AMD increases a child's ability to move about independently early in the O&M instructional process. Most AMDs are simple to use, can detect curbs and other drop-offs, and provide information about the walking surface. Some AMDs have rollers or casters, while others slide across the walking surface as they are pushed. An AMD provides the same kind of protection as the long cane, but does not require the conceptual or motor skills needed for the long cane. A child is protected from obstacles in his travel path as he pushes the AMD in front of himself. Depending on the child's problem solving abilities, he may be able to interpret both auditory and tactual information to discriminate between walking surfaces such as carpet or tile.

Long Cane

The long cane is becoming increasingly popular for use with preschool children. There are varying philosophies as to the best age for a child to learn long cane skills. Some O&M instructors think cane skills should be introduced at the earliest possible age. Others prefer to wait until the child has developed fine motor and conceptual skills such as the ability to correctly grip the cane and the ability to follow instructions using basic spatial concepts (in front, behind, over, and under). Your child may benefit from cane instruction now, or he may not need a cane until he is ready to go places himself and has developed prerequisite skills. Ask your O&M instructor to help you decide when and if your child should use a cane.

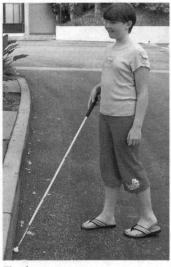

Fig. 6

Two of the more common types of canes are the long, straight cane with or without a crook, and the folding cane. Long canes can be made of many materials including aluminum and fiberglass. Most of the shaft is usually covered with a white reflective material, while a small portion of the lower shaft is covered with a red reflective material (Figure 6). The tips of both long and folding canes can be made of nylon or metal, and come in different types, such as a roller, marshmallow, or narrow tip.

Several different cane techniques and modifications may be used, depending on the environment and age of the child. The O&M instructor introduces, teaches, and monitors these techniques, over a period of time. Before deciding whether your child needs to use a cane, several factors should be considered. These include your child's amount of vision, need for a cane, maturity level, and ability to manipulate a cane while walking. You should also consider whether your child needs to get around better in his current travel environment or is at the age where he needs to travel to new places on his own within the neighborhood.

Dog Guides

Even though the public often envisions most blind people as using dog guides for assistance with mobility, this is not the case. The decision to use a dog guide is highly individual and it is necessary for dog guide users to be capable of independent orientation and mobility prior to the use of a dog. In addition, most dog guide schools have minimum age requirements and only accept applicants who are in their late teens or older.

Choosing the Best Mobility Technique and Device for Your Child

There is not a single mobility technique or device that is best for children with visual impairments. What will work for your child depends on several factors, including your child's specific needs, the complexity of the environments through which he travels, his physical and problem solving capabilities, and his motivation and attitude toward independent travel. Children may use several different mobility techniques and devices at different stages in their development. For example, a young infant may start with a walker and then progress to using push toys and then to a specific AMD or the long cane. Another child may use the cane exclusively as his main mobility system, once he is able to walk. There are many options. The O&M instructor can provide useful information and help with this decision based upon your child's needs and capabilities.

▪▪ Techniques to Facilitate Orientation

Orientation skills include the problem solving and perceptual skills that enable a child to determine his position and relationship to significant objects in his environment. To establish his orientation, the child must first have a concept of self, or body image—he must understand his body parts, including the function of each part and how they move in relationship to each other (self-to-self awareness). He must also understand the environment and his relationship to the environment (self-to-object relationships). Finally, he must be able to understand how different aspects of the environment relate to each other—such as where the bathroom is located in relationship to his bedroom (object-to-object relationships).

Because orientation skills are very closely related to mobility skills, the two are generally taught at the same time. The more formalized orientation skills your child may learn include:

1. Trailing,
2. Systematic Search Patterns, and
3. Route Travel.

Trailing

The purposes of trailing are to establish and maintain a straight line of travel by following along a "trailing surface" such as a wall or the edge of a table; and to locate specific objectives such as the third doorway or a book on or along the trailing surface. This can begin very early, for example, when an infant is encouraged to crawl along the edge of a mat or carpet to locate a familiar toy. A toddler may be encouraged to trail a wall with his hand fisted and slightly ahead of his body. With refined motor control development, the preschooler is able to extend his arm at an angle of approximately 45 degrees out in front and to the side of his body. With the fingers relaxed and slightly cupped, he maintains light contact with the trailing surface with the side of his pinkie finger. Even adults with visual impairments continue to use this technique in some situations.

Systematic Search Patterns

Systematic search patterns are used to locate objects and/or to explore a space. There are two basic types of patterns. The first type

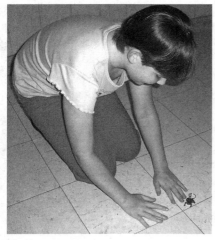

involves using the hand(s) and arm(s) to find a nearby object such as a toy or an item on a highchair tray, or to retrieve a dropped object. Using this type of search pattern, the child establishes a starting point and then can use a variety of patterns (fan, circular, etc.) to locate the object. (See Figure 7.)

The second type of search pattern is used to search larger spaces. It is done while walking and uses the whole body.

Fig. 7

One whole-body search pattern called the "perimeter" search method involves establishing a starting point for the search and then walking around the border of the area back to the starting point. The perimeter method provides information about the size and shape of the area, and about objects along the border. To learn where objects in a room are located, it is helpful to have the child travel to and from a familiar object and a reference point in the room, typically the door. Through repeated movements between objects in the room and relating them to a reference point your child will begin to understand where objects are located in relation to himself and other objects.

Route Travel

Young children typically learn to travel toward an objective by following a sequence of known stationary objects, called landmarks, in familiar areas. The first routes learned are those that have particular meaning for the child, like going to the kitchen for something to eat, or finding the toy basket in the living room. As your child repeats the same route daily, and with encouragement from you to locate each step (or landmark) along the route, your child will easily begin to learn the path to certain locations.

When a child enters a preschool program, the O&M instructor can further assist you and your child's teachers in determining natural landmarks and placing tactile markers to signal specific locations. Such locations may include your child's hook or cubby, the door to the classroom or playroom, and the bathroom. Initially, teachers and parents may need to provide verbal and/or physical assistance for young children to move along these routes. With repeated exposure and experience with the route, young children begin to move with more confidence and speed. Consequently, they begin to travel along longer, more complex routes, adding to their independence.

■■ Who Needs O&M Training?

It is likely that your child will easily and safely maneuver through familiar areas such as his home and preschool. If he does not have trouble locating or moving around objects at home or school, you may wonder whether he really needs O&M training. The fact is, most children with visual impairments learn to get around familiar places quite well. However, this does not mean that they could not benefit from O&M services.

A child capable of good mobility in familiar places will likely still have some orientation needs, such as learning to travel in unfamiliar places and understanding environmental concepts such as neighborhood, street corner, intersection, etc. Even children with low vision can often profit from training in concept development, sensory skills, and orientation. For example, a child with some vision may not automatically understand what he is seeing, and may therefore have trouble understanding concepts such as playgrounds, stores, neighborhoods, and intersections. Allowing a child to experience concepts in a variety of ways involving all the senses helps him to better understand what he sees. This same child could probably improve his orientation skills by learning what, when, where, and how to look for important landmarks and features around him. For example, he might be taught how to systematically scan and visually search for the swing set in his backyard. Additionally, learning how to use optical devices such as telescopes to locate important objects and landmarks is helpful for some young children with low vision.

In short, regardless of how much vision your child has, he could probably benefit from some O&M training. A comprehensive O&M assessment will help determine the nature and extent of need for O&M services. This assessment might take place when your child is being assessed for early intervention for the first time. Alternatively, it might be conducted after your child has been receiving services for some time. This may be the case if his eye condition has deteriorated, affecting his ability to travel safely and independently. As a parent, you may also request an O&M assessment at any time.

The O&M instructor takes the lead role in assessing formal orientation skills and formal mobility skills; determining the appropriate mobility techniques and tools (in particular, AMD, the long cane, etc.); and analyzing the home and school environment to determine what assistance parents and teachers will need in teaching safe and efficient O&M skills. The O&M instructor also works with preschool and elementary school teachers to assess a child's needs and abilities in concept development, motor development, and sensory skills development. Other professionals such as occupational and physical therapists and a speech-language pathologist should be consulted and involved in the assessment if the child also has a physical disability or other special needs.

If your child is found to need O&M services, he will be periodically reevaluated to find out whether he still needs the services or whether his need for services has changed. Often, a child receives O&M instruction throughout his entire educational career. Sometimes O&M instruction is short-term to meet specific needs, is terminated, and then reactivated as the child's needs change. For example, parents of an infant may need consultation from an O&M instructor to learn how to enhance the use of their child's senses and encourage him to use purposeful movement patterns. Later, toddlers and preschoolers may need to learn techniques of basic guiding skills, self-protective skills, trailing, or how to use an AMD to travel at home, in the community, or at preschool. Once a child has successfully learned functional routes, the teacher can be responsible for monitoring correct skills. As the child gets older and needs to move independently through more environments, the O&M instructor would resume training and introduce more advanced skills such as cane techniques or provide support for orientation to a new school building.

▪▪ Working on O&M at Home

When your child is young, there are a number of ways you can help him develop O&M skills. Many of these strategies are simply common sense, and you may already have adopted them without even realizing that you were enhancing your child's O&M skills. Others can be easily incorporated into your daily routine, once you become aware of what helps children acquire O&M skills. What follows are some general suggestions for helping a child develop O&M skills. Your child's O&M instructor will give you specific suggestions tailored to your child's unique needs and capabilities.

Modifying Your Home

How your home is arranged can greatly affect the development of O&M skills. Usually families do not need to go to a great deal of time and expense to modify the home environment for their children. In most cases, common sense changes that benefit all family members can be made. The following factors should be considered when making modifications.

Safety. Families should decide on the amount and nature of "child-proofing" to be done in the home. Many safety considerations for children with visual impairment are the same as those for children with normal vision. For example, most babies love to mouth objects, so make sure your child does not get a hold of objects or toys that are small enough to swallow. Provide optimum natural lighting without glare at critical locations throughout your home. For example, avoid sudden changes in lighting as your child moves from the hallway to the family room by partly drawing the blinds when the sun is brightly shining through the window. A landmark such as a low-hanging picture or carpeted mat can be placed at the end of the hallway to indicate the presence of a staircase.

Protect your child from hurting himself on table corners by using padding or corner buffers and keep closet and cabinet doors fully open or fully closed. Keep all electrical cords out of main travel paths to prevent tripping accidents. Use nonslip guards under area rugs and runners to prevent your child from slipping or tripping over curled corners. Have family members push in chairs at tables after use.

Spatial Arrangement. How organized, complex, and consistent is your home environment? Sometimes rearranging furniture to create accessible travel pathways for a young child makes it much easier for him to move about the house and develop confidence. For example, when your child is first learning to travel from his bedroom to the kitchen, he may need to travel through the family room. Instead of expecting him to travel through a large, empty space, you could initially arrange the furniture along the walls so that he could travel along the furniture without having to move out into open space.

As your child becomes more motivated and proficient, you could rearrange the furniture and provide landmarks. For example, when your child contacts the coffee table, instead of continuing in the same direction along the wall, he would turn left, trail the edge of the coffee table to the end, continue across two feet of open space to the big chair, walk around the chair to the wall, and turn the corner into the kitchen. As your child becomes still more proficient, you can challenge him to continue to use his O&M skills by creating a more complex environment. That is, increase or decrease the amount of furniture or rearrange it to encourage him to problem solve how to safely and efficiently make his way through the environment.

Accessibility to Items. Your child's clothes, toys, personal belongings, and other personal objects such as a potty chair should be placed within easy reach. Making items accessible will encourage your child to explore his surroundings and enhance early movement.

Familiarity/Novelty. It *is* important to establish some consistency in the environment so that your child becomes familiar with the spatial arrangement and develops confidence in his mobility. Sometimes, however, children do not use proper O&M skills because they are "too familiar" with the environment. For example, if your child knows where all the furniture is, he may stop using self-protective techniques. Therefore, you should continually assess and adapt the environment to provide appropriate novelty and stimulation. For example, you might move the toy chest to a different corner of the room so your child has to use his self-protective techniques to travel the new route from the doorway to the toy chest.

Taking Advantage of Community Resources

Most communities offer a rich array of opportunities for enhancing O&M concepts and skills. For example, taking your child grocery shopping is an excellent opportunity to teach many new concepts. If your child is sitting in the grocery cart, hand him the items you select and let him explore them and make comparisons. Talk about their size (big, little), weight (heavy, light), texture (rough, smooth), temperature (cool, very cold), shape, etc. For example, as your child is examining a package of bacon, you could talk about it being cold, shaped like a rectangle, packaged in a smooth covering, etc. Upon arriving home, have your child help you unpack the grocery items and place them in their appropriate places. This, again, is an excellent opportunity to teach spatial arrangement and concepts in the home. When it is time to cook the bacon, let your child get the bacon out of the fridge, locate the appropriate size frying pan, and help to place the bacon in the pan, noting the texture, smell, and shape of the bacon.

Spending time at a neighborhood park is another excellent activity for introducing and reinforcing many O&M concepts and skills as well as language skills. When pushing your child in the swing, you can tell him he is going high or low, up or down, fast or slow. You might also take him to a slide and have him experience those same concepts in a different manner (going up and down the slide).

Riding in the car provides opportunities for your child to develop environmental awareness and for you to teach specific spatial concepts. For example, you can play games with your child by having him keep track of left turns, right turns, and full stops. When taking trips in the community, you can have him compare the time and distance it takes to get to different places. For example, going to the post office from home is a shorter trip than going to the bank.

Motivating Your Child to Explore

Children need a reason to move. Infants with sight may pick their heads up to look at someone's face or crawl across the room to get an appealing, colorful toy. Children with visual impairments also use their senses to find motivating reasons to move. You can help motivate your child by using sounds he likes, such as your voice or a musical toy, to encourage him to move across the room. Instead of placing a rattle in his hand, shake it to one side of him and help him reach for it. Stand a few feet from him, and have him move toward you when you approach him. Help him explore the cupboards, crawl up and down steps, and get up on a stool to see what is higher than his reach.

Encourage your child to be as mobile as other children his age. Most infants are allowed to crawl about on the floor, so be sure to encourage your child to do so too.

Leaving a "good" baby content for a long period of time in the crib or playpen is not always the best thing for him. As a toddler and preschooler, allow plenty of opportunity for your child to experience movement on scooter boards, swings, slides, and climbing equipment. Encourage him to refine his balance skills and move in and out of different positions while interacting with toys and play equipment. Using music, rhymes, and games will help your child learn smooth, coordinated movement patterns as he relates sound and language to movement. Like all children, your child will fall, bump into things, and cry. These experiences are a normal part of growing up, and your child should be allowed to have them.

Focusing on Everyday Learning Opportunities

You can help lay the foundation for your child's O&M skills by involving him in everyday activities that help him learn about environmental and sensory information. It is especially important to help him learn about sounds. Talk about the way things sound (loud, soft, high, low). Also, help him learn about the sources of sounds. Tell him what or who is making the noise when the phone rings, when someone comes into your home, or when the water is running. If possible, allow him to touch the source of the sound. Recognizing the source of sounds will be critical later for such activities as crossing the street, when it is essential to know the position of passing cars. It is helpful if all family members become aware of the importance of discussing sounds and incorporate this discussion into the daily routine.

Help your child learn about other sensations just as you help him learn about sounds. Talk about how things feel (hard, soft, smooth, bumpy, wet, dry), look (dark, light, what color), and smell (strong, sweet, and dangerous). When your child is in a new place or gets a new toy, describe the way it looks, sounds, feels, and smells. During bath time, talk about the smell of the soap and powder and have your child help rub lotion onto his body. Point out and name the textures on the walking surface (carpet, wood, tile, grass, dirt, and sidewalk) and connect these textures to a specific location or activity. For example, tell your child that the bathroom has a tile floor and that the grass is in the backyard.

Remember that your child depends on you and others to show him what he might not learn naturally on his own. Children without visual impairments learn a great deal by watching their parents. For instance, young children learn how clothes become clean by seeing their mother or father take the dirty clothes from the hamper, put them in the washing machine, move them to the dryer, and then fold them and place them in drawers. A child with a visual impairment may only be aware that every morning he is handed his clothes from mid-air and that at night when he takes them off, his mother or father takes them away. By having your child help with the laundry, you can teach him where dirty and clean clothes come from and go to, what the concepts of wet and dry mean, and how to identify clothes by touch. Think of all the things that you can teach your child while shopping at the grocery store, planting flowers in the yard, housecleaning, or washing the car.

Teaching about Spatial Relationships

It is important to teach your child position words that will enable him to understand his relationship to objects or other people around him. Tell your child where he is as he moves or is carried from place to place. For example, tell him that he is *in* the living room, *in front of* the couch; his blocks are *behind* his back; and you are sitting *on* the rocking chair. Have him touch the couch, blocks, and you to reinforce what these position words mean. Help him learn that his bed is *next* to the wall and that the bathtub is *in* the bathroom. When he drops a toy or is looking for something, tell him it is to his *left, under* his foot, or *in front of* him. Help him reach *to his left* to find the toy. Ask him questions about where objects are located.

When your child is just learning to use a new position word such as *behind,* be sure to use this word every time you describe an object in that particular location. Once he knows what it means, you can tell him that other words, such as *in back of,* mean the same thing. Remember that verbal directions are not enough. Hands-on experiences will reinforce your child's learning of all these position words.

It is also important to teach your child to look for or explore objects in an organized way. If he drops a toy, he should listen for the sound of it hitting the floor and look for it in that particular direction, first searching closer to him, then further away. At lunchtime, he can figure out what kind of food he has by systematically exploring his tray and the tabletop surrounding it. If his cup is always placed in the same location, he will learn to anticipate this and can reach the same distance in the same direction each time. This can help him avoid accidental spills as well as frustration.

■■ Working with the O&M Instructor

Although the O&M instructor will provide suggestions, information, and ideas about your child's development and O&M needs, family members are a child's best teachers. You, your child's family, have the most love, concern for his best interests, and time to teach and reinforce O&M skills. This means you can really help your child learn and grow by forming a partnership with his O&M instructor.

As a parent, you can work with the O&M instructor in several ways. First, you can help the instructor and others who work with your child in developing short- and long-term goals, as well as reasonable time limits for completing the goals. Second, you can expect the O&M instructor to work with you to develop specific activities that you and other family members can do at home to make sure there is continuity of instruction. These activities should be designed so that you can incorporate them into everyday and recreational activities. For example, at the supper table, you can ask your child to pass you the butter with his right hand and pass the peas with his left hand. In your back yard, you can ask your child to kick the ball with his left foot and pet the cat with his right hand.

Third, you should expect the O&M instructor to keep you informed about your child's progress, possibly through a notebook, regular (biweekly or possibly monthly) phone calls, or written progress reports (perhaps every six or eight weeks). In addition, you should feel free to observe O&M lessons whenever possible. Showing confidence in your child's travel abilities both at lessons and out in the community can help give him the assurance he needs to develop his skills to the utmost.

Finally, as your child grows older, the O&M instructor can let you know when your child has the skills to go places by himself or with friends and how you can encourage him to use his O&M skills. It is understandable that you might be concerned about his safety when using O&M skills. Remember, though, there is a certain amount of risk for all of us in moving about the environment. Orientation and mobility instructors are specifically trained to monitor the safety of children with visual impairments and to intervene when necessary.

❚❚ Conclusion

Early O&M instruction is critical to enabling your child to successfully move about his environment throughout his life. Your involvement in your child's O&M program is equally important. The O&M instructor is responsible for providing you with an ongoing parent education program that will help you actively participate in your child's O&M instructional program and reinforce important O&M concepts and skills on a daily basis. An O&M instructor can assist you in understanding your child's strengths and needs and provide you with the skills necessary to reinforce his strengths and compensate for his needs. At the same time, the O&M instructor should encourage you to participate in the decision-making process regarding your child's O&M program and should respect your wishes or suggestions for instruction. Ultimately, the focus of the O&M program should be on providing your child with appropriate O&M instruction at the earliest possible age through an ongoing partnership between you and the O&M instructor.

❚❚ Parent Statements

Zachary crawled, then trailed walls, and then at fifteen months, took his first steps unassisted into space. It was thrilling to watch! He used several different push toys in the house and outside. The O&M instructor suggested we make what is referred to as a "t-cane," usually made from PVC pipe. That worked fine for Zach as a sort of pre-cane, but now we think we could have skipped that and gone straight to a regular cane.

❦

When the orientation and mobility specialist brought Nakisha's cane to her, I thought she was too young but she really took to it easier than I thought.

❦

I know I should encourage my son to use his cane but it is so much easier just to hold his hand as we walk. If he uses his cane, we walk so slowly.

❦

I'm just getting used to my son using a cane. At first I didn't know how much information I should give him and how much I should allow him to discover on his own.

❦

It seemed to me Brandon felt comfortable using his cane from the first day it arrived. Knowing nothing about proper technique, we pulled it out of the box together, and I told him, "Tap, tap, tap, and roll, roll, roll!" He looked so handsome with his first real white cane, and instead of being sad as I had feared I would be with such a visual reminder of his blindness, I was immensely proud.

❦

There is a person who is blind in our town who takes the bus everywhere. He shops by himself and goes to work. He visits friends and goes to church. All on a city bus. I am really encouraged by this when I think about Matthew's future.

❦

I hate when somebody "pulls" my child. I know they don't understand, but it still makes me mad.

❦

How will my child get around in school? Will he have trouble in the lunchroom?

❦

We prepared for the cane travel portion of our next team meeting diligently, searching for information on the web and asking a number of blind adults when they got their first cane and when they wish they had gotten their first canes. We heard a resounding response of "I wish I'd gotten it when I first started walking!" The meeting time came and we laid out our reasons, fully expecting to hear, "No." Instead, we were told they were willing to try it. We measured Ethan for his first cane—a full 22 inches—and it arrived two days before his second birthday.

❧

My child has great mobility. He runs around outside and plays with the other kids just fine. He has trouble when he tries to look at things close up, but he doesn't have trouble walking around. Sometimes that is confusing for people—they doubt that he has a visual impairment.

❧

I've asked the orientation and mobility specialist about guide dogs. It seems like a good option for the future.

❧

I have been stopped at the mall or at the grocery store by people who think I am being mean to Beth by making her walk by herself with a cane. They just don't understand.

❧

By the time Madison was 20 months, we began to wonder why she wasn't being given a cane. We'd read accounts of blind and visually impaired children not getting canes until they were 5 or 6 years old at the earliest, but did not understand the reasoning behind that. We thought that if she was mobile, she needed the tools necessary to navigate her space. While we certainly realized there were perhaps children her age not ready to handle that responsibility, we believed Maddy was. The swinging and correct cane-travel techniques were responsibilities we were willing to help Maddy undertake.

❧

I know that a big part of independence for Joey will be his ability to get around by himself. So, even though it is hard sometimes, we try to encourage him to be independent now. It would be so much easier and faster to take his hand or guide him, but that won't really help him.

Children with Multiple and Visual Disabilities

Jane Erin, Ph.D.

It was time for breakfast! Eric knew this because he could hear the coffeepot dripping and the clatter of the bowls as his sister got them out of the cupboard. As his mother lifted him into his special chair and buckled the strap around him, he began to chuckle with anticipation. "Time to eat, champ," his father commented from across the table.

Mr. Harris thought about how much had changed since Eric was born four years ago. Then, doctors had said that his son might not live: he was three months premature, and so tiny that his father could have held him in one hand if they had been allowed to hold him at all.

They knew from the beginning that Eric might have some disabilities. But they were so happy that he had survived that it was a long time before they considered how Eric's differences might affect the family's life. Doctors had talked about the possibility that he might have cerebral palsy and intellectual disabilities, but no one had mentioned blindness. Mrs. Harris had been the first to notice that Eric's eyes didn't seem to follow people walking in front of him. When they took him back to the doctor and learned that Eric could only see light, it seemed like the ultimate irony. After all of the medical crises that Eric had survived, it was difficult for his family to accept that he would never enjoy the visual beauty of the world that he had struggled to enter.

During the first two years, there were times that the Harrises wondered whether Eric's disabilities were more than they could handle. He had difficulty eating, was often ill, and needed frequent hospitalizations. It became apparent that he had cerebral palsy and that he would learn very slowly. But after the second year, things began to change. Gradually, Eric was becoming a member of the family. His laugh was contagious, and his brother and sister learned that he enjoyed roughhousing and listening to music. And it was obvious that he could learn: in the last year he had started sitting up by himself and searching for toys when they disappeared. He could imitate sounds that others made, and now used special sounds for "cup" and for rides in the car. Although Eric was very different from what the Harrises expected their third child to be, they were often glad that he had introduced them to an unknown world.

There are many children like Eric who have a visual disability in combination with one or more other disabilities. Disabilities commonly associated with visual impairment include cerebral palsy and other movement disorders, mental retardation, and hearing impairment. As many as 40 percent of children who have these physical and mental disabilities may also have some visual impairment. Conversely, as many as 50 to 60

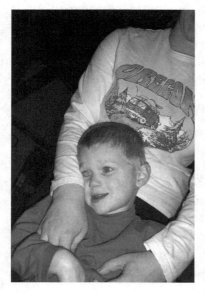

percent of children with visual impairments have other disabilities.

Most children who have a visual impairment in combination with another disability have low vision. Although their vision may not provide as much detail or information as it does for others, they can still use vision as a means of learning. A smaller number of children are functionally blind and learn mainly through touch and hearing. They may be aware of light or the location of lighting, but cannot see detail and form well enough to use sight to learn about the world around them.

The term "multiply disabled" is frequently used to describe a child who has more than one condition that affects learning. Under the current version of IDEA (formerly Public Law 94–142), a child is considered multiply disabled if she has several impairments that result in educational problems that are not accommodated if the child receives special education for one disability. According to this definition, a child who has cerebral palsy which makes it impossible for her to write with a pencil and who also has low vision which makes enlarged print necessary for reading would be considered multiply disabled. A child with the same visual condition whose reading skills are delayed for no identifiable reason would not be considered to have multiple disabilities.

Some states define multiply disabled a little differently. For instance, some specify that a child must have major delays in several developmental areas in order to qualify for educational services as multiply handicapped. (Although many people today prefer the term "disability" to "handicapped," you will probably still hear the term "handicapped" if your child is identified as having multiple disabilities. This is because some legal and legislative documents use the term "multiply handicapped" to refer to children who may receive certain specialized services.)

Each child with multiple disabilities is unique. Each child has her own temperament and her own set of experiences and may be affected in different ways by a medical condition or physical disability. This makes it almost impossible to predict how much any child will learn and what she will be able to do as an adult. For parents of children with multiple disabilities, facing this uncertainty may be the greatest challenge. No doctor, therapist, or educator can predict just what to expect for the future, and coordinating information and experiences from many sources may sometimes seem overwhelming. Ultimately, you will become the expert on your own child.

This chapter discusses the types of disabilities that sometimes accompany a visual impairment. It also examines the effects these conditions can have on a child with a visual impairment, as well as some ways to help minimize these effects on learning and growing.

▪▪ Visual Conditions That Often Occur with Other Disabilities

Any of the visual conditions described in Chapter 2 can occur with or without additional disabilities. Several visual conditions, however, almost always occur with another disability. These visual conditions are discussed in this chapter to help you understand why.

Cortical Visual Impairments

Cortical visual impairments are caused by an abnormality in the brain. The eyeball and other optical structures are often normal, but for some reason, the brain has difficulty processing and interpreting visual information. The damage that causes the visual impairment may result from loss of oxygen to the brain, bleeding in the brain, or other types of trauma. This same injury to the brain may also result in cerebral palsy, mental retardation, seizures, or language difficulties.

Although some children with this condition are totally blind, most have some vision, and their use of vision often improves over time. Children with cortical impairments may behave in puzzling ways. For example, their vision may seem to change at different times of the day, they may seem to stare straight ahead or "through" things, and they may seem to use vision to confirm information discovered through other senses rather than as their primary sense. Many children with this condition pay more attention to colorful or moving objects and to bright, primary colors. Associating consistent visual cues with familiar routines and events can help the child to link meaning with what she sees.

Optic Nerve Atrophy and Optic Nerve Hypoplasia

These conditions affect the optic nerve, the bundle of fibers that transmits signals from the retina to the brain. In optic nerve atrophy, the optic nerve has been damaged in some way; in optic nerve hypoplasia, the nerve has not developed. This may mean that the child may have some vision or may be blind, depending on how much of the optic nerve is intact.

These conditions often occur in children whose brains are impaired in other ways. A child's optic nerve may fail to develop properly because of something that occurred early in pregnancy. These events, such as a mother's exposure to a toxic substance or an accidental change in the genes, can result in damage to other parts of the brain. Children with optic nerve hypoplasia may have other disabilities such as cerebral palsy or growth problems, since the optic nerve is located close to the pituitary gland. Septo Optic Dysplasia is a condition in which the nerves between the eye and brain are underdeveloped, resulting in optic nerve hypoplasia, growth and metabolism problems related to the pituitary gland, and other difficulties related to brain structure and function.

Some children with optic nerve atrophy or hypoplasia have a loss of peripheral vision and can only see objects that are straight ahead of them; others lose central vision and may notice objects to the sides more easily. If your child has either diagnosis, it is important to observe her carefully to discover whether her central or peripheral vision is better and whether she prefers using one eye over the other. This is important so you can teach your child to pay attention to things on the side where the visual field is not as wide. In addition, children who mainly use one eye do not see depth as easily as other children, and may have particular difficulty walking down stairs or catching a ball, especially one that is moving fast.

Other Conditions

Various other conditions can also affect both the brain and the visual system. Cytomegalovirus is a common virus that can damage a child's brain before birth, resulting in such disabilities as mental retardation, hearing impairment, and visual impairment. Toxoplasmosis is a parasite commonly transmitted by cats which can invade the brain and eyes if the mother is exposed to it during pregnancy. The resulting brain damage can cause mental retardation, seizures, cerebral palsy, and visual impairment, alone or in combination. Rubella, or German measles, can affect the developing fetus if the mother has the illness early in her pregnancy. Depending upon when in the pregnancy the illness occurs, the baby may be born with conditions such as mental retardation, cerebral palsy, seizures, heart defects, and visual impairment. A very common cause of visual and multiple disabilities is a loss of oxygen to the brain (anoxia), either during delivery or as a result of an accident later in childhood. Again, loss of oxygen can lead to brain damage and a wide variety of disabilities, including learning disabilities, mental retardation, cerebral palsy, and visual impairment.

The vision loss caused by these conditions can range from a mild impairment to complete blindness. Most students do have some vision and should be encouraged to use it. However, children with visual disabilities and brain damage may seem to use their vision differently at different times of day. In addition, these children often have trouble with perceptual responses such as perceiving depth, remembering visual information, reaching for objects they see, and identifying important visual information.

While it is helpful to know the cause and implications of your child's visual condition, it is important to keep in mind that the amount of functional vision varies greatly among children with most conditions. It is impossible to predict how a child will function based on a medical diagnosis. Even the information provided by complex medical tests cannot describe exactly the amount and nature of a vision loss for a child with multiple disabilities. This is because parts of the brain have different purposes in different people. The amount of vision that a child has depends on how old she was when the brain damage occurred, as well as on other factors such as the child's maturity and learning experiences.

Most of the methods of assessing vision in children require the child to speak or to match pictures. When a child cannot do these things because of a physical or other disability, it is important to watch the way she acts when there are things to see. Some eye specialists or educators will test vision using procedures that depend on eye movements. One example is called preferential looking. Using this method, a trained professional shows the child a large card with two shapes on it. One shape has very narrow stripes on it, and the other is plain gray. If the child looks at the stripes instead of the plain shape, the specialist can estimate how much detail she can see. A child does not have to talk or follow directions for this method to be used.

Careful observation of your child in many different situations will provide the best information about her vision. Sometimes you will notice things that don't fit in with the doctor's description of your child's vision; for example, the doctor may describe your child as "blind" but you may notice that she finds toys and reaches for them using vision. It is important for you to describe what you notice to doctors and educators because you have the best opportunity to see your child every day, in different situations. Sometimes professionals may not know how to assess a child with multiple disabilities and they may not want to do an evaluation. As a parent, you can advocate for the importance of knowing what your child can see and having a thorough vision assessment, regardless of other disabilities.

⠿ Common Conditions Associated with Visual Impairments

Several disabilities frequently occur with visual impairments. They include mental retardation, cerebral palsy, spina bifida, physical impairments resulting from trauma, speech and communication disorders, and hearing impairments.

In combination with a visual impairment, these conditions can affect your child's development. First, they may change the rate of learning. For example, if your child has mental retardation, she will require more time to learn most skills than she would if her only disability was a visual impairment. Second, they may change the form of learning. For example, if your child has a hearing impairment, she may need to rely more on touch than on hearing to learn. Third, they may change the content of learning. If your child has a

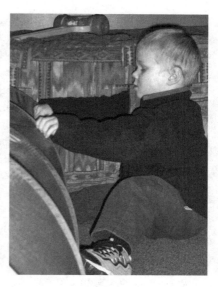

physical disability and a visual impairment, learning the rules of football are not as important as learning how to operate a tape recorder.

Generally, the most important skills for children with multiple disabilities to learn are functional skills. These are the skills that enable your child to do ordinary daily tasks. They may be as simple as grasping a spoon or as complex as traveling to a job independently. But in any case, the skill is something that will require assistance from another person if your child cannot learn to do it on her own. In planning for your child's future, the following are important questions: What does she need to be able to do to be successful now in our household? What might she need to do soon . . . next month or next year? What does our family really want her to learn? The sections below will help you understand the challenges that face children with various types of multiple disabilities so that you can begin to answer these questions for your family.

Mental Retardation

Children with visual impairments often show delayed development during the preschool years because of the learning challenges posed by their vision differences. For example, they may be slow to crawl or walk because they are not aware of interesting things around them to be explored, or they may repeat others' words more frequently than usual because the sounds of speech are more available to them than information about the meaning of language. But these developmental lags usually disappear as language becomes more meaningful to them and as they begin to explore and understand their environment. When a child's slowness in learning is only the result of visual impairment she is said to have "developmental delays."

Other children with visual impairments experience a true limitation in the rate and quality of learning. They do not ever "catch up" with other children their age. Their skills in all areas of development—cognition, language, movement, self-help, and social skills—usually remain significantly below average all their lives. In addition, they have more difficulty learning adaptive behaviors. These are the skills that enable people to independently meet the expectations of their world, such as dressing and feeding themselves, managing money, or talking appropriately with other people. Children with these limitations in learning are said to have mental retardation (referred to as intellectual disabilities or learning disabilities in other English-speaking countries). About 3 percent of all children in the United States have mental retardation, but the percentage among children with visual disabilities is much greater—possibly as high as 40 percent.

Mental retardation is not caused by visual impairment, although either condition can increase the delays normally caused by one of the conditions. That is, children with mental retardation would have significant learning delays even if they did not have visual impairments, but learning may take still longer if they also have a visual impairment. As the preceding section explained, often what causes a child's visual impairment also causes her mental retardation. For example, lack of oxygen (anoxia) can result in both mental retardation and visual impairment. Less often, the two conditions result from entirely different causes. For example, a child may have mental retardation from bleeding in the brain at birth and may be blind as a result of retinopathy of prematurity, a retinal problem that may occur in premature infants. Frequently, the cause of mental retardation cannot be pinpointed, even though over 350 causes of mental retardation have been identified.

It can be very frustrating for parents to see that their child is not progressing rapidly and to wonder whether this delay is solely the result of a visual impairment. Your frustration may be compounded because mental retardation can be especially difficult to diagnose in children with visual impairments. Often, the evaluation procedures used by schools do not take a child's visual differences into consideration. This may result in a child being diagnosed with mental retardation when her delays result from a lack of experience due to a visual impairment. Or a child's mental retardation may not be diagnosed because her learning delays are attributed only to a visual impairment.

Because it is more difficult to assess the true cognitive abilities of children with visual impairments, a professional who is knowledgeable about children with these impairments should be involved in evaluating your child's intellectual function. If the psychologist or diagnostician who evaluates your child is not experienced in working with students with visual impairments, a certified teacher of students with visual impairments should help decide what tests and procedures will give the most accurate picture of your child's abilities. And if the way a test is given is modified because of your child's disabilities, this information should be written in the report. It is also important to gather information about your child's abilities using other methods besides tests and planned activities. For example, observations of your child and interviews with you and other family members can help to provide a more accurate picture of your child's behaviors.

As Chapter 9 explains, if you are concerned that an assessment may not be accurate, you have the right to request a second evaluation by a qualified person of your own choice. Although IDEA 2004 no longer requires evaluations every three years to maintain special education eligibility, parents may request reevaluation if they have concerns about their child's assessment.

If your child is diagnosed as having mental retardation, you may also be told that she has a specific degree of mental retardation. That is, you may hear that her mental retardation is mild, moderate, severe, or profound. Or, if the professional who diagnoses your child is using more recent terminology, you may hear that your child needs intermittent, limited, extensive, or pervasive support. These degrees of mental retardation have been identified because children with mental retardation, like all children, have a wide range of intellectual abilities. Although their development is delayed, some children with mental retardation learn more quickly and easily than other children with mental retardation.

Children who have mild mental retardation (or need intermittent support) may not look or act much differently from others of their age and often learn to read and write up to about the sixth grade level. However, they may have difficulty with complex thinking and reasoning, and as adults may need occasional assistance to live independently. Children who have moderate mental retardation (or need limited support) usually can speak and understand full sentences. They may learn to read the words they need to know to function semi-independently as adults, and with assistance can usually learn most daily living skills such as dressing, grooming, and meal preparation. Children who have severe mental retardation (or need extensive support) have more difficulty with all skills, but with help can often learn to communicate their wants and needs and can learn community survival skills, such as signing their name and behaving appropriately in a variety of situations. Children who have profound mental retardation (or need pervasive support) can sometimes learn some self-help and communication skills with intensive training, and may communicate using manual signs or gestures, or simply through voice sounds. Children with severe or profound mental retardation need a responsible person to care for them throughout their lives, but they can participate in and enjoy many routines and activities with friends and family members.

The world can be a confusing place for children who have mental retardation in addition to a visual impairment. One reason is that it is very difficult for them to make sense of the abstract cues and symbols, such as speech or pictures, that give order and meaning to events around them. An example is understanding the significance of putting on a coat. Although a child with a visual impairment may not see others do this, she learns to associate her own experience of putting on a coat and the conversation of others with the experience of going outdoors. A child who has mental retardation but no other disability will also learn this by noticing others put on their coats, although it may take her longer to make this association. A child with both mental retardation and blindness does not have visual cues (seeing her own and others' coats) and may not understand spoken cues. It may therefore take this child even longer to learn that when she is dressed in a coat she is going outdoors, and she may not learn it at all unless it happens frequently.

If your child has both mental retardation and a visual impairment, it is important to carefully structure her world to help her anticipate events and objects, through touch and sound as well as through sight. For example, using a timer with a bell to signal the end of playtime provides a cue that your child can understand and learn to associate with the change of an activity. Always using the same materials, such as a familiar plastic mug for drinking, provides the best chance for your child to recall the cue, understand its meaning, and learn the related skill.

Children with visual and cognitive disabilities may have extra difficulty understanding the concept of time, including past and future events, since they do not see the visual cues to coming events such as mother getting out a paintbrush to paint or father carrying a book and walking toward his chair. If they do not understand speech, others cannot convey information to them about events as they might with a child who has a visual impairment but no additional disabilities. They need to participate directly in an activity to learn from it, and they need many more repetitions of a new skill in order to master it. The sections below describe some ways that mental retardation can complicate learning in specific developmental areas and offer suggestions for helping children with mental retardation learn. Some organizations that can be helpful to parents of children with mental retardation are the ARC and the TASH (formerly the Association for Persons with Severe Handicaps). Information on how to contact these organizations is provided in the Resource Guide.

Communication Disorders

People usually expect communication to be easy for a child with visual impairments to learn. This is not always the case, however, especially if the child also has other disabilities.

To communicate effectively, your child must understand that she can receive a response from others if she expresses a message or feeling. She must also have a form of communication that she can use and respond to. That form of communication may be gestures, picture symbols, object symbols, sign language, speech, braille, or print. Children with multiple disabilities can have more trouble than usual with either of these elements of effective communication. That is, they may have extra difficulty understanding how language works or remembering specific elements such as words or signs.

Children with mental retardation have more difficulty than usual learning how to understand and use language. This is because mental retardation causes delays in all areas of development, including communication skills. When a child with mental retardation also has a visual impairment, the difficulties are compounded. One reason is that the development of language depends on the child's awareness of *referents*—the objects, events, and people to be talked about. If a child cannot see what others are talking about, it is harder to learn that a specific word refers to a specific object or event. If the child also has cognitive delays, figuring out the relationships between words and objects or events becomes still harder. Using the same words and phrases to refer to familiar routines and events will give the child the best opportunity to match language with its referents, especially if language is used while an activity is taking place.

Echolalia, or the word-for-word repetition of other's speech, is another communication problem common to children with visual impairments, especially those with mental retardation or autism (see below). Children with visual impairments are likely to use echolalia for a longer period of time than other children. This can range from meaningless repetition, in which a child repeats the words, but doesn't understand them, to the meaningful use of echolalia in an interactive situation. For example, when someone asks, "Do you want a cookie?" and five-year-old Mary holds out her hands, smiles, and says, "Do you want a cookie," she is clearly responding, "Yes, I want one!" When a child has mental retardation in addition to a visual impairment, she is even more likely to persist in using echolalia. This may be because the child's ability to speak has outdistanced her understanding of words and concepts.

If your child often uses echolalic speech, it is best to respond as if she has made an appropriate attempt to communicate. For example, when Mary responds to the questions about a cookie using the same words, handing her a cookie and saying, "You do want a cookie!" is one way to let her know that her message is understood. Ignoring echolalia or correcting it may make your child feel that her communication is not effective, and she may try to speak less often. Only if your child has proven that she is a competent speaker should you suggest, "Try it again," when she uses echolalia. It is also not very useful to suggest, "Say it this way: 'I want a cookie'" because you are asking the child to imitate your sentence. The goal is to teach the child that she or he can think of the right words and use them for different reasons in different situations.

Some children may speak infrequently, or, in some cases, not at all. This may result from a lack of understanding of the function of language, an inability to remember words and meanings, or from lack of motivation. Specific drill or practice is not as important as establishing a meaningful, motivating language environment in the natural setting of home or classroom. This is especially true for children whose language is in the early stages of development. Speaking to your child in short, simple sentences about things happening around her will provide opportunities for her to build bridges between words and experiences. Doing routine task using the same objects and words will help the child associate sounds with experiences.

Movement Skills

Most children with mental retardation—with and without visual impairments—have motor delays. As a rule, they learn to sit up, stand, walk, climb stairs, draw with a crayon, cut with scissors, throw a ball, ride a bike, and so forth later than typically developing children do. Depending on their level of mental retardation, they may never learn to do some of these things at all, or may not be able to do them as proficiently as someone who doesn't have mental retardation.

Having a visual impairment along with mental retardation can cause even greater delays in motor skills. For example, many children with mental retardation are slow in learning to crawl or walk. When a child also has a visual impairment, she may be less motivated to learn these skills, because she may not know what objects are available to be explored or may not be curious about something she hears that is out of reach. It also may be more difficult for her to recall an experience or activity that has brought her pleasure in the past, so she may not make the effort to begin it again. For example, it may take many repetitions of hitting a mobile to ring a bell before a child understands that the sound is the result of her own movement.

You can encourage your child to move by positioning objects or people just out of reach. A music box or the voice of her grandmother will remind your child that there is someone or something interesting out there to be discovered. At first, the sound should be constant: the music box or grandmother's voice singing or talking motivates your child to move forward. Later, just calling your child's name once or twice will require her to remember where the sound came from as she moves.

Play activities can also encourage different movements and positions. Physical play on the floor with pillows and on hard and soft surfaces, as well as body contact with others, will teach your child how it feels to push and move against gravity. The feeling of physical contact is pleasurable for many children and should be introduced according to your child's preference. Many children prefer firm touches to light ones. Physical play with familiar people provides a chance to discover how others move their bodies and teaches children that others have body parts similar to their own. This can help extend your child's understanding of the world beyond her own body and discourage the repetitive behaviors that some children develop because their own body is the most available source of stimulation.

These repetitive motions, such as rocking or head banging, may occur in part because children do not know what else to do with their bodies or because they do not know how to communicate that they are frustrated. Some children rock or poke their eyes when they are tired or anxious, and others do this when they are working or relaxed. Others can sometimes discourage these behaviors by telling the child that they do not look nice and by providing praise or a small treat when they notice the child is sitting still. Providing plenty of opportunity for physical activity can also show the child new ways of moving that will take the place of repetitive behaviors.

Social and Emotional Skills

Because vision brings us information about how others act and react, a visual disability can make it more challenging to learn social skills. If your child also has mental retardation, it may take longer to understand information that is available through nonvisual means. Identifying a person who is speaking or remembering names requires memory of voice sounds, and understanding social rules such as when to shake hands means that a child must know when this is appropriate.

It is important for you to describe and model social behaviors so that your child can learn about them: "I shook hands with Mr. Green because I want to be friendly. Let's try shaking hands the way I did with Mr. Green." Another way you can help your child develop social skills is to make sure she learns that other people are enjoyable and can make interesting things happen. So as not to overwhelm or confuse her, it is best to start out with a few familiar people in her circle of acquaintances. These people should be reminded to let her know when they are approaching, especially if your child does not have enough vision to see them coming. If your child cannot understand words, you may want to think of a consistent way to help her identify familiar individuals by touch. For instance, placing your child's hand on her sister's long ponytail or on grandmother's ring will help her learn to expect the voice and manner of that person.

Later, you can arrange for play activities with groups of other children. It may be helpful to explain to other children what your child can and cannot do: "Sharon doesn't see with her eyes, but if you put the clay in her hand, she likes the cold feeling on her fingers." You can help choose materials that will interest your own child as well as other children of the same age, even though their interests and capabilities are different.

It can be particularly challenging to teach children with visual and mental disabilities how to protect themselves and follow safety rules. Skills such as walking on sidewalks rather than in streets or not going away with strangers can be learned through role playing and practice. To be sure that your child remembers what you have taught her, provide frequent opportunities to repeat the role playing. Because children with disabilities interact with many different adults and may become very trusting, also be sure to explain to your child when others should *not* be trusted.

Children with multiple and visual disabilities need systematic teaching to help them understand ideas and behaviors related to sexuality. Many concepts related to sexuality are visual; examples are clothing styles, nonverbal communication, and physical characteristics. It is important that children learn to refuse inappropriate touches and suggestions from others and to get help when needed. It is also important to answer your child's questions at a level that she can understand, and to encourage her to make age-appropriate decisions about relating to others. Some people with visual and multiple disabilities have adult relationships, and they need to receive information as teenagers that will help them to make appropriate decisions.

Although some children will not be able to interact with others using speech, they should be encouraged to develop their communication skills in normal social situations. Attending parties and social events, going to the grocery store, attending religious services, and visiting friends can be very satisfying to children and can give them practice with social routines that will make them more pleasant companions and family members.

Like other children, your child must also learn that there are limits and rules that apply to daily routines. Your approach to discipline should be as similar as possible to the approach you take with other children in the family. Sometimes you may need to provide extra opportunities to practice a rule so that you can be sure your child understands it. Then you can give your child praise and occasional rewards when she behaves appropriately.

Occasionally, you may need to discipline your child by withdrawing a privilege. When you do this, be sure that your child understands why you are taking something away, and make the punishment fit the behavior. For example, if your child does not put a toy away, you might tell her that she may not use the toy for a week. Show her where the toy will be stored, and each time she asks to use it, remind her that she will be able to use it again on Monday. Then be sure that you praise her for putting the toy away until that becomes a habit. Many children with mental retardation do not understand complex reasoning, and scolding or lecturing will not change their behavior. It is more effective to arrange their world so that good things happen when they behave appropriately.

Autism Spectrum Disorders

Some children with visual impairments are diagnosed with autism spectrum disorders (ASD), and others show characteristics of ASD even though they do not meet the diagnostic criteria. Autism spectrum disorders are estimated to occur in about 1 to 6 children out of every 1000 in the general population. Many professionals believe the incidence is greater among students with visual impairments, although no data are available to verify this.

Children with ASD show differences in social interaction, communication, and behaviors. They may repeat behaviors or routines rigidly, demonstrate physical mannerisms, and become preoccupied with objects. Social communication and imaginative play are often limited, and children may not make eye contact with others or seem to notice that people are different from objects.

About 80 percent of students with autism spectrum disorders also have mental retardation, but some children are of average or above average in intelligence. Children who have some autistic symptoms despite high intelligence and relatively good communication skills are often diagnosed with Asperger syndrome, and they often do well in academic achievement even though social interactions are difficult for them. They also tend to have intense interests in one or two specialized or unusual areas (such as train schedules or hockey statistics).

Over the past ten years, there has been a great increase in the number of children diagnosed with autism spectrum disorders. In 1990 autism was designated as a separate category under IDEA, and the increase in children diagnosed with autism may in part be due to the fact that the condition is now separately identified under educational law.

Education of children with ASD emphasizes the development of positive behavioral support to ensure desirable consequences for appropriate responses. This means that the child is rewarded for using appropriate behaviors and communication as a substitute for inappropriate behaviors, and that this is done consistently so that the child understands what is expected. Many of the behavioral difficulties displayed by students with autism can be changed when the children learn to communicate appropriately. For example, a child who screams and runs away when she hears a loud sound like a vacuum cleaner may be taught to gesture that she wants to leave the room when she sees the vacuum. Knowing that she can change the situation reduces her inappropriate screaming.

Children who have visual impairments and autism spectrum disorders often use echolalic speech past the preschool years, and they may depend on other people's directions and prompts to complete basic routines. They may be easily upset by changes in routine and may repeat movements or sequences of movements again and again. Familiar routines are the basis for learning, with opportunities for communication and choice included in routines so that students can take greater initiative. For students who are blind, the use of objects as cues to predict events and activities can be a helpful way to establish structure.

Physical and Motor Impairments

For a child with a visual impairment, the ability to move out into the world, to explore with hands and feet, and to experience changes in temperatures and texture are important in building concepts about what the world is like. If a child also has a physical disorder that limits her ability to move and explore, she may have trouble learning directly through discovery. A child with "normal" intelligence who has both a physical and visual handicap may learn to rely excessively on words and sounds for information and stimulation. She may play with rhyming words or may prefer listening to the radio to any other activity. A child with mental retardation may withdraw into a world that does not extend beyond her own body and physical needs. Because she does not know that there are other people and objects to be explored, she may repeat behaviors such as rocking or making interesting sounds that have no meaning.

Several types of physical disabilities, including cerebral palsy and spina bifida, often accompany visual impairment. The sections below discuss how these conditions can further complicate learning and development in children with visual impairments.

Cerebral Palsy

Cerebral palsy is the name for a variety of disorders that affect a child's motor abilities, including movement, balance, and posture.

The condition results from a difference in the early development of the brain or from an injury to the brain before birth, during birth, or shortly after birth. Types of injuries that can result in cerebral palsy include: infections; head trauma during or after birth; toxic injuries from maternal drug or alcohol use; too little oxygen before, during, or after birth; bleeding in the brain. Cerebral palsy is not a disease. It does not become worse with time, and it is not contagious.

How cerebral palsy affects a child's motor skills depends on the location and extent of the brain injury. But all children with cerebral palsy have problems with *muscle tone,* or the amount of resistance to movement in a muscle. Types of muscle tone problems that may be present include:

- **High tone** (*hypertonia, spasticity*). Children with high tone have muscles that are "tighter" or more resistant to movement than usual. As a result, their movements are stiff and awkward.
- **Low tone** (*hypotonia, floppiness*). Children with low tone have muscles that are "floppier" and less resistant to movement than usual. Consequently, it requires a great deal of effort for them to move and to maintain a position.
- **Fluctuating** (variable) **tone.** Children with fluctuating tone sometimes have low tone and sometimes have high tone.

Besides having problems with muscle tone, some children with cerebral palsy also have involuntary movements. Involuntary movements are uncontrolled movements in the face, arms, legs, or elsewhere in the body. Cerebral palsy is also frequently associated with mental retardation and seizures.

A child with cerebral palsy may have motor problems throughout her entire body. That is, she may have involuntary movements or high or low tone in her head, trunk, arms, and legs. This is known as *quadriplegia.* Then again, motor problems may affect only the upper extremities, the lower extremities, or one side of the body.

As mentioned earlier, some children with cerebral palsy have cortical visual impairments. In addition, about 50 percent of children with cerebral palsy have difficulty controlling the muscles of the eyes. This lack of muscle control usually results in *strabismus.* In this condition, the eyes are misaligned so that one or both eyes turns inward or outward. The eyes may be misaligned all the time, or only when the child looks in a particular direction. *Amblyopia,* or loss of vision in one eye due to disuse, may occur as a result of strabismus. Both of these conditions are described in greater detail in Chapter 2.

To correct strabismus, sometimes the doctor will try surgery to tighten the eye muscles or put a patch over the stronger eye. For many children with cerebral palsy, however, the problem is never completely corrected. Instead, these children learn to use their eyes selectively in order to get the most visual information. Many children with strabismus rely mainly on one eye for visual information. This means that they may have difficulty judging depth. They may, for example, have trouble anticipating a ball rolled toward them or difficulty inserting coins into a piggy bank. They also have a small field loss on the side of the less useful eye. This means they may turn their head slightly toward that side to make up for the missing information. Some children learn to use one eye for near tasks and the other for distance tasks. Watching your child carefully when she is using her eyes will help you decide what she is seeing and whether she is using one eye more than the other.

United Cerebral Palsy (UCP) and its many local affiliates can provide helpful information and support to parents of children with cerebral palsy. See the Resource Guide for contact information.

Other Physical and Motor Impairments

Although cerebral palsy is the most common cause of visual and motor difficulties in children, there are other reasons why a child with a visual impairment may also have a physical disability. Spina bifida, for example, is a physical disability that can indirectly cause a visual disability. In this condition, a child is born with an opening in the backbone and skin around it, so that a portion of the spinal cord protrudes through the back. Sometimes the child also has hydrocephalus, or excess fluid in the brain. The exact cause of spina bifida is still unknown. Children with spina bifida may be unable to walk or experience sensations, often in the lower part of the body. They often have optic nerve atrophy or cortical visual impairment as a result of extra pressure within the brain. This can cause a visual impairment or complete blindness.

Occasionally children are injured in accidents which result in visual disabilities. Very often, this is due to a head injury, and children may experience a cortical visual loss as well as physical disabilities in various parts of the body. Some children who acquire physical and visual disabilities as the result of accidents rapidly recover their visual and physical abilities during the first year or two after the accident.

Others improve more gradually for years after the accident occurred. And some never fully recover.

How Physical Disabilities Affect Learning

Most young children do a great deal of learning by watching and doing. For example, they learn about the concept of cause and effect by smacking a tower of blocks and then watching it fall over. They learn about the concept of object permanence by watching a ball roll under the couch and then retrieving it. They learn the difference between hard and soft by touching or chewing on a variety of different objects.

Obviously, when a child has both visual and motor handicaps, she may have trouble learning by watching and doing. And yet, she still needs immediate and concrete opportunities for learning, with plenty of emphasis on doing rather than just listening. As a parent, there are many ways you can provide these opportunities to your child. For example, if your child cannot see a toy or reach forward to get it, you can make her aware of its presence some other way. Although technology has expanded the options for children with combinations of disabilities, the best solutions to problems such as retrieving a toy are not always technologically complex. Your child's cue to an object's existence may be a ticking timer or her brother's voice calling; her means of getting the object may be a string or a stick with a T-hook. What is important is that your child experiences the result of her own actions.

If your child has some vision, it is important for her to be positioned in a way that will help her to see efficiently. Sometimes the positions that promote good physical development do not provide the best visual information. For example, a child positioned on her stomach with a wedge for support may see only objects directly in front of her and may not be able to raise or turn her head to see other parts of the room. Your child's physical or occupational therapist should work closely with the vision specialist to help you decide what positions are best for your child. They can also help you decide how much time your child should spend in different positions.

If your child cannot walk or crawl, there are many ways you can help her experience movement through space. When she is young, you can carry her in a sling or backpack as you move around the house. This way, she can experience the immediate sensations that go along with routine activities. She can hear and feel water coming out of the faucet or the breeze blowing in when you open a window.

As your child gets older, physical and occupational therapists can work with your family to obtain an appropriate travel chair or wheelchair. There are wheelchairs that require very little movement and control to operate, and children with severe physical disabilities can often learn to control their own movement using an electric wheelchair. Your child's wheelchair should provide comfortable, symmetrical positioning that allows 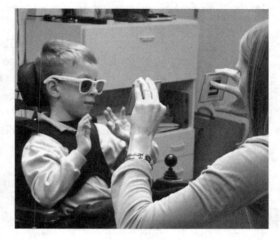 her maximum control over the position and the movement of the chair. If your child has vision, take care that the side panels on the head support of the chair do not restrict head movement or reduce visual field.

If your child does not have enough vision to anticipate landmarks in a route of travel, devices can be attached to her wheelchair or travel chair to provide feedback. For example, an antenna attached to the right wheel can act as a trailing device and provide an auditory cue about your child's distance from the wall. Some children are able to use devices such as the Mowat sensor™, a small box that is held in the traveler's hand and vibrates to tell her that she is approaching an object. The orientation and mobility instructor can work with the physical and occupational therapist to devise the most effective adaptations for your child. See Chapter 11 for more information on orientation and mobility.

The following sections describe some ways that having a physical disability can affect specific areas of development. They also include suggestions to help your child learn and grow in these areas.

Communication Skills

Many children who have cerebral palsy in addition to a visual impairment also have added problems in learning to use speech and understand language. The physical process of producing speech may be affected by the child's difficulty controlling muscles of the face, mouth, throat, and chest. Some children may produce speech that is difficult to understand, partly because they cannot close their lips to produce clear consonant sounds. A child who also has a visual impairment may not see the lips of others moving, so imitating the movements that produce specific sounds may be difficult.

Physical disabilities can also affect a child's ability to understand language. Movement limitations may reduce opportunities for new experiences and for interaction with others. Others may assume that the child understands a word or idea that relates to something the child has never done. For example, words that refer to a farm, a circus, or forest animals may have little meaning to a child who lives in a city and spends most of her time indoors, especially if she does not have enough vision to learn from pictures.

Obviously, it can be frustrating if your child can understand others' speech but has difficulty making herself understood. To help your child communicate, an augmentative device may therefore be recommended. As the term implies, an augmentative device is one that is meant to *augment,* not replace, a child's speech abilities. Although parents sometimes worry that using an augmentative device will prevent their child from learning to speak, this is not the case. Most studies show that using an augmentative device encourages a child to use other forms of expression, such as speech.

Your child's augmentative device will be selected based on her communication needs, developmental level, and useful vision. For a young child who has some vision, picture symbols or photographs might be arranged on a language board. The child could then point to or touch pictures of objects and actions to express her thoughts and needs. Contrast, color, background, and size should be considered in choosing pictures or symbols that the child could best see. Pictures can be too large as well as too small for a child to view comfortably. For most children with visual impairments, pictures of three inches or smaller are large enough.

For young children with little or no vision, object cues or language boards often use real objects or parts of real objects as cues to meaning. For a child who does not know the meaning of symbols, learning will occur best if the object is regularly associated with a routine. For example, a cup that is used at snack time can be touched to her hand and placed on the table before the meal begins, and she can help in putting it into the sink after the meal. Later, the handle of the cup or the clapper from the bell can be included on a language board to represent the whole object.

Some children eventually learn to use language boards on which words are indicated with braille or with a symbol that has no relationship to the real object. There are also a variety of computerized devices available, including some that can produce a synthesized voice.

If your child uses augmentative communication or a gesture or sign system, remember that she may not see when others are looking at the device or at the signs she makes. Consequently, she needs to learn ways of establishing the presence of others, such as touching others' arms before beginning to communicate. Your child also needs to receive a response whenever she makes an attempt to communicate.

Whatever system your child uses to communicate, it is important that you don't just communicate with her in commands or questions. Your child needs to learn to take an active role in conversations—to initiate them, as well as to participate in them. She needs to learn that through communication, she can gain more control over her world. For example, she may not be able to walk over to the stereo and turn it on herself, but she can ask somebody to do it for her. Likewise, she may not be able to open the refrigerator and pour herself a glass of juice, but if she asks appropriately, you may do it for her.

You can encourage active communication by presenting choices whenever possible. In addition, you can be sure that your child has enough time to express ideas and a communication method that does not just limit her to answering questions. Pausing when talking is important because it lets your child know when it is her turn to speak. Responding to any movement or behavior that seems to communicate will help your child understand that communication includes at least two people. If you comment, "I'll bet you're hungry" when your child moves her mouth or looks at her spoon, she may later learn to use one of these gestures to request food or to answer the question, "Are you hungry?"

Movement Skills

Motor dysfunctions such as cerebral palsy or spina bifida can put some real limits on how well and how quickly a child is able to master motor skills. For example, depending on the location of nerve damage, a child with spina bifida may have trouble learning to roll over and sit up, and may never be able to stand or walk unaided. Depending on the location and severity of brain injury, a child with cerebral palsy might have these same problems, as well as difficulty using her arms and hands to reach and grasp. Like other children, however, children with motor disabilities can develop the physical abilities they have to the utmost. With the right kinds of encouragement and help, they can improve their strength, coordination, and endurance, and can master many important motor skills.

As Chapters 8 and 11 explain, your child can receive a great deal of assistance in learning movement skills from physical therapists, occupational therapists, and orientation and mobility specialists at school. As a parent, you can encourage movement by positioning playthings so that your child must move to reach for them, and by making sure she participates in daily routines that involve movement.

Social and Emotional Skills

For a variety of reasons, children with multiple disabilities may make slower progress than usual in social and emotional development. Physical, mental, or hearing impairments may make it harder for them to hone their social skills by initiating interactions with others. And others may interpret their lack of interaction to mean that they do not want to have social contact, and therefore leave them alone. Compounding the problem, parents may not correct inappropriate behavior because they feel sorry for their child or think she cannot understand what is expected of her. To get along in society, however, all children need to understand social conventions and safety rules. Your child, like all children, can pick up much of this understanding at home.

One way you can help with your child's social skills is to discourage any repetitive behaviors such as eye poking, rocking, finger chewing, or head banging. Children with multiple disabilities may sometimes have these mannerisms because they are not aware that there are things to be explored beyond their own bodies. If a child is blind, she may not be aware that others do not have the same habits. You can discourage these behaviors by a gentle reminder or a signal such as a tap on the shoulder. You can also offer your child toys or other objects to draw her attention away from the repetitive behavior.

Another way to boost your child's social skills is to prepare her for visits and social events. If your child understands words, this may mean talking to her about what she will do and who will be there. If she does not understand words, it may help to show her pictures of people she will see or to give her an object to remind her of a special event to come. For example, she may hold an inflated toy as you drive to the swimming pool or an overnight bag with her pajamas on the way to her grandparents' house. This will help her to be aware of the people and objects around her and to feel good about being with other people.

Deaf-Blindness

Less than 5 percent of all children with visual impairments also have hearing disabilities. Although these children are often called "deaf-blind," most of them do have usable vision, hearing, or both. In some areas of the country, the term "dual sensory impairment" is used to describe a reduction in both vision and hearing.

Deaf-blindness in children can be caused by several conditions: neurological complications that accompany premature birth; infections and viruses such as toxoplasmosis, meningitis, or cytomegalovirus; and maternal rubella are among the most common causes.

There are two types of hearing losses: sensorineural and conductive. A sensorineural loss means that the nerves that receive sound and carry it into the brain are damaged or have not developed. This kind of loss can result from any condition that damages the brain, such as infection before the baby is born, premature birth, or the effects of drugs or medication. Some sensorineural hearing loss is inherited. Sensorineural losses are often more severe than conductive losses. Sometimes hearing can be improved through use of a hearing aid, but other times hearing aids are not helpful.

A conductive loss occurs when something interferes with the passage of sound through the ear canal or the structures of the middle and inner ear. This can be a permanent condition, and may be caused by something like a growth of tissue in the ear, or it may be temporary and caused by a cold or a middle ear infection. Often this type of hearing loss can be improved by surgery or by the use of a hearing aid.

Children with hearing losses may hear some frequencies of sound better than others. Frequency refers to how high- or low-pitched sound is, and is measured in hertz. The loudness or volume of a sound, measured in decibels, can also affect how well it can be heard. When your child's hearing is tested, the degree of hearing loss she has at each frequency will be measured. A reading of 0 to 15 decibels at any given frequency means your child has normal hearing at that frequency; anything higher than 15 generally means she has a hearing loss.

A variety of tests can assess hearing, but finding one that is appropriate for a child with both a hearing and vision impairment can be difficult. You may need to work with professionals to teach your child an action such as dropping a block in a can to signal that she hears a sound. There are also medical tests that can provide general information about whether your child is receiving sound in the brain, even if she is too young or otherwise unable to signal what she hears. In an auditory brain stem response (ABR), for example, clicks or other sounds are produced in the child's ears and a computer recording made that tells whether the brain has received the sound signals. This test does not provide information about the quality of sounds that a child hears, but it does tell whether the brain has received the sounds. If she is given an ABR, your child may need to be sedated.

You can also learn about your child's hearing on an informal basis by watching her reactions around the house. Does she pay attention to the stereo but ignore water running? Does she notice her father's voice more than her mother's? Her use of hearing in everyday situations is often the best way to learn whether sounds and voices will be meaningful to her.

Some children with hearing losses can be assisted by hearing aids, which increase the loudness of the sounds they hear. Sometimes children initially reject the hearing aid, because louder sounds may be unpleasant at first and they may not know what the sounds mean. In the beginning, it may therefore be better for the child to use the hearing aid for short periods of time. The speech-language pathologist or vision specialist can also help the child become accustomed to the hearing aid. Some children do not benefit from the use of a hearing aid, and will be encouraged to make sense of sound in other ways if they have some hearing. For example, games in which the child listens to one sound at a time and then learns to recognize that same sound with other noises in the background can help a child tell important sounds from unimportant sounds.

If your child is deaf-blind, her senses bring her limited information about the world around her. This makes it easy for her to become withdrawn and to be most interested in her body or in inanimate objects that are readily accessible. For example, she may prefer to bang two blocks together again and again because they make a loud sound she can hear. She may not know that blocks can be stacked, placed in containers, or used to create structures.

With appropriate instruction, most children who are deaf-blind can make steady progress in all areas of development. Children with deaf-blindness usually learn best when they have immediate contact with a few familiar caregivers in a predictable environment. Educational programs that use methods such as the Van Dijk procedures are especially effective with some deaf-blind children. This program emphasizes learning language through movement and the use of predictable routines. For example, a child can be taught to imitate the movements of an adult by moving with her along a mat or balance beam. Later, the child learns to anticipate events of the day through the use of a "calendar box," a sectioned box or shelf which contains objects representing each activity of a child's day in the order that the activities occur.

Sometimes children become deaf-blind as the result of an accident or illness later in childhood. Educational programs for these children focus on retaining their current communication skills while developing additional ones. For example, speech-language pathologists will work on helping the child continue to speak clearly, but professionals may also introduce sign language so that she can easily receive information from others.

It is crucial that all children with deaf-blindness be encouraged to communicate and to socialize. Having regular opportunities to interact with others is vitally important, both at school and at home. The next sections offer some strategies that can enhance development of communication, social, and motor skills in children with deaf-blindness. There are also several organizations, including the Deaf Blind Coalition, based at Perkins School for the Blind, that you can contact for more information on deaf-blindness. See the Resource Guide for addresses.

Communication Skills

How well a deaf-blind child is able to communicate depends on several factors, including how much vision and hearing she has. How she communicates is also influenced by her mental ability, including her memory and ability to apply words and ideas in different situations. In addition, a child's motivation has a big impact on learning to communicate. Some deaf-blind children are very motivated to communicate, but others are not very interested in other people.

If your child is deaf-blind, an important step in building the foundation for communication skills is to make the environment more meaningful. For example, you can make a habit of tapping her on the palm of the hand to let her know that you are there and that you will respond to her efforts to communicate. You can also work out cues to help her recognize familiar people. For instance, you could place your child's hand on Dad's beard or Mom's curly hair to aid in identification. You could hand her a spoon before you guide her to the table to eat, or place the same cap on her head each time you take her outdoors. When using signals like these, make sure that the event happens immediately after your child is aware of the object, especially if she is young or has a short memory.

If your child is not very motivated to communicate, it is important to help her see how others are involved in her favorite activities. For example, if she enjoys eating or swinging on a swing, help her understand that these good things happen because another person is there to provide the things she likes.

Some deaf-blind children learn to use gestures, body movements, or sign language as their primary form of communication. Your child may begin communicating through natural gestures. These are gestures she chooses for herself to stand for people and events in her world. For example, she may touch her mouth when she is hungry or tug at her socks when she wants to walk in bare feet. You should accept and respond to these gestures until she is ready to move on to a more complex sign language system. At that time, you should plan to learn sign language yourself so that you can begin to show her some of the accepted signs when they are needed. Some children will learn formal signs as toddlers, but many deaf-blind children take years to reach that point, and others use natural gestures all of their lives.

If your child is blind as well as hearing impaired, she may learn "covered" or tactile sign. That is, she will lightly cover the hand of the signer with her own hand so she can feel, rather than see, the signs being made. If she has sufficient vision to see signs, you will need to take her visual differences into account when presenting signs. It is helpful to present the signs against a background that contrasts with your hand, and at the most appropriate distances for her visual field and acuity. Although the classroom teacher and speech-language pathologist may be the team members who instruct your child in sign, it is important for all family and team members to learn sign language so that she has plenty of opportunities for real communication.

However your child learns to communicate, it is important that everybody at home and school provide her with consistent input in the chosen form of communication. Using words and signs related to activities such as dressing, eating, and using the toilet are especially important since these are things that your child will do every day.

Movement Skills

Children who are deaf-blind can learn the same movement skills as other children. However, many learn more slowly. Because their hearing and visual impairments make it difficult for them to know what is around them to be explored, they may not have the motivation to move through space. And like children with visual impairments alone, they cannot imitate the movements of others around them. You will need to keep your child close to you as you move so that she can notice your movements. You may need to guide her as she moves from one position to another, such as sitting to standing, so that she will feel secure while doing this. Many deaf-blind children enjoy repeated movement activities such as rocking or swinging. You can encourage these for short periods of time, but help your child find ways to add variety to them and to use movement to explore, not just stimulate herself.

It is also important to give your child cues to help her understand where she is going when she moves. For example, using an object that stands for an activity, such as a cake of soap to be carried to the bathroom, will help your child understand that she is moving toward the same room where she took a bath the day before.

Social and Emotional Skills

Children who are deaf-blind may have more difficulty learning social skills because they cannot easily perceive others' responses or imitate others' behavior in social situations. Some social skills will be learned gradually. For example, waiting in a store line or taking turns with a toy may be difficult if your child cannot understand the reason, so you will need to start by providing a reward for just a little cooperation. In other situations, you may decide that the skill is too difficult for your child and that it is not important to learn right now. For example, you may take your child along for a meal at a fast-food restaurant, but leave her with a family member or babysitter while the family goes out to a more formal restaurant.

Some deaf-blind children have behaviors that are difficult to deal with at times. This may be because they cannot communicate their real feelings and thoughts, but it can also be because their brains have been affected by the same condition that caused their hearing and vision impairment. To deal with a difficult behavior, you can begin by writing down what happens just before the behavior usually occurs. For example, if your child always cries and throws toys at mealtime, then you can begin to explore the cause. Does she dislike a food? Does she dislike having her hand held with a spoon in it?

Once you know why your child behaves as she does, you can try rewarding her during or immediately after the difficult time if she controls her behavior. For example, if your child does not like riding in the car but plays quietly with a toy during a car ride, you could reward her with a favorite activity like rocking in the rocking chair or watering plants right after the car ride. This helps your child learn that good things happen when she works to control her behavior. If your child regularly does things that hurt herself or other people, request that her educational team include someone who is knowledgeable in managing difficult behaviors.

▪▪ The Importance of Routine

For all children with multiple disabilities, it is important to have regular routines that provide opportunities to repeat and apply new skills and to learn to anticipate events. Otherwise, a child with multiple disabilities may not realize that there are connections between what happens at different times or at different places. For example, she may not understand that putting on a coat has any connection with the cold outdoors unless she always puts her coat on right before going out.

Your child should have routines for functional activities such as eating or preparing for bed, as well as routines for recreation or play. Routines should always occur in the same place using the same materials. And they should require that your child and at least one other person take roles understood by each. For example, at mealtime someone should always give your child a signal that helps her understand what will take place next. Handing her a bib or a placemat to carry to the kitchen or showing her a picture of a plate of food are examples of such signals. When your child understands what will happen next, she is more likely to cooperate in a routine.

Many people look for new technology that will help their children learn. However, too much complex technology can separate a child from others or cause frustration if it is not right for the child. Your child is more likely to learn if she can use technology in a meaningful way during the course of regular routines. Technology will only be useful if it is regularly accessible and allows a child to do a regular or interesting activity more effectively.

You can establish routines around interactive play to help your child learn communication and social skills. For example, if you rock your child to a song and then pause, she can learn to use a gesture or word to ask to continue. If you hide a toy in a box with a latch, your child can tap on the box to signal you to open it. The success of such activities depends on your child's interest in achieving the result, and your ability to read the response and elaborate on it.

For most children with multiple disabilities and major learning delays, routines must be repeated frequently and consistently in order to be effective. They should occur daily or several times a day until they are well established. After your child has learned her role in the routine, you can vary it somewhat and make the routine more elaborate. The routine can then act as a framework for presenting new information and for teaching your child to deal with novel occurrences, as well as expected ones. For example, if your child bounces on your knee as a signal that she wants to be bounced up and down, then you can encourage her to use new signals to indicate that she wants to rock, swing, or do other movements she enjoys. When your child has thoroughly learned a routine, you may introduce an unexpected object to encourage her to communicate. For example, you may give her a comb instead of a spoon at breakfast so that she will notice the difference and request the appropriate item for her routine.

▪▪ Conclusion

If your child has multiple disabilities, she may learn many skills at a slower rate than she would otherwise, and she may need to learn about the world through a different medium. She will also need more support from a wider range of people to make progress at home, school, work, and play. The key is to establish predictable routines that provide the framework to expand learning and give her a sense of control over events around her.

Regardless of your child's strengths and needs, she should receive the message that she can make things happen. Lifting a spoon, calling out to a friend, protesting about a wet diaper, or moving her own wheelchair are everyday events that may help her understand that she can take action. With the support of an effective, consistent educational team, your child can make steady progress toward becoming a participating member of her family and her community.

■■ Parent Statements

Our daughter's grandparents could not understand why she was born with disabilities, but they have grown to love and care for her so much. Her disability is just not an issue now.

❧❀❧

Kelsey's sister tries to help and sometimes has to stick up for her in front of other children. This may be a little difficult for her, but I think it is good preparation for life.

❧❀❧

Our daughter has both blindness and cerebral palsy. The cerebral palsy has been much harder for our family to understand and accept.

❧❀❧

Having more than one disability really seems to complicate matters, especially with the school. I never know which problems they should be focusing on the most.

❧❀❧

It has been a real battle to get David to wear his hearing aid and in the process we seem to have lost the battle with his eyeglasses. But we haven't given up yet.

❧❀❧

At first I was very angry and bitter, and I blamed God. I have since learned to adjust to my son's disabilities. Every day seems to come with new challenges and I don't always have the patience I wish I had, but I know I will continually adjust.

❧❀❧

Nicky has so many problems; blindness is the least of our worries right now.

❧❀❧

I hate to admit it, but I sometimes resent parents of children who have only one disability.

❧❀❧

My biggest pet peeve is people who stare. Don't just stare at my child. Come and talk to me. I am proud of him and I can talk about him all day long.

❧❀❧

One thing I have trouble with is how to separate being a parent from teaching my daughter things. I know that my most important job is to be Kayla's mother, but I keep thinking of everything she needs to learn and I want to help her learn the things she needs to learn to be ready to go to school in two years.

❧❀❧

We are learning something new every day.

❧❀❧

From my child, I have learned to love unconditionally. My life has been opened up to include experiences I never would have considered before Heather was born.

The Years Ahead

LaRhea Sanford, Ph.D., &
Rebecca Burnett, Ed.D.

Even though your child is young now, you probably already have many questions about his future. Will he be able to finish high school and go to college? Will he date? How will he be able to get to work when he is living on his own? What about grocery shopping and laundry and balancing his checkbook? All parents have questions and concerns about their children's future. Your questions and concerns are more complicated, however, because you may not know how your child's vision loss will affect his future.

Today it may be frightening for you to think of your child (who may now be four years old) ironing his own clothes. But by the time he is a young adult, he will be ready to learn to do such things with adaptations. You and his teachers will make sure that he will have learned the prerequisite skills to make these activities much easier. Taking time now to think about some of your concerns and questions can help you identify ways to help your child accomplish future goals.

⁜ Educational Issues

As Chapter 8 explained, you will probably be actively involved in your child's schooling when he is young. You will be consulted about what you think is important for your child to learn, how you think he would learn it best, and where you think the learning should take place. You may be asked to help your child work on educational goals at home, and you may have direct contact with teachers and other educators fairly frequently. As your child grows older, the intensity of your involvement may diminish. One reason, of course, is that your child will learn skills that enable him to be more independent. Another reason is that he will probably take on more responsibility for his own education. He should have increasing involvement in the IEP process and decisions as he gets older and becomes more independent.

Despite all the gains your child will make, you will still be more involved in his education than you would be if he did not have a visual impairment. If he continues to need special education services, you will continue to help plan his IEP every year. You will also want to make sure: 1) that he is placed in, and remains in, the most appropriate educational setting; 2) that all adaptations necessary to help him learn are made; and 3) that there is an appropriate balance between the general education curriculum and expanded core curriculum (specialized skills that are needed specifically to help compensate for loss of vision).

Placement Decisions

Throughout your child's elementary and high school years, a wide variety of placement options will be available. These range from full inclusion in a regular classroom with consultation services from a teacher of students with visual impairments (TVI) to placement in a residential school for the blind, with a variety of options and combinations of options between the two extremes. (See Chapter 8 for a description of these options.)

Often, children with visual impairments do not stay in the same type of placement from kindergarten through high school. They may need more intensive and specialized services in the early years when basic skills and concepts are being developed. So, they may start out in a self-contained classroom or residential school that provides intense specialized services. Then, once they have acquired skills and learned to compensate for their visual impairment, they may move to a placement that requires more independence. It is also possible that a child may periodically need more intense specialized services at various times in his educational career. This may be the case if he has a sudden loss of vision or a change in his educational needs.

To make sure that your child's needs are being properly met by his educational placement, his needs must be reevaluated at least once a year at the annual IEP meeting. His placement can also be reviewed any other time you request it. Some questions you may want to ask are:

- Is my child making progress as expected—academically, socially, and physically?
- Is he challenged academically?
- Is he learning the specialized skills he needs?
- Are his vocational needs being met?
- Are services available in all the areas needed (for example, orientation and mobility, speech, occupational therapy)?
- Are adapted materials available in a timely manner? (Your child's textbooks and classroom materials should be available at the beginning of each school year and as needed throughout the school year.)
- Do my child's teachers receive appropriate and timely consultation with the TVI about his special needs? This may be essential to providing effective instruction.

Successful placement depends on the flexible use of a variety of placement options for different periods of time. The length of time your child spends in a particular setting may vary from as little as six to twelve weeks to as much as several years, depending on his needs and how well they are being met. For example, your child might be in a public school program during the school year. In the summer, however, he may attend a residential program for a specified period of specialized and intensive training in orientation and mobility, adaptive technology, or self-help skills. Or a child placed at a residential school may attend public school for certain classes. This might give him more opportunities for social interactions as well as academic variety.

If you believe that your child's needs are not being met or that his placement should be changed, you should request an IEP meeting to discuss your concerns. Putting your request in writing and sending it to the teacher of students with visual impairments (TVI) and district special education administrator should help you get a timely response, as required by law.

Classroom Adaptations

Whatever your child's placement, he will likely need at least some specialized materials, equipment, techniques, or curricula to benefit fully from his education. For example, Chapter 10 describes adaptations that can enable people with all kinds of visual impairments to read and write.

As your child grows older, he may need additional adaptations, or he may learn to use more sophisticated equipment. For instance, in the primary grades, your child might be able to read the print in regular textbooks. But in about fourth grade, when the print becomes smaller, he may require larger print. Print size in handouts and class materials might be increased by actually making the print larger with a copier or a word processor, or by using a magnifying device, such as a hand-held magnifier or closed circuit television.

Your child may also need to have assignments modified so that he is not inadvertently penalized for having a visual impairment. One common reason for modifications is that students who are visually impaired and blind usually read at a slower rate than their sighted classmates. Some students' eyes tire more easily and may require brief rest periods or alternating periods of near and distant visual tasks. Students can be given extra time to complete assignments or standardized tests or they may be allowed to use adaptive equipment such as a talking calculator. Some people may incorrectly assume that making assignments shorter (assigning only half of the mathematics problems, or a three- instead of six-page paper) would be a good strategy to use with children who have visual impairments. Actually, shortening assignments should not routinely be done. It is important to hold children with visual impairments to the same standard as their sighted classmates.

Children with visual impairments participate in literacy activities using a wide variety of tools including print and braille. As he grows older, your child will also learn to use other types of technology that will give him access to the world of communication. Most likely, he will learn to use computers to produce documents that can be printed in both braille and print and also to access the Internet. Many students use taped books to read their assignments and a tape player to take notes in class. They may also use specially designed machines that scan and read a book using computerized speech output. Books such as encyclopedias are also available on computer software to use with voice output.

The teacher of students with visual impairments is responsible for adapting and ordering any special materials and equipment your child needs, as well as for informing teachers about appropriate techniques to meet your child's needs. Additionally, the TVI will observe your child in the classroom, and talk with you, your child, and his classroom teachers to determine appropriate adaptations. This process is continuous throughout the school years, and changes are made as needed.

Not all school systems are as able and willing as others to provide expensive adaptive equipment. Generally, however, schools are responsible for providing the technology necessary to meet a student's needs at school. Federal court cases have upheld that school systems must provide needed equipment and materials, but are not required to provide "Cadillac" (very expensive and advanced) services or equipment. However, energetic teachers and parents can often find funding sources to provide more equipment and materials.

Curricula

Most students with visual impairments receive instruction not only in the usual general education curriculum, but also in expanded core curriculum skills (ECC)—specialized skills that are needed specifically to help compensate for poor vision or the loss of vision. Because students with visual impairments have more to learn than other students, they should not be pushed through the grades just so they can graduate with others their age. Under federal law, students with disabilities are eligible for educational services through their twenty-first birthday. You and your child should take advantage of this provision, if necessary. The additional skills your child needs to learn because of his visual impairment may require additional time in school.

General Education Curricula

A visual impairment, per se, does not affect a child's ability to learn academic skills. But a visual impairment usually does affect how a child is taught academic skills, to a certain extent. Often textbooks and other instructional materials designed for typically sighted children are transcribed into braille or large type or recorded on tape. Sometimes instructional methods and materials need to be adapted in other ways. The sections below describe some typical differences in the ways academic subjects are taught.

Language Arts. Your child may learn to read using reading programs designed for sighted students. How materials and teaching techniques are adapted will depend on your child's need and age. After he has developed literacy skills and is a proficient reader, taped books may be provided for extensive reading assignments, especially at the high school level. CD/

ROM and computer software with voice, large print, and braille output capabilities will help your child conduct research. Technologies of today and the future will put your child on the Information Super Highway.

The American Printing House for the Blind has developed a special reading curriculum called *Patterns* for students learning to read braille in kindergarten through third grade. The series is designed to eliminate or minimize braille reading problems for beginners. This basal-type reading series takes into consideration such factors as the sequence of difficulty of the braille code and the frequency of occurrence of specific braille characters. The texts emphasize acquisition of experiences through senses other than vision. After completing the program, students are provided with the same reading materials that sighted students use that are transcribed into braille.

Spelling books are transcribed into braille with no changes in format or content, except that words are first presented in contracted form, then spelled out letter by letter. Keyboarding may be taught as early as first grade. Keyboarding helps strengthen spelling skills because each word must be spelled letter by letter, instead of using braille contractions. See Chapter 10 for a description of the writing methods a child with visual impairments might learn.

Mathematics. Your child will learn mathematics using the same curriculum designed for sighted students. Adapted materials and manipulatives (concrete objects that can be handled) will help him learn mathematical concepts.

The primary adaptation used to teach mathematics to braille readers is called the Nemeth Code, the braille symbol system for mathematical and scientific notations. Students usually learn the Nemeth Code at the same time other students are learning the symbols for addition, multiplication, etc. To help your child make calculations, he may use several aids and devices. These include the braille writer, which is used to write numbers and math problems; the abacus; and the talking calculator. Talking calculators are relatively inexpensive and are quite helpful in solving complex problems in advanced classes, especially after the student has memorized the basic facts in mathematics and understands computational processes.

Science. Students with visual impairments should be encouraged to explore their natural curiosities related to science. While the techniques used to support students as they learn scientific concepts may be different, the expectation for success in this area should be the same as with their sighted classmates. Students with visual impairments can learn the concepts underlying all sciences through adapted reading materials and hands-on experiments. Your child will be able to conduct experiments using specialized and adapted equipment, materials, and techniques. The classroom teacher should incorporate a hands-on approach utilizing all the senses—sight, hearing, touch, and smell. For example, your child may plant a bean seed in a container filled with water instead of soil so he can touch and feel the root system as it grows.

Social Studies. Much of social studies is verbal in nature, so students with visual impairments can easily learn the information and participate in discussions. The main challenge that arises in social studies classes is using pictures, maps, globes, graphs, and diagrams. The TVI will make sure that your child understands the concepts and acquires the skills needed to interpret maps and other materials, and that materials are available in bold line or tactile form. The classroom teacher will provide verbal descriptions of adapted materials and of pictures and diagrams that have not been adapted.

Physical Education. There are several reasons why it is important for children with visual impairments to participate in physical education. First, they often lag behind in developing mobility skills and tend to be less physically active than other children. This may be due to fear of the unknown and an inability to observe and imitate motor skills. Second, poor posture can be a problem for children with disabilities. Sometimes students must hold their heads or bodies in unusual positions in order to use their vision most efficiently.

Adapted techniques and materials may be needed for your child to participate safely in physical education. One or more of the following modifications might be required:

1. adapted methods (for instance, maintaining physical contact at all times when wrestling);
2. adapted equipment and materials (such as the use of a rail during bowling to help students with balance and directionality, or a beeping or brightly colored ball and bold boundary markers for certain kinds of ball games);

3. omission of activities such as ping pong which require good vision; and

4. modified versions of activities, such as having a sighted student run with a student who is blind.

While your child will be able to participate more easily in individual activities than in group sports, he should be given as many opportunities to join group sporting activities as possible. He may need special instruction in some skills such as gymnastics, especially if he cannot observe and imitate these skills. Many different people may help your child during physical activities, including classroom teachers, adaptive physical education teachers, physical therapists, teacher assistants, adult volunteers, and other students.

The TVI should consult with the physical education teacher and let him know about your child's visual needs and concerns. For example, if your child is extremely sensitive to sunlight, protective clothing, a sun visor, and sunglasses should be available at school for use during outside activities.

Foreign Languages. Most students with visual impairments do not have any more trouble than their typical peers in learning to *speak* a foreign language. But learning to *read and write* a foreign language may present a few more challenges for braille reading children because not all foreign languages use exactly the same braille code as is used in English. Although the symbols for most letters are the same as in English, there may be symbols for accents and other symbols not present in English. The TVI will need to refer to the *Code of Braille Textbook Formats and Techniques* to teach your child the braille code used in reading and writing the language.

Art and Music. Many children with visual impairments enjoy expressing themselves artistically. It is sometimes difficult to predict what art activities any given student will enjoy. Individuals who are visually impaired enjoy and participate in the wide range of art activities from photography to sculpting. Allowing and encouraging artistic expression is important for your child.

Children with visual impairments can usually participate fully in a variety of music activities. Adaptations for music may be as simple as providing lyrics to songs in large print or braille. If your child sings in a chorus, he may need to be given some kind of cue (an introduction played on the piano or a nudge from another student) so he knows when to begin singing or is aware of other gestures the instructor may be using. Students who are interested in learning to play a musical instrument should be encouraged to do so. Children with visual impairments usually have all the motor skills necessary to play any instrument in the band or orchestra, as well as piano. Students who are blind, however, will learn a special braille music code if they wish to read music. They must also be prepared to memorize their music prior to performing it since most instruments (except some of the brass ones) require two hands on the instrument to play.

Expanded Core Curriculum

The Expanded Core Curriculum (ECC) is the umbrella term for a variety of specialized skills that can help individuals with visual impairments lead satisfying lives and get along independently in the real world. These skills are taught in addition to the general education curriculum. The kind and amount of specialized instruction your child receives in these skills will depend on his abilities and needs, as well as his background experiences at home and in the community.

The members of your child's education team should evaluate his needs in the expanded core curriculum at least once a year. To document your child's progress and identify future needs, checklists and task analyses (breaking a skill down into small steps) may be used. The TVI is then responsible for either teaching your child these skills or for coordinating the services and activities your child needs.

When scheduling and planning for instruction, you, your child, and his education team members should not underestimate the importance of expanded core skills. Academics are important, but the expanded core skills are also a necessity. *The Expanded Core Curriculum for Blind and Visually Impaired Students, Including those with Additional Disabilities* includes the following areas (see Chapter 8 for more information):

- Visual Efficiency
- Compensatory Skills
- Technology
- Orientation and Mobility
- Social Interaction Skills
- Independent Living Skills
- Recreation and Leisure Skills
- Career Education
- Self-determination

Specialized skills in these areas can help children compensate for a visual loss and develop their skills and concepts more completely. Training in any of these skills should be available to your child if he needs them, no matter what his educational placement. Some examples of areas in which your child may need instruction are:

- Sensory development (visual, auditory, tactile, olfactory)
- Concept development (such as directionality, size, positions, time)
- Prevocational skills (such as on-task behavior, task completion)
- Visual efficiency training (learning to use vision to the greatest extent possible to identify and discriminate objects)
- Listening skills
- Braille reading and writing (See Chapter 10)
- Nemeth code (the braille math and science code)
- Mathematical devices (such as an abacus or talking calculator)
- Orientation and mobility (such as protective technique, sighted guide, and cane travel); See Chapter 12
- Handwriting (such as learning to sign checks and other documents in cursive, even if the child is totally blind; using adaptive writing materials and equipment such as raised line paper and writing guides)
- Keyboarding
- Study skills (such as using reference materials, note-taking)
- Organization skills (such as keeping an assignment notebook or organizing and packing a school bag)
- Activities of daily living (such as personal grooming, eating, and meal preparation)
- Using technology such as a tape player or computer
- Low vision devices (such as hand-held magnifiers and closed circuit televisions)
- Using resources (such as Recording for the Blind & Dyslexic, Library for the Blind, the local public library)
- Social skills training
- Counseling (such as in dealing with unwanted attention in public or changes in vision due to a deteriorating eye condition)
- Sex education

- Leisure activities
- Career education
- Vocational education
- Use of sighted readers

Vocational Education

As your child grows older, you will probably wonder, "What will he be when he grows up?" The job options available to people with visual impairments are numerous and should not be limited by misconceptions, misinformation, and low expectations of others. It will be exciting for you and your child to find opportunities to get involved in work-related activities. As he gets older, your child may want to baby sit younger children, or volunteer at a nonprofit agency in your neighborhood. One blind student in high school became proficient at raking leaves. He used a systematic grid, working his way from one corner of the yard to the opposite corner and was known for not leaving a single leaf on the ground. He had a great after school and weekend job in the neighborhood during the fall months! Another had his first job as a receptionist in a special education department at a university during the busy summer months. Having these early work experiences are important for preparing your child to enter the workforce after he leaves school.

Whether or not they are aware of it, all children receive vocational education throughout their school years. They learn how to follow directions, how to organize their work, and how to be on time. Students with visual impairments need to learn these skills, too. Simple adaptations such as using a braille Dymotape™ labeler, a talking watch, or compartmentalized containers for school supplies can help your child acquire these skills.

It is sometimes hard to separate vocational skills from skills that will help your child be a good student. Under IDEA 2004, however, his IEP must include goals that will help him make the transition from school to the next phase in his life, whether that is work or college. By law, beginning in the first IEP after your child turns 16, the IEP must contain appropriate measurable postsecondary goals and address other issues (including assessment, training, and education) related to the transition goals.

∷ Social and Emotional Concerns

As your child grows older, his social and emotional well-being will increasingly depend on his feelings about his own worth. These feelings, in turn, will be influenced by whether or not he feels that others value him. Generally, if your child feels good about himself he will get along better with others and have an easier time fitting into society. The reverse is also true. If his relationships with others are good and he is well integrated into society, he will feel good about himself. The following sections discuss some important social and emotional concerns that can help or hinder your child's ability to relate to others and get along in society.

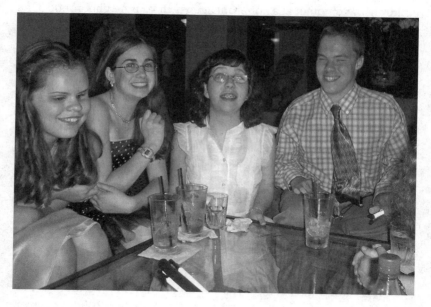

Fitting In

In later childhood and adolescence, most young people want to dress like, talk like, act like—*be* like—everybody else. Being part of the crowd will probably be equally important to your child. And so it should be: social acceptance is essential to successful integration into society.

Fitting in *can* be difficult for children with visual impairments, but it does not *have* to be difficult. Merely having a visual impairment—being physically different—can make your child stand out from the crowd. Your child may also appear different if he has not learned social behaviors such as head movements, facial expressions, gestures, and use of body space that most children learn through visual imitation. And if he has any mannerisms such as eye poking or rubbing, rocking, or hand or object flipping, he can draw even more attention to his differences. Delayed communication skills can also impede your child's social acceptance. Because they have trouble reading facial expressions and other social cues, some children with visual impairments have difficulty knowing how and when to interrupt in a conversation, taking turns, and resolving conflicts.

Because of these common obstacles to social acceptance, children with visual impairments often need formal training in social skills. But these things are not learned quickly or in only one context, so this training should be included in your child's IEP for as long as he needs it. This is true whether or not your child is included in a class with sighted students. Just being placed with sighted children does not necessarily mean that your child will develop and learn appropriate social behaviors.

At school, teachers can be instrumental in helping your child develop social skills. For example, they might help sighted classmates feel comfortable initiating interactions with your child, use role playing, give your child assertiveness training, model appropriate behavior, and give your child feedback about appropriate and inappropriate behaviors. The techniques used will depend on your child's age and abilities. Keeping interactions as natural as possible is preferable, but sometimes it helps to do a little role playing. For example, it might help your child to practice what he will say when he wants to ask someone out for the first time. This is a scary experience for all of us and giving your child support to feel confident in these situations can help him develop his own unique ways of interacting socially with others.

At home, there are many techniques you can use to help your child develop appropriate social behaviors. The following is not an all-inclusive list, but some suggestions you can use before your child enters school and continuing through the school years.

1. *Be aware that your child's openness and comfort level about his visual impairment will go a long way in helping others feel comfortable around him.* Help him to understand his visual impairment without overemphasizing it. Encourage the attitude that your child can do the same things as sighted peers, but may do them in a different way. If your child has albinism or other obvious physical differences,

he may need special support and counseling from the teacher and the TVI to help him deal with any problems he has being accepted by other children.

2. *Talk with your child on his level and tell him what is and is not socially appropriate.* For example, a fourth grader may need to be reminded to clean his prosthetic eye daily, and a high school girl may need to be reminded to check her feminine hygiene more often. To prevent your child from being set apart from others even more, it is essential that he be well groomed. Make sure he presents a neat and clean appearance, and, as he grows older, let him know what is "in style." It is also important to emphasize good eating habits—most people feel uncomfortable with someone who has poor table manners. As your child gets older, encourage him to find a friend who can give honest feedback about social appearances and behaviors.

3. *Use verbal and physical prompts to show your child how to make certain gestures, how to use eating utensils correctly, and procedures for proper table manners.* Provide as many opportunities as possible for hands-on experiences with games, sports, and audio and video equipment while explaining and demonstrating proper use.

4. *Provide opportunities for your child to be involved with other children in a variety of activities such as clubs, the YMCA, and Boy Scouts.* Do not constantly hover over him, but give him room to explore. Overprotectiveness will make your child more dependent and will prevent interactions that allow healthy growth and development.

5. *Praise your child for behaving, or attempting to behave, in socially acceptable ways. Give him gentle reminders when necessary.* For example, say, "If you face me when you talk, I can hear you better." Remember: you must consistently expect him to behave appropriately if you want him to develop good social skills.

6. *Help and encourage your child to know when and how to request assistance and when and how to decline it.* No one likes to be around someone who is rude. Well-meaning people will sometimes offer unneeded assistance and it

is important that your child respond in a polite and man-
nerly fashion.

7. *Continue to discourage or prevent mannerisms, as described in Chapter 5.* Not only can mannerisms physically
harm your child, but they can also make him appear different from typical children.

Recreation and Leisure

Having opportunities for recreation and leisure-time pursuits is
just as important, if not more so, for your child as it is for other children.
Recreational activities help children grow up to be well-balanced and
well-adjusted human beings by helping them hone gross and fine motor
skills, learn about social rules such as turn taking, stay fit and healthy,
make friends with similar interests, express themselves, make decisions,
and last, but not least—have fun.

Sighted children often develop recreation and leisure interests
and skills naturally and effortlessly. Children with visual impairments,
however, may not be able to observe and imitate others participating in
recreational activities. This can make it harder for them to cultivate such
interests and skills. Parents and teachers may need to provide encouragement, deliberate exposure, direct teaching, and modeling to help
children with visual impairments learn to make good use of leisure time.
The eventual goal is to enable your child to make informed, voluntary
choices about recreational activities and how to spend his leisure time,
as well as to fully participate in the activities he chooses.

Your child, like other children, will probably first learn about leisure activities from his family. He will begin to lay the foundation for the
development of recreational skills during infancy and early childhood
by playing with toys and other children. As time goes by, you can help
him develop interests in hobbies, games, and passive leisure activities.
Your child's passive leisure activities will probably be very similar to
other children's, and may include listening to radios, records, tapes, and
compact discs; reading books and magazines; watching television and
going to movies; and attending sporting events. A variety of adaptations
can make these activities more enjoyable. For example, a family member
or friend can sit beside your child to describe the action of movies and
television shows. Or your child might prefer using descriptive video—a
spoken, prerecorded description of actions on the screen that can be
heard through a special simultaneous radio broadcast or directly from

video or DVD. Descriptive video is becoming more available for television shows and movies. Your child may get more out of sporting events if he listens to the play-by-play action on a radio or Internet broadcast.

With modifications and adaptations, your child can also play many table games and ball games. A number of table games are available in tactile and enlarged formats. Examples include Monopoly, cards, checkers, and dominoes. Ball games can be adapted by using beeping balls and other modifications described under the section on physical education. Your child can also pursue a wide range of hobbies—with or without

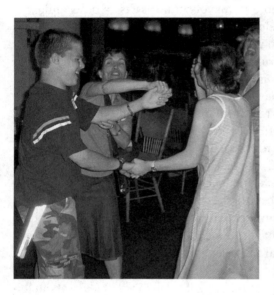

adaptations—ranging from indoor activities such as arts and crafts, pet care, and collecting, to outdoor activities such as gardening, hiking, and biking.

When introducing a new activity to your child, there are several ways you can make learning easier. First, help your child become oriented to the environment of the activity. For example, allow him to explore game boundaries, game pieces, equipment, or other materials with his hands, and verbally explain the object of the game, the rules, equipment, and procedures. If necessary, provide a hand-over-hand demonstration. For some activities, you may need to develop signs and cues to tell your child when to start, stop, change directions or actions. During a kickball game, for instance, the basemen might provide sound cues so your child can find the bases. Some activities lend themselves to buddy systems, which should be used as appropriate. For example, during the kickball game, your child might prefer to have a sighted player run the bases with him. Activities may also need some minor environmental modifications (a bright red or yellow kickball) for your child to successfully participate. For guidance in adapting rules, procedures, or equipment for your child, consult his TVI .

You may also want to inquire about recreational activities in your community. As Chapter 9 explains, your child should be allowed to participate in any activity that can be adapted to his needs, thanks to the Americans with Disabilities Act (ADA). If your child is old enough, let him choose an activity to try. After you enroll him in the chosen activity, make sure that he receives appropriate support from you or someone familiar with visual impairments, so that he and the other participants have positive and successful experiences.

Special groups, organizations, and agencies in your community might also offer activities specifically for children who have disabilities. Groups such as those organized for blind skiers can provide role models and tremendous opportunities for your child. You can find out about recreational opportunities for children with disabilities from the TVI, state schools for the blind, parent groups, or community organizations such as the ARC or Easter Seals.

Whatever modifications or adaptations your child needs, he should be involved in a variety of activities. This will prepare him to make choices of leisure-time activities based on knowledge and experience rather than on ignorance and feelings of inadequacy. Eventually, your child should choose his own activities based on his enjoyment, satisfaction, and pleasure.

Sex Education

People with visual impairments have the same desires for intimacy and love and the same sexual urges as other people. Children with visual impairments therefore need the same information about sex as any sighted child.

Ordinarily, even very young children pick up basic information about sex through visual observation. But because your child may use the sense of touch to gather much information, and touch is often discouraged in learning about sex, access to information may be more limited. Your child may ask fewer questions about sexual matters because he sees fewer things to ask questions about. And what he does see or hear he may misunderstand or misinterpret.

With your direction, your child can learn much about sex, even with limited or no vision. When he is young, you can point out gender differences during normal family interactions and activities, such as bathing, dressing, and diaper changing. Later on, you can give your child factual information about gender differences, body changes and processes, and sexual behaviors, habits, and diseases. You should provide this information in the way that seems most comfortable to you—just as you would with any other child. To help your child understand, you might let him tactually examine anatomically correct dolls, personal hygiene items, and birth control devices. Commercially available books and tapes may also be useful in helping you with the how-to and what-to of your child's sex education. In addition, some agencies serving individuals with visual impairments have developed and adapted sex education materials.

Just as other students do, your child will participate in class discussions and activities regarding sex education. The education team may also determine that your child would benefit from additional instruction. If so, this should be included in his IEP.

As you would with any child, you should share your own value system and standards for moral conduct, discuss the consequences of behaviors, guide your child in making good choices, and make sure he understands the impact of his choices on his own and others' lives. Especially as your child grows older, he needs to have someone—a family member, relative, or close friend—that he can confide in about personal matters. Being able to ask personal questions, accept feedback about personal and social matters, and discuss and share feelings, doubts, and experiences all contribute to the development of a healthy, well-adjusted human being.

Of course, all parents worry about their children's safety. Children with visual impairments may be more vulnerable to exploitation. You will need to talk openly with your child about dangers and how to protect himself. This may be uncomfortable and difficult for you, but the more openly you discuss these matters, the more aware your child will be and the more willing he will be to share concerns and fears.

Dating

The adolescent years are both exciting and troubling for most children, in part because this is when they enter the world of dating. Like other teenagers, your child will likely have mixed feelings about dating at first. He may want to date because he feels attracted to the opposite sex, because he feels social pressure to do so, and because dating is often essential to peer approval. At the same time, however, he may have fears and anxieties about his own physical attractiveness, sexuality, or the process of dating. These are common feelings for everyone during these adolescent years.

Your child will need to resolve many of these fears and anxieties himself, simply by taking the plunge into dating and confronting his feelings head on. But you can also help prepare your child by helping him acquire the basic building blocks needed for successful socializing. These include conversational skills, good grooming habits, appropriate table manners, and interests and abilities in activities that others enjoy talking about or doing. Helping your child develop a healthy sense of self-esteem, as described in Chapter 7, is also critical. In addition, you may want to ensure that your teenager has the opportunity to meet, interact with, and share experiences with peers and successful adults who are also visually impaired. This will allow him to talk about problems and concerns and to hear how others have handled difficult situations.

When your child is just beginning to date, you may want to suggest that he start with group boy/girl activities and dates in familiar environments (for example, parties in your own home). Your child may find these types of dates more comfortable at first. Group activities and double dating with sighted friends can also solve your child's transportation needs. Few teenagers—sighted or not—find that being chauffeured around by a parent is conducive to romance! In these situations, your child can help out with travel expenses by paying for gas.

Unfortunately, even if your child has good social skills, he may sometimes run into dating difficulties due to ignorance, prejudice, or fear. You may need to help him realize that he will encounter rude and insensitive people and that he should not let this affect the way he feels about himself. Ultimately, you and others who care about your child will help him realize his self-worth. These types of problems seem to decrease after the adolescent years, possibly because older people are more mature and better educated, or because there are often opportunities to get to know others on a deeper level before dating.

▪▪ The Transition to Independence

Generations of children with visual impairments have grown up to be successful, productive, independent, happy adults. The factors that contribute to independence for children with visual impairments depend a great deal on expectations, family and community support, and education and training. In addition, advances in technology are opening up more opportunities for independence. Thanks to technol-

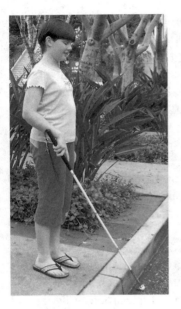

ogy, adults with visual impairments can participate in more activities than ever before and have an increasing number of career opportunities.

To be independent as an adult, your child needs to acquire self-help skills in many areas, including travel, personal grooming, housekeeping, food preparation, money management, and shopping. He also needs to learn good work habits and specific job skills and become informed about creating and maintaining a comfortable, healthy home. Your child can receive training in all of these areas at school if his education team agrees that it is necessary. But it is also important for you, other family members, and other significant adults to work *together* to help your child develop the skills needed for independence. You should make sure that training toward independence begins when your child is very young and that he has plenty of opportunities to practice and form good habits early on.

Travel

In many states, some people with low vision are able to obtain driver's licenses, with or without the use of low vision devices. However, for most people with visual impairments, driving is not a reality. This can be very difficult to accept. Other methods of transportation may not always be as convenient, and driving is often regarded as a critical step in making the transition to independence.

If your child will be unable to drive, he will need to learn that he can be independent without a driver's license. With training and experience, he can learn to use a variety of transportation modes. While he is still in high school, transportation needs can be met through group activities, double dating, or having a sighted friend, date, or relative drive, with the understanding that he will help defray expenses by paying for gas. In adulthood, he can achieve true independence in transportation by using a car pool (paying instead of driving), a paid driver, or a bus, taxi, subway, train, or other forms of public transportation.

Personal Grooming

Chapter 5 covers personal grooming for parents of younger children. As your child grows older, he will become more independent with his personal grooming skills. Following are some questions you may ask:

1. *How can my child distinguish personal care items?* Items such as perfume, lotion, and shampoo can be distinguished by their weight, size, odor, and shape of container. Similar objects can be labeled or placed in separate locations so they can be distinguished. Bits of tape and rubber bands can be used to identify items, if necessary. For example, shampoo and cream rinse can by distinguished by placing a rubber band around one container, and a piece of tape on a lipstick tube can help distinguish it from another similar tube.

2. *How can clothing be distinguished?* Some clothing can be identified by texture, seams, pockets, buttons, and shapes. Knots of thread can be sewn inside matching pieces of clothing. For example, a matching suit coat, pants, shirt, and tie may all have three knots. In general, learning which colors, types of patterns, and fabrics match requires input from a relative or friend.

3. *How does my child know whether his hair needs brushing, combing, or cutting?* Are there any special considerations in choosing hairstyles? Teach your child to wash his hair frequently. Have a friend, family member, or hairdresser help select an easy-to-care-for, attractive hairstyle. Morning hair care should generally suffice, although you should teach your child to brush or comb his hair more often in bad weather. He should also learn to ask a friend for feedback.

4. *How does a girl learn to use cosmetics?* Department stores often offer free advice and training about selection and use of make-up. Daily practice and feedback from a friend or family member will increase skill and competence in make-up application. Your child can learn that when in doubt, neutral colors are often best.

5. *How will my child handle shaving?* When your son starts shaving, it may be easier to use an electric razor at first. Mustaches and beards may need to be trimmed by a

friend, family member, or a hairdresser. Similarly, girls can begin shaving their legs using an electric razor as they get used to the process, and progress to using a razor if necessary or desired.

6. *How does my child know whether his clothes are wrinkled, stained, worn, or dirty?* Teach him to launder his clothes after he wears them once. Wrinkle-free fabrics make laundering easier. Dials on washers and dryers can be easily marked for use by a person who is blind. Most likely, your child will be aware of spills which cause stains on clothes. Teach him to either send stained clothes to the laundry or to ask for help in treating the stain. Your child can learn to iron his own clothes by first beginning with a simple garment and a cool iron. To prevent burns when a hot iron is used, your child can purchase a specially made guard for the iron.

Many of the same techniques used by children and adolescents who are sighted can be very effective for those who have visual impairments, but children with visual impairments may need to learn some specific grooming skills. Even so, there is no substitute for the honest feedback of a family member or a good friend where personal grooming is concerned.

Housekeeping

Children with visual impairments are usually able to do most housekeeping chores with minor adaptations. You can introduce your child to these chores at the same age you would if he did not have a visual impairment. Giving your child these responsibilities will not only prepare him to be independent, but will also increase his sense of self-worth.

When teaching your child to clean surfaces such as a countertop or floor, it is helpful to show him how to follow a systematic pattern. For instance, have him wipe a countertop length-wise across the entire surface and then width-wise. Using a systematic pattern also works for vacuuming and dusting and prevents spots from being missed. Teach your child to clean spots and spills immediately to prevent slipping or staining. As with toiletries, cleaning products may need special labels or markings so they can be distinguished if your child cannot identify them by weight, size, fragrance, or shape.

Tidying up should be done methodically. Your child should learn to put items back where they belong as soon as he is through with them. Otherwise, he may not be able to find them again or they may create obstacles in his path.

Food Preparation

Like any child, your child should be actively involved in food preparation at an early age—pouring a drink, getting a bowl of cereal, making a snack. As with all children, safety is an issue in the kitchen. Some precautions to keep in mind include:

1. Teach your child the location and purpose of kitchen equipment, food items, and cleaning supplies, and keep a well-organized kitchen.
2. Keep items in the same location and label them with brailled Dymo tape to help your child identify them.
3. Make sure pot handles point inward over the stove and not out where they can be a hazard.
4. Use heavy pots and pans and teach your child to approach handles slowly and cautiously when stirring or attempting to remove pots from the stove.
5. When pouring liquids into glasses, measuring cups, etc., teach your child to place an index finger slightly inside the top of the container to determine when it is full. This can be tricky when the liquids are very hot. A better method in this instance would be to measure the amount of liquid needed and then use the microwave to heat it.

Labeling dials and controls with raised lines or dots can enable your child to use kitchen appliances. You can file notches, make braille dots on Dymo tape, or use drops of glue or puffy paint to mark items. Usually at least one reference point is placed on a dial and one on the background. For example, on the stove, marks may be placed at the off position, 300 degrees, and 500 degrees. To avoid confusion, it is usually best to use a minimum of marks. Before using any unfamiliar appliances or equipment, your child should examine them to become familiar with the way they are constructed and the way they operate.

With minor adaptations to equipment, your child should be able to participate in the standard curriculum in a high school home economics class. To help him succeed in class, the TVI should:

- demonstrate adaptive techniques to your child and the teacher;
- provide books and recipes in large print, braille, or recorded form, or provide a low vision device;
- advise or assist in labeling equipment and packaged food;
- assist during certain activities such as sewing;
- order or obtain adaptive devices needed in the kitchen;
- recommend safety precautions such as keeping doors opened flat or closed;
- suggest ways of storing utensils and food for ease in locating.

Before your child is in high school, your child's teacher of students with visual impairments can advise you about adaptations in the home or sources of adapted cooking equipment. It is advisable that *all* students, male and female, take home economics. The home economics curriculum is usually extremely useful in helping students develop independent living skills.

Money Management and Shopping

Most adults who are blind find that it is most time effective and less stressful to rely on someone else to help them when shopping in a store. You can and should, however, acquaint your child with the basics of shopping at an early age. Stores can offer wonderful learning opportunities for young children. Take him along on trips to grocery, clothing, drug, and other stores and describe the environment, the products, and the process of buying to him.

Once your child begins to shop and make his own selections, he can decide whether he would like a friend, relative, or store employee to help him. Federal law requires that stores provide assistance upon request to people with disabilities. Often, however, it is wise to call ahead or shop during less busy times when using a store employee for assistance. Teach your child how to politely request and refuse assistance, and how to be assertive in getting his shopping needs met.

While some people love the hustle and bustle of a shopping trip, others find that ordering by telephone, home shopping from the television, and using a computer to shop electronically can be helpful and convenient. To shop using these methods, your child should know specifically what items he needs when ordering by phone; listen to detailed descriptions given on television; and have a computer with voice output.

With a few adaptations, your child should be able to pay for his purchases himself. If he cannot identify coins by sight, he can identify them by feel. He can identify them by their size, thickness, and their smooth or ridged edges—pennies and nickels have smooth edges, while dimes, quarters, and half dollars have ridged edges. If your child cannot visually identify paper money, he can learn to fold different denominations different ways. For example, dollars can be left unfolded, fives can be folded in half, and tens can be folded lengthwise. Or he can place different denominations in different places in his billfold. If your child ever is not sure that he is receiving correct change, he can always ask that he be given all one-dollar bills so he can be absolutely sure that he has been given the correct change. This is rarely necessary, but it is a good strategy for your child to know!

Although more and more people are conducting banking activities online, including paying bills, writing and signing checks is still a necessary activity for most adults. Your child will need to learn to sign his name, using a signature guide if needed. This is a small cardboard or plastic card, about the size of a credit card, with a rectangular slot cut out. The card is placed on the paper with the slot over the space where the signature is required. A trusted sighted friend might help prepare checks for your child by filling in the date, payee, and amount ahead of time. Your child can also fill out the information himself on a raised-line check, or he can use a computer program that fills out checks after he types in the information.

▪▪ Career Opportunities

Unfortunately, there is a high rate of unemployment among adults with visual impairments at present. You can, however, do a lot throughout your child's life to prepare him for being successful at a job, and there are good reasons to believe that the job outlook will brighten in the near future. Career opportunities for workers with visual impairments have grown tremendously in recent years. These expanded opportunities are due in part to new technology, such as computers with speech output, portable electronic braillers, and print-enlarging devices. The Americans with Disabilities Act, which prohibits discrimination on the basis of disability, is also opening the door to more and better job opportunities. Today, career opportunities should no longer be limited by misconceptions, misinformation, and negative attitudes of family members and the general public.

Some adults with visual impairments are fully capable of working on their own along with nondisabled employees in "blue collar" or "white collar" positions. This is known as competitive employment. Sometimes before an adult can be competitively employed, he needs to work in a supported employment setting. During supported employment, a job coach accompanies the worker to his job and helps him adapt to the environment and learn skills needed to work independently. Adults who have visual impairments and additional disabilities may work in sheltered workshops. Here they work alongside other employees with disabilities and receive supervision and training in job-related skills. Some adults with visual impairments may work in sheltered workshops throughout their working career, but others learn skills that enable them to move on to supported or competitive employment.

:: Living Arrangements

Where your child lives as an adult depends on many factors. These include the level of his personal, social, and financial independence; personal preference; safety; options available in your community; and community resources and support. Providing they have received appropriate support, adults with visual impairments and no additional disabilities are able to live on their own, with a roommate, or with a spouse and family in an apartment or house. Even those who need more support or supervision have options for living with a level of independence in the community. Residential options generally available include: semi-independent living; group home; family home; and residential facility. Most individuals with visual impairments progress from living at home with their parents to living alone or with a roommate or spouse with no difficulty. For some, though, this transition is more difficult. The following list includes the variety of alternative options for individuals of all ability levels.

Semi-independent Living. This option includes living in a boarding-house type situation in which meals are provided for residents. It could also involve living in a house or apartment with a roommate/assistant. This roommate could be a family member, friend, or someone who is paid to help with certain activities.

Group Home. Group homes for adults with disabilities are operated by state and community agencies. Trained employees provide supervision and involve residents in housekeeping and meal preparation to the degree possible. Costs vary, but are usually very expensive.

Family Home. Some adults with visual impairments and their families may choose to continue to live together. Living arrangements, individual responsibilities, and so forth naturally vary from family to family.

Residential Facility. Some adults with severe multiple disabilities may live in a residential facility such as a nursing home or facility just for adults with disabilities where supervision, housekeeping, meal preparation, and other types of care are provided by the staff. Generally, states are phasing out these facilities. This option is very expensive and usually funded by the state.

For information about residential options in your community, contact the local ARC, Easter Seals, or other community agencies serving people with disabilities. You can also contact Rehabilitation Services for the Blind, a federal and state agency, for information. (See the Resource Guide.) These federal, state, and community resources can advise you about financial assistance in providing living options.

■■ Working with Other Parents

Because visual impairments are relatively rare, the resources and support your child needs in order to maximize his independence may not be readily available in your community. As a result, you may need to help develop some of your own resources. For example, you may want to help develop better living arrangements, or educate prospective employers about the abilities of persons with visual impairments. Often, the best way to accomplish these types of goals is to work together with other parents. Finding other parents to join with is easy if there is already a parent group in your community. You will often find parents who share your concerns in the state, as well as local chapters of organizations such as the National Association for Parents of the Visually Impaired (NAPVI). NAPVI hosts conferences and regular meetings that provide parents with pertinent information and opportunities for sharing.

If there is no local chapter in your community, you may want to help form your own group. Your child's TVI or other vision professional may be able to give you the names of parents who might be interested in starting a group. Your group can then receive guidance in advocacy and the important issues confronting adolescents and adults with visual impairments from such national organizations as NAPVI, The Council for Exceptional Children (CEC), The American Foundation for the Blind (AFB), The American Printing House for the Blind (APH), and The National Federation of the Blind (NFB). All provide helpful publications for parents, and are listed in the Resource Guide at the back of this book.

▪▪ Conclusion

Many parents of young children have their hands full just taking care of their family's day-to-day needs. And when your child is young, most of your efforts probably *should* go toward taking care of his current needs. It is also important, however, to remember that someday your child will grow up. And because his transition to independence may be more complicated or at least different from most children's, you will probably be more directly involved in helping him make the transition.

Taking the time now to get an idea of your child's future needs can help you anticipate where and when trouble spots may arise. This will help prepare you to deal with potential difficulties and to plan ways around them.

▪▪ Parent Statements

Hope is a key word for me. Even though my child is having difficulty now, I have to believe that everything will turn out all right for him.

❧

If we do not work on things now, Janie won't be ready for her future.

❧

Evan has a bright future. He can do anything he sets his mind to do.

❧

I know it sounds crazy, but I have spent a lot of time since Paul was born worrying about what his life will be like in high school. I focus a lot on driving—I guess because I like to drive and I can't imagine a life in which driving wasn't possible. Will he date? Will he have friends? My wife thinks

I should stop thinking about that and just concentrate on today, but I have trouble doing that. I want some answers to the bigger picture.

✥

We visited a summer program at the school for the blind and saw lots of kids. They were laughing and joking around at lunch just like any school-aged children will do. It helped me a lot to see that things were so "normal" for them.

✥

I want the same thing for both my child with visual impairments and her brother: to be happy with the way their lives turn out. I'm willing to do whatever it takes to support and help them along the way.

✥

I hate thinking that there are doors that might be closed for my child because of his blindness. It's hard for me to accept that there are things that we won't be able to do. I mean, what if he wanted to be a major league baseball player?

✥

My daughter is pretty stubborn. That is difficult to deal with now, but I think it will help her in the future.

✥

Before Donna was born I never noticed anything about blindness. Now it seems that every time I turn around there is something in the paper or on the news or a magazine article about someone who is blind. Now I know that there are many more successful blind adults than Stevie Wonder and Ronnie Milsap.

GLOSSARY

Academic goals: what a student is expected to learn in educational areas such as reading, mathematics, and science.

ADA: The Americans with Disabilities Act of 1990. It prohibits discrimination against individuals with disabilities in the areas of employment, public service, and public accommodations.

Accommodation: the focusing ability of the eye.

Adaptive behavior: the ability to take care of personal needs independently and to act appropriately in social situations.

Adaptive goals: the overall plan for learning specialized skills (such as orientation and mobility) needed because of a child's visual impairment or other disability.

Advocate: to speak up on someone else's behalf.

Albinism: an inherited condition which causes decreased pigment either in the skin, hair, and eyes or in the eyes alone.

Amblyopia: a visual impairment which is the result of a child not using her eyesight in one eye during the developmental period (until the child is about 9 years old).

Americans with Disabilities Act: see ADA.

Aniridia: congenital absence of an iris of the eye, resulting in some degree of visual impairment.

Anisometropia: a significant difference in the refractive power of the right and left eyes.

Anoxia: lack of oxygen to tissues (including the brain), which causes cell death or damage. May be a complication of a difficult birth.

Anterior chamber: the space between the cornea and the iris near the front of the eye.

Apert syndrome: an inherited disorder in which skull bones fuse prematurely and there is underdevelopment of facial bones, wide-spaced and bulging eyes, and webbed fingers and toes.

Aphakia: the condition in which an eye has no lens.

Aqueous: the fluid which fills the anterior chamber of the eye.

Astigmatism: blurry vision caused by abnormal curvature of the cornea.

Attachment: the process by which infants and parents learn to care for and love one another and form a human bond.

Augmentative communication: the use of nonspeech techniques such as signs, gestures, or pictures to supplement a child's speech abilities.

Avascular: without blood vessels.

Bilateral: relating to or affecting both sides of the body—for example, both eyes.

Binocular vision: the ability of the eyes to fuse their separate images into one single three-dimensional image.

Blind: having a loss of vision, typically referring to total loss of vision but also used to refer to any level of vision loss.

Blindisms: movements or behaviors that are repetitive and not purposeful. Examples include body rocking, head swaying, and eye rubbing.

Book behaviors: behaviors which children use as they read books, such as turning pages of the book, holding the book right-side up, reading from left to right.

Braille: a system of reading and writing in which letters and words are formed by patterns of raised dots that are felt with the fingers.

Braille, Louis: the inventor of the braille system.

Calendar box: a sectioned box which contains objects representing each activity of a child's day.

Cataracts: cloudiness of the lens of the eye.

Categorization: the ability to organize objects according to characteristics such as color, size, group, function, etc.

Cause and effect: the understanding that certain actions can make certain things happen (for example, stacking too many blocks in a tower will cause it to tumble down).

Cell: the unit in braille which consists of six dots, two across and three down.

Center-based program: special instruction provided in any of a variety of centers (schools, offices, hospitals) for preschoolers.

Central nervous system: the brain and the nerves which travel along the spinal cord to and from the brain.

Cerebral palsy: a disorder of movement, balance, and coordination resulting from damage to the brain before the age of three.

Choroid: the second layer of the eye that is rich in blood vessels and carries nourishment to the eye.

Chromosomes: the microscopic rod-shaped bodies that contain genetic material and are located in every cell of the body.

Clinical low vision specialist: an optometrist, ophthalmologist, or university-trained professional specializing in helping children with limited visual ability optimize their remaining vision.

CF: counts fingers.

Cognitive development: the acquisition of the ability to think, reason, and problem-solve.

Conductive hearing loss: a temporary or permanent hearing loss which occurs when something (such as fluid) interferes with the passage of sound through the ear canal or middle ear.

Concave: thinner in the center and thicker at the edges.

Cones: cells located in the center of the retina that enable us to see detail and color.

Continuum of services: the variety of placement options available in special education (from placement in a typical classroom with no extra support to placement in a school solely for children with disabilities).

Contractions: words or letters represented by one cell in the braille code.

Converge: come together.

Convex: thicker in the center and thinner in the edges.

Cornea: the clear, curved, smooth structure at the front of the eye.

Cortical blindness: *See* cortical visual impairment.

Cortical visual impairment: a visual loss due to damage to the part of the brain that interprets visual information.

Counts fingers: a measurement of visual ability indicating that a person can determine how many fingers are being held in front of him.

Crouzon syndrome: an inherited condition in which the sutures between the bones and the skull close prematurely. Other characteristics include bulging eyes due to shallow orbits, hearing loss, and underdevelopment of the upper jaw bone.

CV: color vision.

D: diopter.

Daily living skills: a term referring to the set of abilities needed to accomplish functional, everyday tasks. Examples include making a bed, preparing a meal, dressing, hygienic care.

Deaf-blind: sometimes called dual sensory impairment, this term refers to a combination of hearing and vision problems that require educational modification.

Depth perception: the ability to see 3-D, to tell the differences in surface heights, made possible through binocular vision.

Development: the process by which children grow physically and mentally and learn increasingly complex skills.

Developmental disability: a lifelong condition that begins before adulthood and prevents a child from developing normally. Often used to refer to conditions that result in mental retardation.

Dilate: to widen.

Diopter: the unit of measurement of the strength or refractive power of lenses.

Diverge: move apart.

Dog guides: dogs that receive extensive training and then are matched with a person with a visual impairment to help the person travel safely and efficiently while locating familiar landmarks and negotiating obstacles.

Domains of growth: the areas of cognitive, communication, motor, self-help, sensory, and social development.

Due process hearing: one of the procedures established to protect the rights of families during disputes under IDEA. The hearing is held before an impartial person to resolve disagreements about a child's identification, evaluation, placement, or special educational services.

Early intervention: individualized programs of instruction and therapy developed for children aged birth to three to help minimize the effects of conditions that can delay development and learning.

EC: eyes closed.

Echolalia: word-for-word repetition of other's speech.

Emergent literacy: early literacy.

Enucleation: removal of the eye.

Epilepsy: a condition that causes recurrent episodes of seizures—abnormal electrical discharges in the brain that result in involuntary movement and/or changes in consciousness.

Esotropia: a type of strabismus in which one or both eyes turn inward.

Etiol: etiology (cause).

Exorbitism: a condition in which the eyes appear to bulge because the bony areas around the eyes (orbits) are too small and shallow to contain them.

Exotropia: a type of strabismus in which one or both eyes turn outward.

Expanded core curriculum: designed to go beyond the core academic curriculum required by all students, the expanded core curriculum includes unique skills that students with visual impairments need as a result of the visual impairment. Expanded core curriculum skills are not taught in the general education classroom, but are typically the responsibility of the teacher of students with visual impairments.

Expressive language: the ability to use gestures, words, and written symbols to communicate.

Extraocular: outside the eyes.

Farsightedness: a condition in which objects are focused at a point behind, rather than on, the retina. As a result, the child must strain excessively to focus, especially on nearby objects.

FC: finger counting.

Fine motor skills: the ability to use small muscles such as those in the hands and face (for example, drawing, using a fork, drinking from a straw).

Fixate: focus.

Fluctuating tone: muscle tone that is sometimes high, sometimes low.

Fluctuating vision: visual ability that changes from time to time depending on time of day, fatigue, characteristics of particular eye conditions, and other factors.

Functional goals: educational goals related to increasing skills for living independently (for example, cooking, handling money, using public transportation).

Functional vision: how well vision is used to accomplish daily tasks.

Functional vision assessment: a procedure used to determine how well a student sees and how well he uses his vision in a wide variety of educational and daily tasks.

FVA: functional vision assessment.

Generalization: the ability to apply previous learning to new situations (for example, if one furry animal that has four legs, wags its tail, and barks is a "dog," so are all animals with the same characteristics).

Genes: the material in the chromosomes that contains the chemical directions that determines a person's physical, intellectual, and other traits.

Genetic: related to something that is caused by one or more of a person's genes. Genetic conditions may be inherited (due to genetic material passed on by one or both parents) or may occur due to spontaneous changes or mutations in a child's genetic material.

Glaucoma: a condition in which the pressure from fluid inside the anterior chamber of the eye is too high.

Gross motor skills: Skills that involve large muscles such as those in the arms, legs, and abdomen (for example, throwing a ball, walking, sitting up).

Hand movement: a measurement of visual ability indicating the distance at which a person can recognize the movement of a hand in front of her eyes.

Handicapping condition: one of the disabilities listed in IDEA as qualifying a child for special education services.

HM: hand movement.

Home intervention: Special education provided at home.

Hydrocephaly: a condition in which excess fluid collects in the ventricles of the brain.

Hyperopia: farsightedness.

Hypertelorism: a condition in which there is an unusually wide space between two paired body parts, such as the eyes (orbital hypertelorism).

Hypertonia: increased tension or spasticity of the muscles; also known as high muscle tone.

Hypertropia: a condition in which the gaze of one eye is higher than the other.

Hypotonia: decreased tension of a muscle, resulting in floppiness; also known as low muscle tone.

Hypoxia: insufficient oxygen to the tissues of the body, including the brain.

IDEA: The Individuals with Disabilities Education Act—the law that guarantees children with disabilities a free, appropriate education in the least restrictive environment (this law was originally called Public Law 94-142; the current version of this law is called IDEA 2004).

IEP: Individualized Education Program. The written plan that describes the special education program the local education agency has promised to provide a child with disabilities aged three to twenty-one.

IFSP: Individualized Family Service Plan. The written document that describes the early intervention program to be provided for a child with disabilities aged birth to three.

Incidental learning: learning from observation or experience.

Inclusion: an educational term that may be used to mean that a child with disabilities is taught with children without disabilities for some or all activities of the school day. The term "fully included" indicates that the child with disabilities is in a general education classroom for all activities.

Intersensory coordination: the process of taking information obtained through one sensory system and using it in another.

Intraocular lenses: artificial lenses permanently implanted after cataract surgery.

IOP: intraocular pressure (pressure inside the eye).

IQ: the score from a standardized test of intelligence indicating a person's overall level of cognitive functioning relative to other people of the same age. Often scores between 80 and 119 are considered to be in the "average" range of intelligence, while scores between 70 and 80 are considered "borderline" average.

Iris: the colored part of the eye that regulates the amount of light that enters the eye.

Laterality: knowledge of right and left.

Lazy eye: *See* Amblyopia.

Lea Symbol Acuity Test: a test for assessing visual acuity which uses symbols instead of letters and allows children who are nonverbal or very young to match symbols at near and far distances in order to obtain an acuity measure.

Learning disability: a condition that causes a child to have more difficulty learning in one or more specific areas (such as reading or math) than would be expected based on the child's overall cognitive abilities. In the United Kingdom, the preferred term for mental retardation.

Least restrictive environment (LRE): the setting which allows each child the most contact with typically developing children while still allowing the most opportunity for educational progress.

Legal blindness: a visual acuity of 20/200 or less in the better eye after correction (e.g., eye glasses), and/or a visual field of no greater than 20 degrees.

Lens: located behind the iris, the lens helps focus light on the back of the retina.

Light perception: the ability to detect the presence or absence of light.

Light projection: the ability to tell where light is coming from.

Lighthouse Flash Card Test: a test for assessing visual acuity which does not depend on the ability to recognize words or letters, but uses a circle, an apple, a house, and a square.

Literacy: the ability to use written language (both braille and print) to communicate with others. This includes the ability to both receive and transmit messages.

Locomotion: the ability to move independently from place to place.

Low incidence: not very common in the general population. Visual impairment is a low incidence disability among children.

Low vision: vision that is impaired, but sufficient to read print with or without magnification.

Lowe syndrome: a disorder that affects only males and is characterized by congenital cataracts, poor growth, developmental delays, low muscle tone, and sometimes glaucoma.

Macula: the area of sharpest vision in the retina, responsible for central vision and seeing detail.

Marfan syndrome: a genetic disorder characterized by tall, thin stature, long, thin limbs, loose joints, heart abnormalities, and sometimes low vision.

M.D.: Medical doctor.

Mental retardation: cognitive functioning (thinking abilities) below the average range (generally defined as an IQ below 70), resulting in difficulties and delays in learning and adaptive behavior. Some people do not like using the term "mental retardation" but prefer terms such as "cognitive disabilities," "intellectual disabilities," or "developmental delay" instead.

Micropthalmia: abnormally small eyes.

Mobility: the ability to move safely and efficiently through the environment.

Mobility system: a guide or device (such as a cane) that permits an individual with a visual impairment to move independently through the environment.

Motor development: acquisition of the ability to move effectively and efficiently.

Muscle tone: the amount of tension or resistance to movement in a muscle.

Myopia: nearsightedness.

Nearsightedness: a condition in which images of distant objects are not focused precisely on the retina, but in front of it. This results in blurred vision, with distant objects usually appearing more blurred than near objects.

Nystagmus: a rhythmic oscillation or jerking of the eyes which cannot be controlled by the child.

O: eye (Latin: oculus).

O2: both eyes.

OD: right eye (Latin: oculus dexter).

O.D.: Doctor of Optometry.

O&M: orientation and mobility.

Object constancy: the concept that objects that look different can still be the same thing (for instance, even though a ball looks red in bright light and grayish in near darkness, it is the same object).

Object permanence: the concept that things continue to exist even when they can no longer be seen, heard, or touched (the mother is still there even though she is hiding behind a blanket playing peek-a-boo).

Occupational therapist (OT): a professional who specialized in improving the development of fine motor and adaptive skills.

Ophthalmologist: a medical doctor (M.D.) who has specialized training in diagnosing and treating diseases and conditions of the eye.

Optic nerve: the structure consisting of millions of nerve fibers which carry the message from the light receptors in the retina to the brain.

Optic nerve atrophy: damage to the fibers of the optic nerve which interrupts transmission of signals from the retina to the brain.

Optical system: the parts of the eye which receive light rays and focus them.

Optician: a technician who grinds lenses to make glasses

Optometrist: a doctor of optometry (O.D.) who is qualified to measure visual acuity and visual fields and to prescribe eyeglasses.

Orientation: knowing where you are, where you are going, and how to get where you want to be by interpreting information available in your environment.

OS: left eye (Latin: oculus sinister).

Osteogenesis imperfecta: a genetic disorder in which bones are unusually susceptible to fractures. Other features include hearing impairment, cataract, blue sclera, and short stature.

OT: occupational therapy.

OU: both eyes together (Latin: oculi unitas).

Partially sighted: a term used to describe individuals who have sufficient vision to read print.

Peripheral vision: side vision.

Perseveration: continuing or repeating an activity or thought to such an extreme that it interferes with other activities.

Photophobia: sensitivity to light.

Physical therapist (PT): a professional who specializes in improving motor skills (especially gross motor skills) and posture.

Preferential looking: a technique used by eye doctors to determine an approximate visual acuity in infants or children who are not able to easily communicate what they are seeing.

Ptosis: droopy eyelids.

Pupil: the black dot in the center of the eye created by the doughnut-shaped iris.

Receptive language: the ability to understand spoken and written communication as well as gestures.

Refraction: the process by which the cornea and lens of the eye bend light rays so that they focus on the retina.

Refractive error: an inability of the eye to sharply focus images on the back of the retina. Nearsightedness and farsightedness are types of refractive errors.

Related services: under IDEA, transportation and other developmental, corrective, and supportive services (such as OT, O&M, speech-language therapy) needed to enable a child to benefit from her special education program.

Residential school: a state or private school where students attend classes and live.

Resource room: a classroom where students spend part of the school day to learn or practice specific skills.

Retina: the inner layer of the eye consisting of millions of specialized cells which serve as light receptors.

Retinitis Pigmentosa: a disorder which causes the retinas to degenerate and areas of abnormal pigment accumulation to develop. The disorder is usually due to genetic factors and leads to varying degrees of vision loss.

Retinoblastoma: a malignant tumor that develops in the retina of the eye and is usually diagnosed in infancy.

Retinopathy of Prematurity: a condition caused by damage to the retina that can cause vision loss in infants born prematurely.

Rods: the rod-shaped cells in the retina that are primarily responsible for peripheral vision and night vision.

ROP: Retinopathy of Prematurity.

Sclera: the outer layer (white part) of the eye.

Seizure: a temporary burst of abnormal electrical activity in the brain, resulting in involuntary changes in consciousness or behavior.

Self-contained classroom: a room in a "regular" or neighborhood school designed to provide specialized instruction to students with disabilities.

Self-esteem: feelings of self-worth.

Self-help development: acquisition of skills needed to take care of oneself and become more and more independent (for example, eating, dressing).

Sensorineural hearing loss: a hearing impairment that results when the inner ear or the nerves which receive sound and carry it into the brain are damaged or have not developed; usually permanent.

Sensory development: acquisition of the ability to use one's senses to gather information.

Slate and stylus: the slate is a template of several rows of braille cells, and the stylus is a device with a blunt metal tip that is used to punch each dot individually. Together they provide a portable means of note taking.

Snellen Chart: also known as the "E Chart" ; a chart with rows of letters used to measure visual acuity.

Social development: acquisition of the skills needed to interact with others and build relationships.

Special education: a tailor-made program of instruction and other services designed to fit the unique learning strengths and needs of a child with disabilities.

Speech-language pathologist: a therapist who works to diagnose and improve speech and language skills.

Spina bifida: a condition in which a child is born with open vertebrae in the spinal column and sometimes with excess fluid in the brain (hydrocephalus).

Stereoacuity: three-dimensional vision using both eyes together.

Strabismus: misaligned eyes. *See* exotropia and esotropia.

Structural impairment: damage to one or more parts of the eye.

Syndrome: a set of signs and symptoms that occur together due to the same cause and are therefore characteristic of a particular disorder.

Tactile defensiveness: an adverse reaction to or avoidance of touch.

Teacher of students with visual impairments: an educator who has received special preparation and certification to teach students with visual impairments.

Total blindness: no useable vision.

Twin-vision books: books with both braille and print; also called "braille-print" books.

Unilateral: relating to or affecting one side of the body—for example, one eye.

Ushers syndrome: An inherited condition which causes sensorineural hearing loss and progressive vision loss (as a result of Retinitis Pigmentosa). Developmental delays may also be present.

Vision consultant: a teacher who travels from school to school providing technical assistance or support to educators.

Vision specialist (also called vision teacher, teacher of students with visual impairments): a certified teacher who has received specialized training in meeting the educational needs of children with visual impairments.

Visual acuity: a measurement of how clearly one sees.

Visual field (VF): the total area that can be seen without moving the eyes or head.

Visual impairment: any condition in which eyesight cannot be corrected to what is considered "normal." The term "visual impairment" in IDEA 2004 regulations is defined as a condition, including blindness, that, even with correction, has a negative impact on a child's educational performance. This term, according to IDEA, includes both partial sight and blindness.

READING LIST

∷ Chapter 1

American Foundation for the Blind. *Directory of Services for Blind and Visually Impaired Persons in the United States and Canada.* 27th Edition. New York: AFB Press, 2005.

    The most comprehensive and easy-to-use reference for addresses of key agencies and organizations providing support and service to individuals with visual impairments. The current edition of this must-have reference includes an on-line subscription option.

Chen, D., Friedman, C.T. & Calvello, M.A. *Parents and Visually Impaired (PAVII) Infants.* Louisville, KY: American Printing House for the Blind, 1990.

    This classic resource is designed to help parents gather information on how they can fully participate as the most important member of their child's educational team. It was written specifically for parents of babies (birth-3 years).

Warren, D.H. *Blindness and Children: An Individual Approach.* Cambridge: Cambridge University Press, 1994.

    This book is often used in university courses as a textbook. It provides a summary of research findings relating to infants and children with visual impairments.

∷ Chapter 2

Cassin, B. & Rubin, M.L. *Dictionary of Eye Terminology.* 5th edition. Gainesville, FL: Triad Publishing, 2006.

    This little book will help demystify the words that are used in medical reports and conversations with ophthalmologists and optometrists. Parents will find this is a very valuable resource throughout their conversations with doctors, professionals, and other parents.

Goldberg, S. & Trattler, W. *Ophthalmology Made Ridiculously Simple: Interactive Edition.* Miami, FL: MedMaster Publishing, 2005.

    This book provides a brief, simplified explanation of ophthalmological terms and common eye terms. The accompanying interactive CD provides illustrations and video of surgical procedures and common eye conditions.

Iris Medical. *A parent's Guide to Understanding Retinoblastoma.* Mountain View, CA: IRIDEX Corporation, n.d.

This free, downloadable brochure (http://www.retinoblastoma.com/frameset1. htm) contains a great deal of valuable information about retinoblastoma. In addition, it contains a section on general information about the structure of the eye.

Mendiola, R., Bahar, C., Brody, J. & Slott, G.L. *A unique Way of Learning: Teaching Young children with Optic Nerve Hypoplasia.* Los Angeles: Blind Childrens' Center, 2005.

This small booklet contains information about the needs of children with optic nerve hypoplasia, explained in layman's terms with suggestions for supporting preschoolers with this diagnosis.

Roy, A.W.N. & Spinks, R.M. *Real Lives: Personal and Photographic Perspectives on Albinism.* Burnley, Lancashire, UK: Albinism Fellowship, 2006.

Individuals living with albinism provided insight into their lives in this book. Parents of children with albinism will find this an honest discussion about the challenges of albinism and these individuals' journey toward joy and fulfillment.

▪▪ Chapter 3

Gill, B. *Changed by a Child: Companion Notes for Parents of a Child with a Disability.* New York: Doubleday, 1997.

This books consists of very short meditative pieces about topics that parents of children with disabilities often find themselves musing about; for example, Fault, Labels, Losing It, Recurring Sorrow, and In-Jokes. Some end with an affirmation ("Today I will….) but most just provide interesting, empathetic food for thought.

Klein, S., & Schive, K., Editors. *You Will Dream New Dreams: Inspiring Personal Stories by Parents of Children with Disabilities.* New York: Kensington Publishing Corp., 2001.

The 60 parents who contributed to this volume of short essays have children with a variety of disabilities and a variety of perspectives and philosophies on becoming the parent of a child with special needs. Reading this book is a good way for other parents to learn that they are not alone with their emotions, hopes, and fears.

Sullivan, T. *Special Parent, Special Child.* New York: Tarcher/Penguin, 1996.

This book is a compilation of interviews of parents conducted by Tom Sullivan, who is blind. He begins the book by discussing his mother's reaction to his blindness and then focuses on the stories of six families. The stories are inspirational accounts of families' struggles and triumphs.

▪▪ Chapter 4

Fazzi, D.L., & Pogrund, R.L. *Early Focus: Working with Young Children Who Are Blind or Visually Impaired and Their Families.* New York: AFB Press, 2002.

This text was written for professionals but will also be informative for parents of young visually impaired children. It provides important information on development and early intervention strategies for preschool children.

Meyers, L., & Lansky, P. *Dancing Cheek to Cheek: Nurturing Beginning Social, Play, and Language Interactions.* Los Angeles: Blind Childrens Center, 1991.

Based on four years of research with infants with severe visual impairments and their parents, this booklet provides suggestions to support parents and professionals in encouraging babies to be successful in social interactions and play.

Riggio, M., Heyt, K., Allan, M., Edwards, S., Clark, M.J. & Cushman, C. *Perkins Activity and Resource Guide: A Handbook for Teachers and Parents of Students with Visual and Multiple Disabilities,* 2nd edition. Watertown, MA: Perkins School for the Blind, 2004.

This is a practical guide for parents and professionals with valuable suggestions for instructional activities to help young children who have visual impairments and additional disabilities. Topics included in this guide range from development of motor and language skills to using music as a tool for supporting development.

Royal National Institute for the Blind. *Early Years.* London: RNIB, 2003.

Early Years is written for parents of children with visual impairments. It is a set of four books that provides information for parents including topics such as play, movement, and daily living activities.

Schwartz, Sue. *The New Language of Toys: Teaching Communication Skills to Children with Special Needs.* Bethesda, MD: Woodbine House, 2004.

This book explains how to use homemade and commercially available toys to teach and reinforce vocabulary, concepts, and other language skills.

▪▪ Chapter 5

Baker, B.L., & Brightman, A.J. *Steps to Independence: A Skills Training Guide for Parents and Teachers of Children with Special Needs.* Fourth edition. Baltimore, MD: Paul H. Brookes Publishing Co., 2004

Although not written specifically for parents of children with visual impairments, this book provides valuable step-by-step guidelines for teaching self-help skills, play, daily living, and communication skills. The focus of this book is on supporting children with special needs from age three through young adulthood.

Brody, J., & Webber, L. *Let's Eat: Feeding a Child with a Visual Impairment.* Los Angeles, CA: Blind Childrens Center, 1994.

This video (available in VHS or DVD format) and the accompanying booklet provide information for parents as they work with their child on eating and feeding skills.

Glasberg, Beth. *Functional Behavior Assessments for People with Autism: Making Sense of Seemingly Senseless Behavior.* Bethesda, MD: Woodbine House, 2006.

This is another book not specific to visual impairments that can be helpful for parents of children with other disabilities, including visual impairments. Step by step, the book outlines a procedure for pinpointing the causes of a child's challenging behavior as the first step to improving it. Especially useful for children who are not yet verbal or have difficulties expressing their feelings.

Kranowitz, C.S. *The Out of Sync Child: Recognizing and Coping with Sensory Processing Disorder.* Revised edition. New York: Perigee, 2006.

Although not specific to children with visual impairments, this book provides an excellent overview of how sensory processing is supposed to work in children and how difficulties with sensory processing may manifest themselves. The book includes plentiful suggestions for dealing with sensory issues in daily life.

Simmons, S. *First Steps: A Handbook for Teaching Young Children who Are Visually Impaired.* Los Angeles, CA: Blind Childrens Center, 1993.

An easy-to-read resource that addresses basic information about helping young children develop skills that lead to independence.

∷ Chapter 6

American Foundation for the Blind. *Let's Play: A Guide to Toys for Children with Special Needs.* New York: AFB Press, 2005.

Toys are a big part of childhood. Children who are visually impaired enjoy many of the same toys that children without visual impairments enjoy, but there are also some important considerations when choosing toys for these children. This guide is updated regularly and contains helpful information on this topic for parents.

Chapuis, D.K. *In celebration of grandparenting: For grandparents of children with visual impairments.* Watertown, MA: Perkins School for the Blind, 2000.

This book focuses on the unique relationship between children who are blind or visually impaired and their grandparents. The importance of this relationship is highlighted and celebrated.

Fawcett, H., & Baskin, A. *More Than a Mom: Living a Full and Balanced Life When Your Child Has Special Needs.* Bethesda, MD: Woodbine House, 2006.

More Than a Mom explores how women can live rich, fulfilling lives when they have a child who needs more time and attention than usual. The book covers such topics as juggling a job with motherhood, staying physically and emotionally healthy, finding specialized childcare, and nurturing interests and goals.

Gold, D., Editor. *Finding a New Path: Guidance for Parents of Young Children Who Are Visually Impaired or Blind.* Toronto, ON: Canadian National Institute for the Blind, n.d.

This helpful resource is a guide for family members and other caregivers as they create a safe, interesting, and encouraging environment for blind or visually impaired young children.

Marshak, L.E., Prezant, F.P. *Married with Special-Needs Children.* Bethesda, MD: Woodbine House, 2006.

Based on interviews with hundreds of parents of children with special needs, this is a guide to sustaining your marriage or deciding whether it is worth sustaining when you have a child with a disability or significant health care needs. The authors cover such topics as keeping the romance in your marriage, communication skills, and troubleshooting potentially serious marital difficulties.

Meyer, D. *Views from Our Shoes: Growing Up with a Brother or Sister with Special Needs.* Bethesda, MD: Woodbine House, 1997.

This is a collection of 45 short essays from children aged four to eighteen sharing what it is like to have a sibling with a disability, including a visual impairment. Appropriate for children aged 8 to 14.

Meyer, D. *The Sibling Slam Book: What It's Really Like to Have a Brother or Sister with Special Needs.* Bethesda, MD: Woodbine House, 2005.

In this book targeted at teenaged siblings of children with special needs, 81 young people answer short questions related to their own and their siblings' lives. Examples of questions: Does your sib every frustrate you? What do you see for your sibling's future? What do you tell your friends about your sib's disability?

Schmitt, P. *Fathers: A Common Ground.* Los Angeles: Blind Childrens Center, 1999.

The important role of fathers in the lives of infants and preschoolers who are visually impaired is explored in this booklet.

▪▪ Chapter 7

Keef, E.B., Moor, V.M. & Duff, F.R. *Listening to the Experts: Students with Disabilities Speak Out*. Baltimore, MD: Paul H. Brookes, 2006.

The importance of involving students in their own education cannot be overstated. Allowing students to develop independent self-determination will help them become productive and happy adults. This book provides a unique opportunity to hear how special education works, directly from the student's point of view.

Tuttle, D. W. & Tuttle, N.R. *Self-esteem and Adjusting with Blindness.* Springfield, IL: Charles C. Thomas, 2004.

This classic textbook addresses the importance of self-esteem for individuals who are blind or visually impaired. Issues that have an impact on self-esteem are explored as well as suggestions for promoting high self-esteem.

▪▪ Chapter 8

Chen, D. & McCann, M.E. *Selecting a Program: A Guide for Parents of Infants and Preschoolers with Visual Impairments.* Los Angeles: Blind Childrens Center, 1993.

This resource provides parents with information to support their decision-making regarding the choice of appropriate educational programs for their child with a visual impairment.

Coleman, J.G. *The Early Intervention Dictionary: A Multidisciplinary Guide to Terminology.* Third edition. Bethesda, MD: Woodbine House, 2006.

In layman's language, this comprehensive dictionary explains the many medical, educational, and developmental terms parents are likely to encounter when they have a young child with disabilities.

Grisham-Brown, J. & Haynes, D.G. *Reach for the Stars, Planning for the Future: A Transition Process for Families of Young Children.* Louisville, KY: American Printing House for the Blind, 1999.

A first-of-its-kind guidebook about transitioning young children into preschool or kindergarten settings. Designed to help the families of young children with disabilities imagine positive and productive futures. It aids families in working with school personnel to create educational plans

Huebner, K.M, Merk-Adam, B., Stryker, D. & Wolffe, K.E. *National Agenda for Children and Youths with Visual Impairments, Including Those with Multiple Disabilities.* New York: AFB Press, 2004.

This ground-breaking publication outlines a comprehensive plan for systematically addressing the educational needs of children with visual impairments. Parents, professionals, and individuals with visual impairments worked together to create national goals that can be addressed on a local or regional basis in order to increase the quantity and quality of services for this population of students.

Overbrook School for the Blind. *Parent Early Childhood Education Series.* Louisville, KY: American Printing House for the Blind, 1990.

These materials, written by staff at the Overbrook School for the Blind, focus on information helpful to parents of babies (birth to 3 years) with visual impairments. Information related to motor, social, daily living, and cognitive development is included.

∷ Chapter 9

American Foundation for the Blind. *Brief Encounters of the Right Kind...Or, How to Make Your Point as an Advocate in 10 Minutes or Less* (VHS Video). New York: AFB Press, 1997.
This videotape provides a brief introduction to strategies for advocating for the needs of individuals with visual impairments. Parents who want to become involved in local or national advocacy will find this is a helpful resource.

Corn, A.L., & Huebner, K.M. *Report to the Nation: The National Agenda for the Education of Children and Youths with Visual Impairments, Including Those with Multiple Disabilities.* New York: AFB Press, 1998.
This book outlines the efforts of advocates in various locations as they work to implement the goals of the national agenda. This will be an important resource for parents who would like to understand an historical perspective of local or national advocacy efforts.

Crane, P., Cuthbertson, D., Ferrell, K.A. & Scherb, H. *Equals in Partnership: Basic Rights for Families of Children with Blindness or Visual Impairment.* Watertown, MA: Perkins School for the Blind, 1997.
The focus of this handbook is advocacy. Materials included in this book will help parents understand the unique needs of children with visual impairments and ways in which they can access appropriate educational services.

U.S. Department of Justice. *The Americans with Disabilities Act: Questions and Answers* and *A Guide to Disability Rights Laws.* Available by calling the ADA information line at 800-514-0301 or from website: www.ada.gov.
These free booklets are available online for downloading or in standard print, large print, or braille if you call the information line.

Wright, P.W.D., & Wright, P.D. *Wrightslaw: IDEA 2004.* Hartfield, VA: Harbor House Law Press, 2005.
Available in a print and e-book edition, this guide includes the full text of the Individuals with Disabilities Act of 2004 with helpful commentary and annotation by the authors designed to help parents use the law to their children's advantage.

∷ Chapter 10

American Foundation for the Blind. *Connecting the Dots: A Parent's Resource for Promoting Early Braille Literacy.* New York: AFB Press.
This free packet contains information about children's books produced in braille, an overview of braille, and other information to support young braille reading children.

Holbrook, M.C. & Koenig, A.J. *Experiencing Literacy: A Parents' Guide for Fostering Early Literacy Development of Children with Visual Impairments.* Philadelphia, PA: Overbrook School for the Blind, 2006.
Encouraging early literacy begins at birth. This small book provides information about components of literacy instruction including reading aloud, phonemic awareness, use of pictures, and need for rich, varied experiences for concept development. Parents are guided through the what? why? and how? questions for establishing a home environment that supports literacy.

Koenig, A.J. & Holbrook, M.C. *The Braille Enthusiast's Dictionary.* Germantown, TN: SCALARS Publishing, 1995.

This reference book contains approximately 30,000 word in print and contracted braille forms. It was compiled for teachers and parents as a resource for braille transcription.

Mellor, C. M. *Louis Braille: A Touch of Genius.* Boston: National Braille Press, 2006.

This is the most comprehensive book ever written about the life of the person who invented the braille code. Louis Braille lived in France almost two centuries ago but the impact of his life is still felt today.

Miller, D.D. "Reading Comes Naturally: A Mother and Her Blind Child's Experiences." *Journal of Visual Impairment and Blindness.* Vol. 79, 1-4, 1986.

This article tells about early literacy experiences in braille that Mrs. Miller enjoyed with her daughter, Jamaica, who was blind. This is an easy-to-read, fun, and encouraging article that provides a springboard for parents to think of many ways to encourage literacy for their young children.

Trelease, J. *The Read-Aloud Handbook.* 6th edition. New York: Penguin Books, 2006.

This book presents information on the importance of reading aloud to children, as well as many practical suggestions on how to read aloud. It is written for a general audience so adaptations will be necessary before using some of the suggestions with children who are visually impaired.

■■ Chapter 11

Hug, D., Chernus-Mansfield, N., & Hayashi, D. *Move with Me: A Parent's Guide to Movement Development for Babies Who Are Visually Impaired.* Los Angeles: Blind Childrens Center, 1987.

Important considerations for encouraging early movement development are explored in this short, easy-to-understand booklet.

Lyle, L. & Quintana, C. *We're on the Move! O&M Games for the Very Young Child.* Available for free download from Texas School for the Blind (http://www.tsbvi.edu/Education/preschool-om.htm), 2000.

The authors of this resource share the content of a presentation to participants at the international conference of the Association for the Education and Rehabilitation of the Blind and Visually Impaired. Suggestions for games encouraging movement for preschool children are included.

Simmons, S.S. & Maida, S.O. *Reaching, crawling, walking…Let's get moving.* Los Angeles: Blind Childrens Center, 1992.

Parents will find introductory information about orientation and mobility in this booklet along with suggestions for encouraging movement in the home. In addition, this resource provides a discussion about issues related to cane use by preschool children.

■■ Chapter 12

Batshaw, M.L. *When Your Child Has a Disability: The Complete Sourcebook of Daily and Medical Care.* Revised edition. Baltimore, MD: Paul H. Brookes, 2001.

Written by a developmental pediatrician and team of experts, this book contains extensive information about living with and caring for a child with disabilities. It provides information from a medical and legal perspective and addresses long-term issues as well as daily, immediate concerns.

Chen, D. & Downing, J.E. *Tactile Strategies for Children Who Have Visual Impairments and Multiple Disabilities: Promoting Communication and Learning Skills.* New York: AFB Press, 2006.

This manual, written for teachers, early intervention specialists, and families, provides helpful suggestions for supporting children who are visually impaired and have additional disabilities as they learn tactile skills. The authors provide information about creating an environment that will encourage children's use of a wide range of communication options.

Miles, B. & Riggio, M., Editors. *Remarkable Conversations: A Guide to Developing Meaningful Communication with Children and Young Adults Who Are Deafblind.* Watertown, MA: Perkins School for the Blind, 1999.

This book addresses strategies for helping children who are deafblind to communicate.

Sacks, S.Z. & Silberman, R.K. *Educating Students Who Have Visual Impairments with Other Disabilities.* Baltimore, MD: Paul H. Brookes, 1998.

This introductory text provides techniques for facilitating functional learning in students with a wide range of visual impairments and multiple disabilities. With a concentration on educational needs and learning styles, the authors demonstrate functional assessment and teaching adaptations that will improve students' inclusive learning experiences.

▪▪ Chapter 13

Feeney, R. & Trief, E. *College Bound: A Guide for Students with Visual Impairments.* New York: AFB Press, 2005.

This is a "must-have" resource for families who are experiencing the transition from high school to college. There are countless pointers for students to help them navigate this journey. While parents and teachers will find the text informative, students will find it very helpful as they increase their own responsibility for independent decision-making related to the college experience.

Kendrick, D. *Jobs to Be Proud Of: Profiles of Workers Who Are Blind or Visually Impaired.* New York: AFB Press, 1993.

Parents are often concerned about the long-term future for their children. Employment may seem like a long way away when you are rocking your baby to sleep, but this helpful resource will offer valuable information as you begin to think of your child's eventual employment options.

Nielsen, K.E. *Helen Keller: Selected Writings.* New York: New York University Press, 2005.

Most people are aware of the life of Helen Keller who was deaf and blind. The movie "The Miracle Worker" dramatizes Keller's early life with her teacher, Anne Sullivan. This book contains letters and other writings from Keller herself and demonstrates her extraordinary gift for expressing herself. This book provides an insight into Helen Keller's thinking about the world around her and about her disability.

Perkins School for the Blind. *Clean to the Touch.* Watertown, MA: Perkins School for the Blind, 2006.

Daily living skills and independent living are included as a key component of the expanded core curriculum. This book provides a step-by-step guide for supporting young adults in learning how to manage basic housekeeping skills.

Tenberken, S. *My Path Leads to Tibet: The Inspiring Story of How One Young Blind Woman Brought Hope to the Blind Children of Tibet.* New York: Arcade Publishing, 2003.

This is the story of an amazing woman who worked tirelessly through much adversity to help blind children in Tibet. Sabriye Tenberken founded an organization called "Braille without Borders" that continues to work toward literacy for children who are blind around the world. The story of this book is not just Tenberken's dedication to her global mission but also her thoughtful reflections of her life as a blind woman.

Weihenmayer, E. *Touch the Top of the World: A Blind Man's Journey to Climb Farther Than the Eye Can See.* New York: Penguin Group, 2002.

Erik Weihenmayer is the first blind man to ever climb Mount Everest. His memoir provides an honest and inspiring account of facing the challenges of low expectations and discrimination as well as relying on the trust and affection of true friends. This book tells of Erik's adventure but also clearly communicates the importance of believing in yourself and making your own dreams come true.

Resources

:: National Organizations

The national organizations listed below offer a variety of services that may be of help in meeting the needs of children with visual or multiple disabilities and their families.

American Council of the Blind
1155 15th Street, NW, Suite 1004
Washington, DC 20005
202-467-5081; 800-424-8666
www.acb.org

The American Council of the Blind's membership consists of individuals who are blind, family members, and professionals. ACB advocates for civil rights, national health insurance, rehabilitation, eye research technology, and other issues that concern people who are blind.

American Foundation for the Blind
11 Penn Plaza, Suite 300
New York, NY 10001
212-502-7600
www.afb.org

The American Foundation for the Blind works to promote equality of access and opportunity to individuals who are blind or visually impaired. AFB Press, the publishing arm of this organization, produces the *Journal of Visual Impairment and Blindness* and many texts focusing on the topic of blindness and visual impairment.

American Printing House for the Blind
1839 Frankfort Ave.
P.O. Box 6085
Louisville, KY 40206-0085
502-895-2405
www.aph.org

The American Printing House for the Blind publishes literature and textbooks in braille and large print, talking books, microcomputer software, and electronic books. Educational aids for persons with visual impairments are also provided.

The Arc
1010 Wayne Ave., Suite 650
Silver Spring, MD 20910
301-565-3842
www.thearc.org
    A national organization of people with mental retardation and their advocates. It publishes information on all types of developmental delays and has an extensive network of local affiliates which offer support, information, respite care, and other services.

The Association for the Education and Rehabilitation
of the Blind and Visually Impaired (AER)
1703 N. Beauregard St., Suite 440
Alexxandria, VA 22311
703-671-4500; 877-492-2708 (toll-free)
www.aerbvi.org
    This membership organization promotes all phases of education and work for blind and visually impaired persons. AER distributes professional literature and holds a conference every two years, plus additional professional development meetings on various topics.

Blind Children's Fund
311 W. Broadway, Suite 1
Mt. Pleasant, MI 48858
989-779-9966
www.blindchildrensfund.org
    The mission of Blind Children's Fund is to provide parents and professionals with information, materials, and resources that help them successfully teach and nurture infants and children who are blind or visually and multi-impaired and to increase global awareness about the need for early and continuing intervention services for these children. Publishes the VIP newsletter.

Canadian Blind Sports Association
325-5055 Joyce Street
Vancouver, BC V5R 6B2
604-419-0480
www.canadianblindsports.ca
    This organization promotes athletic participation for Canadians who are blind or visually impaired.

Canadian Council of the Blind
401-396 Cooper Street, Suite 200
Ottawa, Ontario K2P 2H7
613-567-0311
www.ccbnational.net
    CCB is a national consumer organization devoted to improving the quality of life for blind Canadians through social, recreational, and advocacy programs. CCB also sponsors activities geared to educating members of the public about the capabilities and talents of people who are blind or visually impaired.

CNIB (formerly Canadian National Institute for the Blind)
National Office
1929 Bayview Avenue
Toronto, ON M4G 3E8
800-563-2642
www.cnib.ca
CNIB is a nationwide, community-based, organization with regional offices throughout Canada. CNIB is committed to research, public education, and vision health for all Canadians. CNIB provides the services and support necessary for people to enjoy a good quality of life while living with vision loss.

Council for Exceptional Children
1110 North Glebe Road, Suite 300
Arlington, VA 22201
703-620-3660
www.cec.sped.org
The Council for Exceptional Children (CEC) is the largest international professional organization dedicated to improving the education of students with disabilities and the gifted. CEC holds an international conference every year and produces professional literature on a variety of topics related to special education. The CEC's Division on Visual Impairments (DVI) focuses on the education of students who are blind or visually impaired.

Council of Families with Visual Impairments
c/o American Council of the Blind
1155 15th Street, Suite 1004
Washington, DC 20005
www.acb.org
This is a support group of parents of children who are blind or visually impaired within the American Council of the Blind.

**DB-Link: The National Information Clearinghouse
on Children Who Are Deaf-Blind**
Teaching Research
345 N. Monmouth Ave.
Monmouth, OR 97361
800-438-9376
www.tr.wou.edu/dblink
DB-link provides resources and personalized services to anyone needing information about or for deaf-blind children. It serves as a centralized hub of information about deaf-blindness and develops and disseminates products related to services for deaf-blind children.

Hadley School for the Blind
700 Elm Street
Winnetka, IL 60093
www.hadley.edu
The Hadley School for the Blind promotes independent living through lifelong distance education programs for blind people and their families. The Hadley School offers free at-home study courses for individuals who are blind and for parents or family members of blind children. Courses include topics related to early childhood and elementary education, independent living skills, and braille.

Helen Keller National Center for Deaf-Blind Youths and Adults
141 Middle Neck Rd.
Sands Point, NY 11050
516-944-8900
www.hknc.org
Helen Keller National Center for Deaf-Blind Youths and Adults provides support services for people who are deaf-blind, their families, and professionals who work with them through a network of regional offices throughout the United States. This organization is committed to work that will enable each person who is deaf-blind to live and work in the community of his or her choice.

Library of Congress
National Library Service for the Blind and Physically Handicapped
1291 Taylor Street NW
Washington, DC 20011
www.loc.gov/nls
The National Library Service for the Blind and Physically Handicapped (NLS) distributes braille and audio reading materials through a system of cooperating libraries to U.S. citizens who cannot use printed reading materials because of a visual or physical impairment. Materials are sent postage free through the U.S. Postal Service.

Lions Clubs International
300 22nd Street
Oak Brook, IL 60523-8842
www.lionsclubs.org
Lions Clubs have a major interest in issues relating to blindness and visual impairments. Sometimes funding is available through local Lions Clubs for equipment or special projects.

National Association for Parents of the Visually Impaired
P.O Box 317
Watertown, MA 02471
800-562-6265; 617-972-7441
www.spedex.com/napvi
This national membership organization for parents and agencies provides support to parents and families of children with visual impairments. NAPVI operates a national clearinghouse for information, education, advocacy, and publishes the newsletter *Awareness*.

National Camps for Blind Children
4444 South 52nd Street
Lincoln, NE 68516
402-488-0981
www.christianrecord.org/blndcmp
This nonprofit, Christian-based organization operates camps for children and adults who are blind or visually impaired.

National Dissemination Center for Children with Disabilities (NICHCY)
P.O. Box 1492
Washington, DC 20013-1492
800-695-0285
www.nichcy.org
NICHCY provides information on disabilities in preschool and school age children, legal issues including IDEA and No Child Left Behind, and research-based information

on effective educational services. NICHCY also publishes fact sheets for each state, listing government offices, disability-specific organizations, and other helpful state organizations. State sheets are available both online and in print versions.

National Federation of the Blind
1800 Johnson Street
Baltimore, MD 21230
410-659-9314
www/nfb.org
    This national membership organization of and for the blind works to improve social and economic conditions of blind persons. NFB holds annual conventions and publishes *The Braille Monitor* and other helpful materials for individuals who are blind and their families. The National Organization of Parents of Blind Children is a division of NFB that provides support for parents and publishes *Future Reflections*.

Prevent Blindness America
211 West Wacker Dr., Suite 1700
Chicago, IL 60606
800-331-2020
www.preventblindness.org
    Through public and professional education, research and service, this organization supports local and regional efforts to promote eye care and prevention of eye disease and blindness.

Recording for the Blind and Dyslexic (RFB&D)
20 Rozel Rd
Princeton, NJ 08540
866-732-3585
www.rfbd.org
    Recording for the Blind and Dyslexic (RFB&D) is a nonprofit agency providing recorded and computerized textbooks, library services, and other educational resources to people who cannot read standard print because of a visual, physical, or perceptual disability.

Senate Printing and Document Services
B-04, Hart Senate Office Building
Washington, DC 20510-7106
202-228-2815 (fax)
orders@senate.gov
http://senate.gov/legislative/common/generic/Doc_Room.htm
    Copies of any U.S. laws or regulations, including IDEA, ADA, and other disability-related laws, may be obtained free of charge by faxing, emailing, or writing to the above address. You must include the document number in your request.

TASH
29 West Susquehanna Ave., Suite 210
Baltimore, MD 21204
410-828-8274
www.tash.org
    TASH is a national membership organization for professionals and parents whose purpose is to advocate for a dignified lifestyle for all individuals with significant disabilities. TASH publishes a newsletter and other publications.

United States Association for Blind Athletes
33 North Institute St.
Colorado Springs, CO 80903
719-630-0422
www.usaba.org
    This national membership organization promotes sports involvement for people who are blind.

▪▪ Schools for the Blind

    Parents often express frustration over the number of phone calls they must make in order to connect with the network of support for the education of their child who is visually impaired. One strategy for circumventing this long process might be to contact your state school for the blind as soon as you feel that you would like some assistance. Schools for the blind often have contact with all educational service providers in the region and access to national and international resources. In addition, many schools for the blind have active alumni organizations and parent groups that might be helpful in your early journey.

    Below are listed the schools for the blind in each state, and the one school in Canada. Please note that calling a school for the blind as a resource does not obligate you to use the services of the school. Many schools today have both residential and outreach programs that provide support to children and families.

ALABAMA
Alabama School for the Blind
205 East South Street, P.O. Box 698
Talladega, AL 35161
256-761-3259
www.aidb.org/asb

ALASKA
No school for the blind; contact:
Special Education Service Agency
3501 Denali Street
Anchorage, AK 99507
907-334-1300
www.sesa.org

ARIZONA
Arizona State Schools for the Deaf and
  the Blind
1200 West Speedway Blvd.
P.O. Box 85000
Tucson, AZ 85754
520-770-3701
www.asdb.state.az.us

Arizona Foundation for Blind Children
1235 E Harmont Dr.
Phoenix, AZ 85020
602-331-1470
www.the-fbc.org

ARKANSAS
Arkansas School for the Blind
2600 West Markham, P.O. Box 668
Little Rock, AR 72203-0668
501-296-1810
www.arkansasschoolfortheblind.org

CALIFORNIA
California School for the Blind
500 Walnut Ave.
Fremont, CA 94536
510-794-3800
www.csb-cde.ca.gov

COLORADO
Colorado School for the Deaf
  and the Blind
33 North Institute Street
Colorado Springs, CO 80903
719-578-2100
www.csdb.org

CONNECTICUT
Connecticut Institute for the
  Blind/Oak Hill
120 Holcomb Street
Hartford, CT 06112
860-242-2274
www.ciboakhill.org

DELAWARE
No school for the blind; contact:
Delaware Department of Public Instruction
John G. Townsend Building
P.O. Box 1402
Dover, DE 19903
302-735-4210
www.doe.k12.de.us

DISTRICT OF COLUMBIA
No school for the blind; contact:
District of Columbia Special Education
  Branch
825 North Capitol Street, NE, 6th Floor
Washington, DC 20002
202-442-4800

FLORIDA
The Florida School for the Deaf
  and the Blind
207 North San Marco Avenue
St. Augustine, FL 32084
904-827-2200
www.fsdb.k12.fl.us

GEORGIA
Georgia Academy for the Blind
2895 Vineville Avenue
Macon, GA 31204
912-751-6083
www.gabmacon.org

HAWAII
Hawaii Center for the Deaf and the Blind
3440 Leahi Avenue
Honolulu, HI 96815
808-733-4999
www.hcdb.k12.hi.us

IDAHO
Idaho State School for the Deaf
  and the Blind
1450 Main Street
Gooding, ID 83330
208-934-4457
www.isdb.idaho.gov

ILLINOIS
Illinois School for the Visually Impaired
658 East State Street
Jacksonville, IL 62650
217-479-4400
www.isvi.net

Philip J. Rock Center and School
818 DuPage Boulevard
Glen Ellyn, IL 60137
630-790-2474
www.project-reach-illinois.org/prc.html

INDIANA
Indiana School for the Blind
7725 North College Avenue
Indianapolis, IN 46240
317-253-1481
http://intra.isbrockets.org/public

IOWA
Iowa Braille and Sight Saving School
1002 G Avenue
Vinton, IA 52349
319-472-5221
www.iowa-braille.k12.ia.us

KANSAS
Kansas State School for the Blind
1100 State Avenue
Kansas City, KS 66102
913-281- 3308
www.kssb.net

KENTUCKY
Kentucky School for the Blind
1867 Frankfort Avenue
Louisville, KY 40206
www.www.ksb.k12.ky.us

LOUISIANA
Louisiana School for the Visually
  Impaired
1120 Government Street
Baton Rouge, LA 70802-4897
225-342-4756
www.lsvi.org

MAINE
No school for the blind; contact:
Division for the Blind and
  Visually Impaired
Maine Department of Human Services
State House Station #150
Augusta, ME 04330-0150
207-624-5950
www.state.me.us/rehab/dbvi/dbvi_pgms.
htm#BEdDescr

MARYLAND
The Maryland School for the Blind
3501 Taylor Avenue
Baltimore, MD 21236-4499
410-444-5000
www.mdschblind.org

MASSACHUSETTS
Perkins School for the Blind
175 North Beacon Street
Watertown, MA 02172
617-924-3434
www.perkins.org

MICHIGAN
Michigan School for the Deaf and Blind
1667 Miller Road
Flint, MI 48503-4720
810-257-1400
www.msdb.k12.mi.us

MINNESOTA
Minnesota State Academy for the Blind
P.O. Box 68
Faribault, MN 55021
507-333-4800
www.msab.state.mn.us

MISSISSIPPI
Mississippi School for the Blind
1252 Eastover Drive
Jackson, MS 39211
601-984-8200
www.msb.k12.ms.us

MISSOURI
Missouri School for the Blind
3815 Magnolia Avenue
St. Louis, MO 63110
800-622-5672; 314-776-4320
www.msb.k12.mo.us

MONTANA
Montana School for the Deaf
  and the Blind
3911 Central Avenue
Great Falls, MT 59405
406-771-6000
http://msdb.mt.gov

NEBRASKA
Nebraska Center for the Education of Children Who Are Blind or Visually Impaired
824 Tenth Avenue, P.O. Box 129
Nebraska City, NE 68410
800-826-4355; 402-873-5513
www.ncecbvi.org

NEVADA
No school for the blind; contact:
Nevada Department of Education
700 East Fifth Street
Carson City, NV 89701
775-687-9171
www.doe.nv.gov

NEW HAMPSHIRE
No school for the blind; contact:
New Hampshire Vision/Hearing Network
117 Pleasant Street
Concord, NH 03301
603- 226-2900
www.nhvhn.org

NEW JERSEY
St. Joseph's School for the Blind
235 Baldwin Avenue
Jersey City, NJ 07306
201-653-0578
www.sjsb.net

NEW MEXICO
New Mexico School for the Visually
  Handicapped
1900 White Sands Blvd.
Alamagordo, NM 88310
800-437-3505; 505-437-3505
www.nmsvh.k12.nm.us

NEW YORK
LaVelle School for the Blind
3830 Paulding Avenue
Bronx, NY 10469
718-882-1212
http://lavelleschoolorg

New York State School for the Blind
24 Richmond Avenue
Batavia, NY 14020
585-343-5384
www.vesid.nysed.gov/specialed/nyssb/
home.html

The New York Institute for Special Education
999 Pelham Parkway
Bronx, NY 10469
718-519-7000, extension 315
www.nyise.org/text/index.html

NORTH CAROLINA
The Governor Morehead School
303 Ashe Avenue
Raleigh, NC 27606
919-733-6392
www.governormorehead.net

NORTH DAKOTA
North Dakota Vision Services School
for the Blind
500 Stanford Road
Grand Forks, ND 58203
800-421-1181;701-795-2700
www.ndvisionservices.com

OHIO
Ohio State School for the Blind
5220 North High Street
Columbus, OH 43214
614-752-1152
www.ode.state.oh.us/ossb

OKLAHOMA
Parkview School/Oklahoma School
for the Blind
3300 Gibson Street
Muskogee, OK 74403
918-781-8200; 877-229-7136 (OK only)
www.osb.k12.ok.us

OREGON
Oregon School for the Blind
700 Church Street, SE
Salem, OR 97301
503-378-3820
www.ode.state.or.us/osb

PENNSYLVANIA
Overbrook School for the Blind
633 Malvern Avenue
Philadelphia, PA 19151
215-877-0313
www.obs.org

St. Lucy Day School for Children with
Visual Impairments
4251 L Street
Philadelphia, PA 19124
www.slds.org

Western Pennsylvania School for
Blind Children
201 North Bellefield Avenue
Pittsburgh, PA 15213-1499
412-621-0100
www.wpsbc.org

RHODE ISLAND
No school for the blind; contact:
Rhode Island Department of Education
255 Westminster Street
Providence, RI 02903
www.ridoe.net/Special_needs/
VisionService.html

SOUTH CAROLINA
South Carolina School for the Deaf
and Blind
355 Cedar Spring Road
Spartanburg, SC 29302
864-585- 7711
www.scsdb.k12.sc.us

SOUTH DAKOTA
South Dakota School for the
Visually Impaired
423 SE 17th Avenue
Aberdeen, SD 57401-7699
888-275-3814; 605-626-2580
www.sdsbvi.sdbor.edu

TENNESSEE
Tennessee School for the Blind
115 Stewarts Ferry Pike
Nashville, TN 37214
615-231-7300
www.tsb.k12tn.net

TEXAS
Texas School for the Blind and
    Visually Impaired
1100 West 45th Street
Austin, TX 78756
512-454-8631
www.tsbvi.edu

UTAH
Utah Schools for the Deaf and Blind
742 Harrison Blvd.
Ogden, UT 84404
801-629-4700
www.usdb.org

VERMONT
No school for the blind; contact:
Vermont Department of Education
120 State Street
Montpelier, VT 05620
802-828-3130
www.state.vt.us/educ/new/html/pgm_
sped.html

VIRGINIA
Virginia School for the Deaf and the Blind
East Beverly Street
P.O. Box 2069
Staunton, VA 24402
540-332-9000
www.vsdbs.virginia.gov

WASHINGTON
Washington State School for the Blind
2214 East 13th Street
Vancouver, WA 98661-4120
360-696-6321
www.wssb.org

WEST VIRGINIA
West Virginia Schools for the Deaf
    and the Blind
301 East Main Street
Romney, WV 26757
304-822-4800
www.wvsdb.state.k12.vw.us

WISCONSIN
Wisconsin School for the Visually
    Handicapped and Educational Services
Center for the Visually Impaired
1700 W State Street
Janesville, WI 53546
800-832-9784; 608-758-6100
www.wcbvi.k12.wi.us

WYOMING
No school for the blind; contact:
Services for the Visually Impaired
Wyoming Department of Education
2300 Capitol Avenue
Hathaway Building, Second Floor
Cheyenne, WY 82002-0050
307-777-6257
www.k12.wy.us/SE/svi.asp

CANADA
Ross MacDonald School for the Blind
350 Brant Ave
Brantford, ON N3T 3J9
519-759-0730
www.psbnet.ca/webs/wrm

CONTRIBUTORS

Tanni Anthony is Supervisor/Consultant on Visual Impairment Project Director of the CO Services for Children with Combined Vision and Hearing Loss for the Colorado Department of Education. She works on developing policies and procedures that support high quality educational services for students with visual impairments.

Bob Brasher is Vice President of Advisory Services and Research at the American Printing House for the Blind. Previously, Mr. Brasher served as Director of Educational Services for Visually Impaired, Arkansas Department of Education/Arkansas School for the Blind.

Rebecca Burnett received her doctoral degree from Peabody College of Vanderbilt University and has worked with children who have multiple disabilities, children with visual impairments, and their families. With LaRhea Sanford, she coauthored the *Functional Vision and Media Assessment for Students with Visual Impairments* and the *Expanded Core Curriculum Screening Record*.

Jane Erin is a professor at The University of Arizona, where she coordinates the program in Visual Disabilities. She has been a teacher of children with visual and multiple disabilities as well as program supervisor at the Western Pennsylvania School for Blind Children. She has published extensively on the topic of educating children with multiple and visual impairments.

Kay Ferrell is currently Professor of Education at The University of Northern Colorado and Associate Director, Policy Research for The American Foundation for the Blind. She is well known for her work and research in preschool services and development of infants and toddlers who are blind or visually impaired. She is the author of various publications, including *Reach Out and Teach*, a program for parents.

Erika Forster is a teacher of students with visual impairments in Coquitlam, BC, Canada. She is currently studying for her doctoral degree in Special Education and School Psychology at The University of British Columbia.

M. Cay Holbrook is Associate Professor of Special Education at The University of British Columbia, Vancouver, BC, Canada. She has prepared teachers of students with visual impairments for the past twenty years. Prior to her work as a teacher trainer, she worked with children with visual impairments in the southeastern United States.

Dr. Robert Knox graduated from the University of Texas Medical Branch and is currently in private practice in Fort Smith, Arkansas.

Until his recent death, **Alan Koenig** was Professor of Special Education at Texas Tech University. His research agenda focused on the literacy needs of students with visual impairments. Dr. Koenig published extensively on the topic and had a significant impact on how teachers assess and teach reading and writing for students who are blind or visually impaired.

Beth Langley is an educational diagnostician for Pinellas County Schools, Florida. She is well known for her expertise in working with children with disabilities. She is the parent of a young man who has a visually impairment and additional disabilities.

Eric and Leslie Ligon are the parents of two boys, one of whom is blind. Leslie designs braille jewelry, and Eric, a graphic designer, has invented a new way of including both braille and print in books for young readers with visual impairments.

LaRhea Sanford has worked extensively with children who have visual impairments in public schools and residential school settings. She has also taught university classes for pre-service teachers at Peabody College of Vanderbilt University, where she received her doctorate in special education.

Tom E.C. Smith is a professor of special education at the University of Arkansas, where he coordinates the graduate program in severe and profound disabilities. He has written many books and articles related to the special needs of children with disabilities and their parents. He is a coauthor of *Teaching Children with Special Needs in Inclusive Settings*.

Kevin A. Stewart received his doctoral degree in special education at Vanderbilt University. He is an orientation and mobility specialist with a focus on the needs of very young children in Toronto, Ontario, Canada. Kevin has had extensive experience consulting and working with parents and teachers who are concerned with preschool services.

Dr. Steven Stiles graduated from Southern College of Optometry and is currently in private practice in Fort Smith, Arkansas. He has a special interest in the needs of individuals with low vision.

Dean and Naomi Tuttle have a distinguished record of providing information and support for individuals with visual impairments and their families. They have both worked with Hadley School for the Blind in developing courses for families. They are coauthors of *Self-esteem and Adjusting with Blindness* and are well known for their work on self-esteem for individuals with visual impairments.

INDEX

Page numbers in *italics* indicate illustrations.

ABOUT THE
EDITOR

M. Cay Holbrook, Ph.D., holds a Doctorate in Special Education from Florida State University. She has educated children with visual impairments and served as an advocate and instructor of teachers for over twenty-five years. Currently, she is an Associate Professor of Special Education and directs the teacher preparation program in visual impairment at The University of British Columbia in Vancouver, BC, Canada.